CHANGING THE COURSE OF AUTISM

CHANGING THE COURSE OF AUTISM

A Scientific Approach for Parents and Physicians

BRYAN JEPSON, M.D.

with Jane Johnson

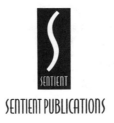

SENTIENT PUBLICATIONS

First Sentient Publications edition 2007
Copyright © 2007 by Bryan Jepson and Jane Johnson

A paperback original

Cover design by Kim Johansen, Black Dog Design
Book design by Timm Bryson and Alfred Hicks

The information in this book in not intended as a protocol for the treatment of individual patients and is not a substitute for professional medical help.

Library of Congress Cataloging-in-Publication Data

Jepson, Bryan, 1967-
Changing the course of autism : a scientific approach to treating your autistic child / by Bryan Jepson.
  p. cm.
ISBN 978-1-59181-061-2
1. Autism in children—Treatment. 2. Autistic children—Rehabilitation. I. Title.
  RJ506.A9J475 2007
  618.92'85882--dc22
    2006038795

Printed in the United States of America

10 9 8 7 6 5 4 3 2 1

SENTIENT PUBLICATIONS
A Limited Liability Company
1113 Spruce Street
Boulder, CO 80302
www.sentientpublications.com

To Laurie, for your love, and for helping me look outside the box; to Ben for being a great big brother and for keeping me laughing; and to Aaron, for your courage, and for reminding me what is important in life.

To Grace, Blakeslee, Whit, and Christopher, with love and gratitude.

CONTENTS

FOREWORD

I STARTED TO LOSE MY SON IN NOVEMBER OF 2003. CHRISTIAN WAS A sweet and loving two-year-old with a big vocabulary and a love of trucks and cars. He would point to trucks on the road and excitedly yell to me: "Mommy! Tractor-trailer! Wow!" Christian loved Barney and was frequently caught sneaking up to the television, remote in hand, trying to play Barney videos. He was extremely attached to his family, telling visitors that his newborn baby brother was "his baby" and soothing his crying brother by saying, "Don't cry, my baby, it's OK, baby." When he felt unsure of a situation he looked at me for reassurance and asked, "Mommy love Christian?" Christian couldn't wait for his dad to come home from work, and would run down the driveway to greet Andreas and ask to drive his car. When Christian was tired or grumpy in the evenings, I would have to wrestle the phone out of his little hand before he went to sleep. He always wanted to call his grandmother and talk about what they would do on their next visit: "Why can't I call Mor Mor? I want her! I go her house, NOW!"

Yes, Christian was somewhat socially anxious, especially at the doctor's office, where his fear frightened me. He would cling to me, howling, refusing to be placed on the white paper of the examining table. He loved other kids, but played a little too roughly and sometimes had a hard time sharing toys. We had ordinary two-year-old problems, or so we thought. The word "autism" never entered our minds.

In November of 2003 Christian got a very serious staph infection and was hospitalized briefly for exploratory surgery. He has never been the same since. After the staph infection came strep, after strep came cellulitis in his eyes, after cellulitis the strep came back, and then by late spring 2004 he had pneumonia. In the midst of all these illnesses came the most damaging sickness of all—constant, truly foul-smelling diarrhea, approximately six to ten times a day, for two solid years. The skin was coming off Christian's backside due to the incredibly high acid level in his bowel movements. Have I mentioned that autism is still frequently classified as a mental health disorder?

Accompanying Christian's illnesses were strange and worrying behaviors. He appeared more and more distant, as if he no longer comprehended what we were saying. In response to questions, Christian would attempt to respond but only garbled bits of language emerged. He quickly started flapping, walking on his toes, refusing to eat, and staying awake all night: symptoms I now refer to as the four horsemen of autism. I took Christian to his pediatrician, routinely rated among the best in the state. I was told that he was likely upset about the birth of his baby brother and "needed time." My repeated requests for a referral to a specialist were brushed aside. To my great regret, we followed this advice for months and things only got worse. Finally, I called the office and demanded a referral, which was given to me with extreme reluctance.

The developmental pediatrician diagnosed Christian with autism after two visits. It was the worst news any parent can hear, other than that their child is dying—although to us that is truly what it felt like. Our next stop was a well-regarded New York City hospital for a full work-up of Christian. The doctors seemed unfamiliar with this sudden onset of autism and rapid regression. His bowel and immune problems were dismissed with a warning to avoid any "alternative therapies." Christian then endured a torturous twenty-four-hour EEG, tethered to a wall. It was horrible and inhumane. As instructed, I pressed the button whenever I noticed strange eye movements or sudden tearful wakefulness that night, which was about every hour. I remember thinking that despite the horror of it all, *finally* we would get some answers regarding what was obviously going wrong in Christian's brain. Wrong. The hospital psychiatrist, who seemed herself to have Asperger's, informed us that Christian had autism and wished us luck with Birth to Three, Connecticut's early intervention program for children with developmental problems. Goodbye. Although the hospital was less than forty miles from our home, they could offer almost no assistance with treatment or information regarding providers or specific treatment modalities best suited to Christian.

The neurologist treating Christian told us that there was "nothing unusual" on his EEG. We were devastated by this news because it was clear that he was having seizure-like activity. Only later when we went to another neurologist for a second opinion did we discover that the treating physician had not studied the EEG results, but had an underling do it for him. When we then requested the results themselves in order to have the second neurologist interpret them, we were told the papers had been "thrown away." Typical. Poor Christian had to endure another EEG. At least this time we were allowed to take him home after the electrodes were attached to a Walkman-like device that allowed him to be mobile. At last the results illustrated that he was, indeed, experiencing seizure-like activity in his brain. We could treat the symptom, but the cause remained a mystery.

My parents, Bob and Suzanne Wright, are very much "can do" people. Through them I had access to the best medical resources in the country for Christian. From reading all the books on autism we could find, we considered ourselves fortunate because Christian was only two-and-a-half, and we were told that if we could get him high quality early intervention therapy, he would be fine. This was a much more difficult endeavor than we could have ever believed. The providers of therapy for autistic children are few and far between. There are waiting lists for waiting lists. The therapy is tremendously expensive, insurance pays for very little, and the vast majority of school systems are unequipped to teach our children. When we discovered autism was an epidemic in this country, with conservatively 1 in 166 children on the spectrum, my family had heard enough. My parents courageously founded Autism Speaks to create awareness and raise money for research.

In the interim, my husband and I put together a home education and behavior program for Christian. We found excellent ABA (Applied Behavior Analysis) therapists and a wonderful RDI (Relationship Development Intervention) speech therapist and added an occupational therapist a few months later, once we got off the waiting list. At first Christian began to make great progress, but after a few months he began to behave very irritably and started lying on tables, chairs, and couches in strange ways. He was always trying to put pressure on his lower abdomen. His diarrhea got much worse and he would start crying for no apparent reason, when no demands had been placed upon him. I read about the GF/CF (gluten-free/casein-free) diet and was intrigued and hopeful—of course this was Christian, addicted to milk and wheat! If we followed the diet, Christian would get better, like all of the children in the books!

We worked very hard to follow the diet and saw some initial improvements. Although Christian appeared less "drugged" after eliminating milk from his diet, he still seemed as if he was in tremendous pain. Yet, the diet did stop the skin on his backside from bleeding and the rashes around his mouth disappeared. We knew the diet was helping when Christian grabbed a wheat waffle and nearly swallowed it whole. An hour later he had the worst diarrhea we had seen in months and the bloody rashes all returned for weeks.

We stuck to the diet religiously, but Christian continued to regress. I remember sobbing as I came across an early vocabulary list of his well-pronounced words. By age three, over half of the words he said easily at two and a half were gone. Whole therapy sessions were spent trying to cajole him off the floor or a tabletop. The therapists were divided: half thought it was behavioral and half believed there was something medically wrong with Christian. This is the worst kind of torture for a parent, watching your child in pain but not being able to understand what is hurting him. We took him to every GI specialist recommended. They instructed us to take most fiber out of his diet and prescribed Prevacid. Later, I would come to understand that that advice is akin to offering a woman in labor a single aspirin. Nothing was helping; Christian was rapidly losing the speech he had left, as well as the new skills he had worked so hard to acquire. Any parent knows that losing a child is the worst possible, almost unsurvivable life event, and as we watched Christian's deterioration we were feeling that fear and dread every minute of the day. The child we once knew had become vacant and racked with pain, crying for most of the day.

Like so many families, we were desperate to turn the corner. After nothing but dead ends with physicians, we seized upon the idea that Christian needed a school with an integrated approach to therapy. We put our house on the market, sold almost all our possessions, and moved into an apartment in the city. Christian enjoyed his new school, but the physical problems persisted. His teachers did not consider his screaming fits and tantrums behavioral, and were bewildered as to their sudden onset and lengthy duration. My husband and I were despondent. Christian would no longer eat anything except GF/CF French fries and yogurt; he looked sick and listless and was barely communicating with us anymore.

My mother was also tremendously frustrated that we could not help Christian. Due to her visibility at Autism Speaks, doctors frequently contacted her offering to help Christian. We went to see dozens of specialists, yet none seemed very knowledgeable about how to relieve his GI distress. One extremely lucky day my Mom called me to ask if I wanted to take Christian to meet Dr. Andrew Wakefield and Jane Johnson. I jumped at the opportunity, knowing little about Dr. Wakefield's work other than that it related to GI problems in autistic kids. Jane is a wonderfully gracious and generous mom, whose own son's learning disability improved dramatically with medical treatment.

Although we had been warned by scores of physicians that engaging in any sort of non-traditional treatment with Christian was dangerous, it seemed far more dangerous to watch his continued decline and do nothing. My husband and I arrived to meet Jane and Dr. Wakefield without any expectations; we had been disappointed so many times before. As we recounted Christian's story, I noticed that we did not get the puzzled looks or doubtful expressions we previously encountered. We still regularly met with physicians who had never heard of regressive autism and seemed to regard Andreas and me as poor, pitiful parents in denial. We were thrilled when *finally*, two years into this horrible odyssey, a doctor seemed to truly understand. Dr. Wakefield was the first physician who was familiar with and knowledgeable about Christian's condition. He told us there was a treatment for his GI problems! He referred us to Dr. Arthur Krigsman on Long Island—very convenient for us considering that parents travel from all over the country to see him. This struck us as insane. Forty to eighty percent of ASD (autism spectrum disorder) kids have GI issues, and there is only one doctor in the country focusing on the bowel symptoms and prescribing effective treatment?

Christian had an endoscopy (a procedure that examines the inside of the GI tract with a specially designed instrument) two years earlier to try to determine the cause of his symptoms and we were told that he did not have celiac disease and that he was "fine." I accepted that he did not have celiac disease, but he was certainly not fine. It turns out that Christian had been inadequately scoped. The doctor had not looked into the terminal ileum, the area of the small bowel where the worst damage was evident. When we finally saw the film of Christian's ileum, I was devastated. One need not be a doctor to understand that those red, inflamed, bulbous intestines had caused Christian terrible pain. Food was not being properly absorbed in his GI system and toxins were leaking out into his bloodstream, affecting his brain. My husband and I were horrified to discover that *Christian's multiple regressions and years of pain could all have been prevented if he had received adequate medi-*

cal care when we first asked for help. We saw Dr. Krigsman in October 2005 and within weeks of starting treatment, Christian's symptoms improved immeasurably. Today, one year later, the tantrums are gone, the strange posturing has almost disappeared, and the diarrhea is 75% better. Christian is also making tremendous progress in his behavioral therapy, because he is no longer in pain!

We still have a long way to go, but Andreas and I feel that finally Christian is on the right track. If we had not met Dr. Krigsman and his colleagues at Thoughtful House, I cannot bear to imagine the state of Christian's health. This book is so sorely needed. I only wish it had existed three years ago. I have read almost every book on autism. Most offer no insight or assistance at all, but hectoring discussions about why vaccines are safe, statements on the genetic nature of this disorder, and advice about accepting the fact that a child is mentally retarded and will need to live in a group home. The books that do address the medical aspects of autism discuss only behavioral strategies such as how to not go insane when your child is up for three hours every single night, or how to lock a child in their room safely. The books about the GF/CF diet were helpful, but the diet and antifungals alone were not enough for Christian.

This book would have answered so many of my questions. I wanted to know why Christian woke up screaming every night, why he clutched his lower abdomen over and over, and why he had ten bowel movements a day. And most of all, I wanted to know what his bowel disease was doing to his brain. No books could answer any of these questions for me. It makes no sense to me that my son has THE most common of all developmental disorders, as well as medical complications that are in no way unusual in kids with autism, and yet Thoughtful House is one of the few centers offering real help to our children.

Our story is in no way unique. Parents of autistic kids all over the country are banging on the doors of pediatricians and pediatric gastroenterologists, looking for answers and finding none. The original GI specialist who performed Christian's first scope is routinely rated the best in New York City. Therein lies the problem—the medical community's unwillingness to address this disease and the related gut condition, autistic enterocolitis, which has left possibly a million autistic children in agonizing pain. Christian's gut disorder is very similar to Crohn's disease, another extremely painful GI disease. Doctors would never dream of not treating a patient with Crohn's, yet they often turn away children with autism. Autism has been misclassified as a mental disorder for half a century. My son has endured two years of extremely debilitating colitis, which nearly destroyed his life.

Every twenty minutes, a family embarks on this terrible journey. I am so tired of seeing so many lives needlessly destroyed, so many families torn apart, and so many doctors without answers. This situation is shameful. I am writing this because I do not want to speak to more parents who have ill, malnourished children, mentally and physically destroyed by autism. No parents should be mopping blood from their toddler's backside for two years. Parents should not be told it is "normal" for their autistic child to stay awake all night, every night. Parents should not have to use the Internet in lieu of a doctor to help their children. Parents should not feel so defeated that they abandon their autistic child in the emergency room, unable to mentally and physically cope anymore, which has happened. We owe so much more to these families. It is my greatest hope that pediatricians all over the country read this book with an open mind.

Katie Wright
Daughter of the founders of Autism Speaks

introduction

COMING TO TERMS WITH AUTISM

MY SECOND SON, AARON, WAS DIAGNOSED WITH AUTISM SHORTLY before his third birthday. The pregnancy and birth were uncomplicated and he seemed to be developing normally for the first year and a half of life. He was an engaged, happy, interactive baby and we had no reason to suspect that anything was wrong. Sometime in his second year, we noticed that he didn't seem to be hearing us when we walked into the room. He no longer noticed me when I came home from work. He did not want us to play with him or read him a book. Our first thought was that he might have a hearing problem, but we knew that he wasn't deaf. He could recite the ABC's. In fact, he did this repeatedly. We were thrilled that he was so smart. He frequently repeated lines from his favorite movie, *Toy Story*. My wife, Laurie, felt that there was something wrong, but I discounted his behavior, attributing it to an independent personality.

When Laurie told our pediatrician that he wasn't developing language at the same rate as our older son Ben, she was told that some boys don't start talking until much later and that we shouldn't worry about it. At that point, the word *autism* never crossed my mind. What I knew about autism was not much more than anyone else who had seen the movie *Rainman*. I'd treated some teenagers with autism in the ER for seizures or injuries. They were severely disabled, minimally verbal people who shrieked whenever they were touched. My son certainly wasn't like that. He was a happy child who loved to be held. He was usually very content and seemed perfectly able to handle breaks in his routine.

I agreed with his doctor that we should simply keep an eye on him, and I fully expected him to grow out of it. But by the time he was two and a half, it was clear that he wasn't getting any better. In fact, he was getting worse. Now he only played with *Toy Story* toys or ABC letters, he spun in circles in the middle of the floor, and he giggled and shrieked for no apparent reason. He wouldn't call us by name and he never looked us in the eyes. Although he knew some words, he never used language to communicate. Shortly before this, our nephew had been diagnosed with Asperger's syndrome, a form of high-functioning autism. This prompted Laurie to begin looking on the Internet, where she found stories of other children with autism. She realized that they were describing our little boy.

We went to the school system for help, tested his hearing, saw a speech pathologist, and were sent to a child psychiatrist. Before we walked into his office, we knew that our child was autistic, but we were not prepared for what he told us. He said that our son met ten of the twelve DSM-IV criteria for autism, and that he carried a poor prognosis for any functional recovery. He told us that their behavioral program could help Aaron gain a few skills or even improve to the point of minimal social functioning, but that we should mentally prepare ourselves for the time when he would need to be institutionalized. He also told us that we would hear about a lot of experimental treatments that many people were trying, but not to waste our time and money, because they were expensive and unproven. Needless to say, we left his office in a state of shock and hopelessness. How could this possibly be the future for our adorable, happy little boy?

Laurie and I dealt with this news in very different ways. I was inclined to view it as one of life's challenges—something that we needed to learn to accept. After all, I was a doctor and I had never heard anything different about effective methods of treating autism. I knew that as long as we were physically able to care for him, Aaron would live with us in our home. We would love him and cherish the opportunity to learn from him and hope that he would be able to reciprocate some of that love, or at least understand that he was loved.

Laurie wasn't willing to accept this bleak prognosis. She immersed herself in the Internet, searching for anything related to autism. She learned about the gluten/casein-free diet and implemented it quickly. She learned about vitamin supplementation, DMG (a supplement that is useful in the treatment of autism), antifungals, and probiotics. This all sounded to me like a good way for vitamin companies to make money on another untreatable illness. I stayed uninvolved and uninterested in these initial interventions because I didn't believe they could affect my son's developmental disorder. However, I figured that the only harm was to my pocketbook, and that was a small price to pay for Laurie's need to *do* something.

But when she told me about the possible link to vaccines, I could no longer be impartial. After all, this was striking at one of the few areas of preventive medicine that physicians are passionate about. Vaccines are good! They eliminate life-threatening disease! I have seen first-hand how vaccines have successfully turned fairly common serious illnesses into rare, interesting cases. Wasn't autism just one more of those coincidental childhood illnesses that the crazy anti-government people were opportunistically using as an excuse to push their agenda?

I looked at the research, largely to prove to my wife that the theory was unfounded. The further I looked, the more interested I became. And before long, I realized that this theory of a vaccine-autism link wasn't driven by the whims of angry activists or the wallets of vitamin manufacturers. Rather, it was based on real science with a strong foundation of biological plausibility, led by knowledgeable and motivated physicians, research scientists, and parents of autistic children, all of whom weren't afraid to question dogma.

I was further convinced after attending a DAN! (Defeat Autism Now!) conference where I heard the scientific presentations of physicians and the stories of families who, like Laurie and me, were looking for answers. There was something different about this conference. They weren't talking about the latest psychotropic medication to be tried in autism. They were teaching biochemistry, and how manipulating it through diet and nutrition in children with autism was changing the course of the disease.

Now, I have always considered myself a mainstream physician. And like most mainstream physicians, I know a lot more about treating disease than truly understanding the origin. In medical school, we spend a lot of time memorizing biochemical pathways, but we easily forget how they relate to normal or impaired body functioning. Much of what we learn is relegated to the hidden corridors of our brains as soon as the exams are completed. Undoubtedly the answers to many of our medical puzzles lie within the confines of these biochemical pathways, but in spite of new technology and thousands of years of study, much of the human body is still very poorly understood.

Pharmaceutical companies develop medications that manipulate our body's biochemistry, and they market their products very aggressively to physicians. It's easy for physicians to become complacent with prescription pads, relying on pharmaceutical companies to work out the details of mechanisms. We just want to know about their risks and if they work. The drug reps show us their company's research, and of course it always shows a benefit over the competitor's product. We know to take it with a grain of salt, but who has time to figure it all out? Just tell us what to write on our prescription pads, or better yet, give us a pen with a product name on it so that we can remember how to spell the name of the drug.

Of course, there are other ways to manipulate biochemistry. There's an entire industry marketing vitamins and herbs to consumers, claiming to modulate disease processes. We physicians tend to discount the importance of nutriceuticals in the treatment of illness. No vitamin reps come to our office to give us all of the details, and we don't have time to research the studies on our own. We consider the doctors who look outside the pharmaceutical box to be "quacks" or "alternative." Doctors, in general, are not very good at admitting ignorance.

As I began to review the literature and learn the biochemistry of autism, I became increasingly convinced that this was much more than a developmental disorder, but that it was in fact a complex metabolic disease affecting multiple organ systems. I realized that autism is a treatable disease and that these children can get better. Soon thereafter, and with the help of my friend Alan Mendel, I established a non-profit medical clinic called The Children's Biomedical Center of Utah, which opened in March 2002. We had a three-part mission: to provide up-to-date medical treatment to people on the autism spectrum, to educate the public and the medical community about the issues surrounding this disorder, and to prevent future cases by participating in research to further understand the disease. Over the next three and a half years, working part-time, I treated nearly four hundred children with autism spectrum disorders (ASD). In January 2006, I joined the staff at the Thoughtful House Center for Children and now work full-time treating children with autism and related disorders. Thoughtful House is an innovative new treatment and research facility in Austin, Texas. It's a collaborative effort among physicians, educational specialists, and scientists who are dedicated to finding the answers to the many questions about autism:

- What is the cause?
- What are safe and effective treatments?
- Can the many therapies that are in use be narrowed and individualized to particular children?

We are coordinating medical treatments with intensive educational programs. I believe we're on the verge of major breakthroughs that will change the way the entire medical community views and treats these diseases. I am excited to be part of it, and I look forward to continuing to serve these courageous children and their families. The vast majority of the children that we treat are making meaningful progress. Some have functionally recovered to the point of completely dropping the behavioral diagnosis. We have not found a cure; it is a chronic disease that requires chronic management, but these children have gone farther than had ever been considered possible.

I decided to write this book to share the medical literature with physicians and families of autistic children, and I hope that it will make a difference in how this illness is perceived. Through my years of medical training I've developed a healthy skepticism of medical dogma. I spent a lot of time in residency learning evidence-based medicine, i.e. the importance of practicing according to the best available evidence rather than relying on historical opinions. Very often, the understanding of a disease that has been passed down through generations in the medical community and accepted as truth or "standard of care" is later proven wrong, or is modified as further research is done. Often this dogma is based on nothing more than the opinions of a few individuals. When the evidence doesn't exist or is incomplete, we must rely on our best judgment, as determined by sound biological principles.

I have also learned that the medical literature must be read with a critical eye. Much of it is biased on several fronts, and often the conclusions do not match the data. Surprisingly, most physicians do not regularly take the time to read the methodology of the studies, and yet will often change how they practice based on faulty conclusions or incomplete evidence. Even worse, many physicians rely solely on the practice patterns of others and never read the literature themselves. It has been frustrating as a physician who spends all day treating children on the autism spectrum to repeatedly hear from patient families that their primary care physicians tell them that there is no research regarding the treatment of autism. I wrote this book to prove that wrong, and more importantly to increase understanding, so that more people with autism will have access to appropriate medical care.

Although my introduction to autism was painful, the years that have followed have been full of rewards. I am rewarded when I see my own son making progress. I'm rewarded with the look of renewed hope on the faces of parents as they tell me how their children are getting better. Autism is treatable.

—Dr. Bryan Jepson

chapter one

AN IMPORTANT NOTE TO READERS

THE STORIES KATIE AND I TOLD IN THE FOREWORD AND introduction are shared by many parents who have searched for answers about their children, only to be rebuffed or even rebuked by the physicians they turned to for help. Instead of finding understanding, information, and direction, parents are all too often turned aside without answers, and without hope.

It's no wonder that many parents of autistic children have turned to the Internet and to parent support groups for answers. Although many times this has led them to useful therapies and resources, these avenues can also lead to treatments that have no scientific foundation, or are inappropriate—possibly even dangerous—for a particular child.

I wrote this book to show mainstream physicians that we need to change our view about autism. It needs to be understood as a medical illness, not just a behavior disorder. It's a disease of disordered biochemistry and metabolism that affects multiple organ systems, and it is treatable. Sound medical research has been published in mainstream medical journals that document these issues, and this information should be shared with families. I have compiled here as much of this medical literature as possible to show that what might seem a confusing miscellany of information on the surface is in fact integral components of a comprehensive disease model. I hope this book will jumpstart other physicians to begin their own study of the disease. If more physicians and researchers are involved in this effort, the answers to the many remaining questions will come more quickly. At the very least, the doctors who read this book should be willing to acknowledge that the viewpoints expressed here have scientific validity and are backed by the research literature.

This book is also written for parents. Much of it will be difficult to understand if you don't have a medical background. But, don't worry if you don't grasp all of the science, especially the first time you read it. Feel free to skip the chapters that feel over your head. I hope that what you gain from the book will be information that will arm you with principles and concepts to discuss with your physician or will direct you to a physician already trained in the treatment of autism. I truly believe that most physicians are willing to do what they can to help you if only they knew what to do or where to send you. The frustrating thing for physicians is that they don't have the answers to your questions about autism and they don't know how to treat children on the spectrum. This is an uncomfortable position to be in as a physician; sometimes it's difficult to admit that we really don't know what to do. So physicians try to protect you from what they perceive as false information, although they often haven't done the research needed to give a truly educated opinion. Some of what they know is outdated, and some of what they've been taught may be inaccurate and misleading. I hope that this book will encourage them to find and use the tools that will help your kids.

You will find that the more complex scientific concepts will become easier to understand over time as you continue to use this book as a reference. Understanding your child's health will make you a much more effective advocate. I explain some of the more difficult terminology as it comes up, but I've also included a glossary and an index at the back.

It is also important to note that when I use the word *autism* in the book, I am generally speaking of the broader autism spectrum (pervasive developmental disorder-not otherwise specified, Asperger's syndrome, Rett's syndrome, childhood disintegrative disorder)—it appears that the medical workup and treatment are the same between the behavioral subtypes. I have also successfully treated children with other disabilities such as ADHD, OCD, non-verbal learning disability (NLD), and Tourette's syndrome using a similar approach.

I purposely avoided writing the book as a step-by-step guide on how to fix your child's autism. Each autistic child is unique, and although there are many common treatment approaches and principles, these are best done under the supervision of a physician who has taken a complete medical history and knows your child well.

The most important point to remember is that with appropriate treatment, autistic children can improve, often dramatically. This represents a profound change in thinking from the historic view of the disorder: that autism is an untreatable psychiatric illness leading inevitably to institutionalization. This traditional dogma has delayed research into the true nature of the disease. Thankfully, over the last few years, a growing body of medical literature has begun to change our outdated view of autism. As more researchers take interest and more studies are published, our understanding of the disease is being refined. There is so much more to learn, and no single book can solve the problem of autism. But I believe that the first step in understanding the disease is to acknowledge the extent of the problem, to be willing to change our thinking, and to work together as parents, physicians, and researchers to provide our children with a brighter future.

chapter two

THE RISE AND FALL OF THE "REFRIGERATOR MOTHER" THEORY

Kanner's Diagnosis

LEO KANNER, A CHILD PSYCHIATRIST AT JOHNS HOPKINS University, first described autism in 1943. His descriptions were published in the textbook *Nervous Child* under the title "Autistic Disturbances of Affective Contact." He reported, "Since 1938, there have come to our attention a number of children whose condition differs so markedly and uniquely from anything reported so far, that each case merits—and, I hope, will eventually receive—a detailed consideration of its fascinating peculiarities."[1]

This, in and of itself, is a remarkable declaration. In the first twenty-one years he practiced child psychiatry, Dr. Kanner had not seen a single case of autism. It wasn't until eight years after he developed the first child psychiatric unit in a hospital in the United States that he saw his first case. Had he or his colleagues identified a medical condition as "fascinating" and "peculiar" as autism prior to 1938, it surely would have been reported. In his discussion, Dr. Kanner comments:

> The eleven children (eight boys and three girls) whose histories have been briefly presented offer, as is to be expected, individual differences in the degree of their disturbance, the manifestation of specific features, the family constellation, and the step-by-step development in the course of years. But even a quick review of the material makes the emergence of a number of essential common characteristics appear inevitable. These characteristics form a unique 'syndrome,' not heretofore reported, which seems to be rare enough, yet is probably more frequent than is indicated by the paucity of observed cases.[2]

He then describes features of the disease without creating specific diagnostic criteria. These include: inability to relate themselves to people and situations; poor (or absent) language skills, echolalia (repetitive verbal echoing); excellent rote memory; sensory sensitivity; perseverative and repetitive behavior (stereotypy); an anxiously obsessive desire for the maintenance of sameness; good cognitive potentialities; and generally normal appearance ("Five had relatively large heads. Several of the children were somewhat clumsy in gait and gross motor performances").

Here are a few of his descriptions:

Case 1: "arranged beads, sticks, or blocks in groups of different series"

Case 2: "when he responded to questions or commands at all, he did so by repeating them echolalia fashion"

Case 3: "did not communicate his wishes but went into a rage until his mother guessed and procured what he wanted"

Case 4: "ran around in circles emitting phrases in an ecstatic-like fashion...took a small blanket and kept shaking it, delightedly shouting, 'Ee! Ee!'...

could continue in this manner for a long time and showed great irritation when he was interfered with"

Case 5: "frequently interrupted with references to 'motor transports,' and 'piggy-back,' both of which had preoccupied her for quite some time"

Case 6: "does not play with other children...does not talk...will amuse herself by the hour putting picture puzzles together"

Case 7: "liked to pull blinds up and down, to tear cardboard boxes in to small pieces and play with them for hours, and to close and open doors"

Case 8: "on several occasions, pebbles were found in his stools...he swallowed some cotton from the Easter Rabbit...swallowed some kerosene"

Case 9: "still not toilet trained"

Case 10: "daily routine must be adhered to rigidly; any slightest change of the pattern called forth outbursts of panic"

Case 11: "language always has the same quality...speech is never accompanied by facial expression or gestures...does not look into one's face...voice is peculiarly unmodulated...never uses the personal pronouns of the first and second persons correctly...does not seem able to conceive the real meaning of these words"[3]

Some other key observations came out of Dr. Kanner's original report that have been ignored or forgotten. Medical tradition holds that children whose symptoms are noted from birth are diagnosed with classic autism or even Kanner autism, as opposed to regressive autism, in which children have a period of normal development followed by a loss of skills. But note that Kanner documents clear regression in two cases and probable regression or, at least, plateau in two others.

Case 3: "In September, 1940, the mother, in commenting on Richard's failure to talk, remarked in her notes: 'I can't be sure just when he stopped the imitation of word sounds. It seems that he has gone backward mentally gradually for the last two years.'"

Case 7: "Seemed alert and responsive as an infant and said many words at eighteen months, but toward the end of the second year she did not show much progression in her play relationships or in contacts with other people."

Case 8: "He has gradually shown a marked tendency toward developing one special interest which will completely dominate his day's activities."

Case 11: "Normal birth, she appeared healthy, took feedings well, stood up at seven months and walked at less than a year. She could say four words at the end of her first year but made no progress in linguistic development for the following four years."[4]

Interestingly, he also identifies gastrointestinal and immunological issues in the children:

Case 1: "Eating has always been a problem for him. He has never shown a normal appetite."

Case 2: "...large and ragged tonsils."

Case 3: "Following smallpox vaccination at twelve months, he had an attack of diarrhea and fever, from which he recovered in somewhat less than a week." "Found to be healthy except for large tonsils and adenoids."

Case 4: "He was born normally. He vomited a great deal

during his first year, and feeding formulas were changed frequently with little success. His tonsils were removed when he was three years old."

Case 5: "She nursed very poorly and was put on a bottle after about a week. She quit taking any kind of nourishment at three months. She was tube-fed five times daily up to one year of age. She began to eat then, though there was much difficulty until she was about eighteen months old." "At camp she slid into avitaminosis and malnutrition but offered almost no verbal complaints."

Case 7: "He vomited all food from birth through the third month."

Case 8: "For the first two months, the feeding formula caused considerable concern." "He had been kept in bed often because of colds, bronchitis, streptococcus infection, impetigo, and a vaguely described condition which the mother—the assurances of various pediatricians to the contrary notwithstanding—insisted was 'rheumatic fever.'"

Case 9: "He has had none of the usual children's diseases." (Children with healthy immune systems get sick occasionally—if they are never sick, it might indicate that their immune system is over-responsive.)

Case 10: "There were frequent hospitalizations because of the feeding problem (could not get food down). No physical disorder was ever found. He suffered from repeated colds and otitis media, which necessitated bilateral myringotomy." "He had two series of predominantly right-sided convulsions, with conjugate deviation of the eyes to the

right and transient paresis of the right arm. Neurological examination showed no abnormalities.
An electroencephalogram indicated 'focal disturbance in the left occipital region.'"

Case 11: "Because of a febrile illness at thirteen months,
her increasing difficulties were interpreted as
possible postencephalitic behavior disorder. For
eighteen months, she was given anterior pituitary
and thyroid preparations."[5]

Dr. Kanner's descriptions and interpretations of the symptoms and
behaviors of both the children and the parents offer a window into the
Freudian bias of the medical community of the 1930s. He believed that
the food-related issues were psychogenic (a psychiatric rather than physiologic cause): "Our patients, anxious to keep the outside world away,
indicated this by the refusal of food…most of them, after an unsuc-
cessful struggle, constantly interfered with, finally gave up the struggle
and of a sudden began eating satisfactorily." He refers to the parents
as "obsessive," "excitable," or "preoccupied with details." He also uses
the terms "frosty" and "inapproachable." In one case, he mentions that,
"Her father hated her ostensibly, and after the parents separated, she
'blossomed out.'" He noted that all of the children came from highly
intelligent families. He comments:

The very detailed diaries and reports and the frequent
remembrance, after several years, that the children had
learned to recite twenty-five questions and answers of the
Presbyterian Catechism, to sing thirty-seven nursery songs,
or to discriminate between eighteen symphonies, furnish a
telling story of parental obsessiveness. One other fact stands
out prominently. In the whole group, there are very few
really warmhearted fathers and mothers. For the most part,
the parents, the grandparents, and collaterals are persons

strongly preoccupied with abstractions of a scientific, literary, or artistic nature, and limited in genuine interest in people... The question arises whether or to what extent this fact has contributed to the condition of the children.[6]

This appears to be the inception of the Refrigerator Mother theory.

The Refrigerator Mother Theory

Based on Kanner's behavioral observations, autism was placed in a category with other strange and unusual psychiatric illnesses. In the 1950s, there was a prominent scholar and educator at the University of Chicago named Bruno Bettelheim[7] (note that he was not a psychiatrist or even an MD—his doctorate was in philosophy). Dr. Bettelheim was also strongly influenced by the psychoanalytical theories of Sigmund Freud. In fact, he claimed to have trained under Dr. Freud in Vienna (later proven to be untrue). Dr. Bettelheim believed that children were not born with autism, but they sensed from a very early age, sometimes only days after birth, that their mothers were withholding love from them. He believed that the mothers, out of a sense of insecurity, felt a need to defend themselves from their children even before birth. The children dealt with this lack of intimacy and affection by withdrawing from society and putting up a wall of defense, resulting in a regression into autistic behaviors. He believed that the only effective way to teach these children was to remove them from the environment that fostered this condition, placing them in a controlled and orderly institutionalized setting away from their families where they could be influenced by positive role models (counselors and teachers) acting as ego supports ("milieu therapy").

As the Director of the University of Chicago's Orthogenic School, Bettelheim implemented his technique for the treatment of autism. Parents were no longer allowed contact and were told that if they had even an ounce of love left for their children, they would not try to see them during their stay at his school. He was possibly the biggest proponent of the theory that the coldness of the mother was responsible for the children's autistic withdrawal. His theories and practices perpetuated and solidified the Refrigerator Mother theory.

In spite of his questionable credentials, Bettelheim was recognized as the leading expert in autism throughout the 1950s and 60s. He was even lauded as a hero by some. In spite of emerging evidence to the contrary, he remained doggedly insistent on attempting to treat this medical disease with psychoanalysis. Even as recently as 1981, Dr. Bettelheim wrote, "All my life, I have been working with children whose lives were destroyed because their mothers hated them."[8]

In the early 1960s, members of the medical community began questioning the prevailing psychoanalytical dogma that autism was a result of poor parenting. Bernard Rimland, a PhD in experimental psychology and the father of an autistic child, published a book in 1964 called *Infantile Autism: The Syndrome and Its Implications for a Neural Theory of Behavior*. He challenged Bettelheim's theories, suggesting that autism was in fact the result of neurological and hereditable factors, its roots deeply embedded in biology rather than psychology. His book was given the 1964 Century Award for "distinguished contribution to psychology." He is largely credited with shifting the medical paradigm toward looking at autism as a biological condition. In 1967, Dr. Rimland founded the nonprofit Autism Research Institute (formerly called the Institute for Child Behavior Research). Over the last forty years, Dr. Rimland and ARI have continued to conduct research and gather information from thousands of parents and physicians about effective biologically based treatments for children with autism (see appendix).

Progress in Behavioral Intervention

Not long after the publication of Dr. Rimland's groundbreaking book, Dr. Eric Schopler at the University of North Carolina pioneered a new treatment program for autistic children, using their parents as cotherapists. This was prompted by his experience as a graduate student at the University of Chicago. He was deeply troubled by his professor's insistence that autistic children climb on a cold stone sculpture of a mother, theoretically helping them to subconsciously understand what their mothers had done to them. Dr. Schopler's innovative program, later named TEACCH (Treatment and Education of Autistic and related Communication-handicapped CHildren), became the first comprehensive statewide program for the education of autistic children.

In 1987, Ivar Lovaas of UCLA published a landmark paper showing for the first time that a group of autistic children could recover functionally when given intensive educational and behavioral intervention.[9] His form of therapy is known as Applied Behavioral Analysis (ABA). It works on the principle of modifying behavior through the positive and negative reinforcement of targeted behaviors. He found that children who received between thirty and forty hours of ABA therapy a week did much better than children who received less than ten hours a week. A follow-up study done in 1993 confirmed that the children who received intensive ABA therapy retained the skills that they had learned and even continued to gain new skills naturally.[10]

This watershed research prompted a move toward early educational intervention for autistic children. Prior to that, most experts did not believe that children with autism could ever improve to any meaningful degree. In 1999, ABA therapy was endorsed by the Surgeon General of the United States as the most appropriate form of behavior therapy for children with this disease. It's unfortunate that most public schools have not implemented this recommendation to a meaningful degree.

The Refrigerator Mother theory was an enormous setback for autistic children and their families. Rather than trying to understand the children's symptoms, decades were wasted in psychoanalytic treatment of the children and their parents. Improved behavior modification techniques have shown us that autistic children can, in fact, get better. It wasn't until recently however, with the emerging understanding of autism as a medical condition, that more large-scale improvements have been seen.

chapter three

AUTISM ISN'T PURELY GENETIC

IN THE 1970S, SIGNIFICANT ADVANCES WERE MADE IN understanding the role of genetics in the cause of disease; it was an exciting new field with a lot of publicity, and autism seemed like a good target. In 1977, Folstein and Rutter published the first of several studies comparing rates of autism in twin pairs.[1] Out of twenty-one pairs, both twins had autism in 40% of the monozygotic (identical) pairs and in only 10% of the dizygotic (fraternal) twins. Subsequent twin studies showed a concordance (both twins affected) of 60%-90% for autism in monozygotic twins, and 10-25% in dizygotic twins.[2][3][4][5] Since the rates of developing the disease were higher in the twins with identical genetics (monozygotic) compared to those twins who only shared a portion of their genetic code (dizygotic), this was taken as evidence that autism is a genetic disease. The risk of non-twin siblings acquiring autism (2 to 4.5%) was one hundred times the estimated prevalence rate for the entire population reported at the time.[6][7] There also appears to be an increased chance of pervasive developmental disorders (PDD), speech delays, and other language disorders in the siblings and parents of children with autism.[8][9][10][11][12]

Although these studies strongly suggest that genetics play a part in this disease, the fact that the incidence in identical twins is not 100% proves that the chromosomal imprint (by definition the same in both twins) cannot be the only factor in developing autism. The genetics of autism are complex, and multiple locations (perhaps fifteen or more) on several genes are likely to be involved.[13][14][15] In fact, as of 2001, all but three of the twenty-four human chromosomes have locations that are suspected to increase the risk of autism.[16][17][18]

The role of genetics in autism appears to extend beyond the neurological system. Genetic abnormalities affecting the immune system have been documented in the families of children with autism. Comi et al. reported that 46% of families with autistic children (16% of mothers and 21% of first-degree relatives compared with 2% and 4% of the controls, respectively) have two or more members with other autoimmune diseases. With three or more members, the risk of having a child with autism triples. The most common autoimmune illnesses reported were type I diabetes, adult-onset rheumatoid arthritis, hypothyroidism, and lupus.[19]

Sweeten et al. compared rates of autoimmune disease in first and second-generation family members of children with autism spectrum disorders (ASD) to children who had other autoimmune diseases and to healthy controls. There was a higher percentage of autoimmune disease in the families of the ASD children compared with both the autoimmune children (p value=0.03) and the healthy controls (p=0.000003; A p-value is a measurement of the possibility that the difference noted between the two groups could have occurred by chance alone. A p-value of 0.05 is considered statistically significant for medical research and means that there is less than a 5% likelihood that the difference occurred because of chance). Interestingly, when they separated out the children with pervasive developmental disorder-not otherwise specified (PDD-NOS) from the children with autism and Asperger's syndrome, the significance rose even higher (p=0.001, p=0.0000004). (PDD-NOS children had about the same rate of autoimmune disease in their families as the control children.) This suggests that there are immune-based genetic subtypes within the broader autism spectrum. The autoimmune illnesses most commonly associated with autism were hypothyroidism, Hashimoto's thyroiditis, and rheumatic fever.[20]

Another study further explored the existence of genetic subtypes in autism by looking at the family history of autoimmune diseases in children with regressive autism versus those without regression. This multi-center study on 308 children found that at least one first or second degree relative had an autoimmune disease in 57% percent of the total group. There was a higher incidence of autoimmune disease in the families of children with regression (odds ratio OR 1.89, p=0.009; an odds ratio of greater than one suggests that there is a higher likelihood for a given outcome in one group compared to the other. The higher the number, the more likely the outcome). Of the common autoimmune diseases, only autoimmune thyroid disease showed a significant association (OR 2.09, p=0.003), and it was more likely to be found in the maternal side of the family (OR 2.40).[21]

Because of a higher risk of autoimmune disease in the mothers of autistic children, Croen et al. did a study to see if the risk of developing autism was temporally related to a maternal autoimmune disease occurring during or near the time of pregnancy. With the exception of a slightly higher rate of psoriasis, they were unable to detect an increased rate of autoimmune diseases within four years of the pregnancy. They did show an increased risk for autism if the mothers had asthma or symptomatic allergies during the second trimester of the pregnancy.[22]

Recently, Campbell et al. found a higher rate of a genetic variant of a cell receptor called MET in families of children with autism (relative risk 2.27—relative risk is the risk of an event relative to a given exposure). This receptor signaling is important for normal growth and maturation of the brain (the cerebral cortex and the cerebellum), for the immune system, and for gastrointestinal repair. This is a good example of a gene variant that can link the physiological abnormalities commonly seen in autism, which involve more than just the brain.[23]

Instead of having a genetic disorder, people with autism are better described as having a genetic susceptibility. The environment is clearly playing a role. Although most researchers acknowledge this in their studies,[24][25][26][27] it appears to have been largely ignored, judging by the direction autism research has taken. Over the last twenty to thirty years, the bulk of research funding in autism has gone to the study of genetics. Until very recently, prevailing opinion continued to promote the theory that autism is a purely genetic disease, occurring as a result of a mutation very early in fetal development; hence, the course of the disease is unalterable. While finding the "autism gene" might allow for in-utero detection and provide the opportunity for counseling parents regarding risk, it is unlikely to make a difference in the outcome for the current generation of children.

Certainly, understanding the genes might someday enable us to modify them, and thereby prevent or correct the problem. Finding the autism genes might help us understand the affected biochemical pathways, which could eventually lead to medications to treat the condition.[28][29] However, understanding the role of the environment and studying the biochemistry of autistic children seems much more likely to lead to effective treatments immediately, and in fact would pinpoint which genes should be targeted. Truly understanding the genetic factors requires understanding the impact of the environment on the genetic code.

chapter four

THE AUTISM EPIDEMIC

BEFORE 1980, AUTISM WAS RARE. PREVALENCE STUDIES DONE BEFORE then consistently estimated the rate to be 2-5 per 10,000 people.[1][2][3] Most general practitioners and pediatricians went through their entire careers without ever seeing a case. If mentioned at all in medical school, it was relegated to part of a lecture on "rare but interesting" psychiatric disorders. In 1958 Kanner wrote, "The fact that an average of not more than eight patients per year [over twenty years] could be diagnosed with reasonable assurance as autistic in a center serving as a sort of a diagnostic clearinghouse, speaks for the infrequency of the disease, especially if one considers that they recruit themselves from all over the North American continent."[4]

Arn Van Krevelen, the first child psychiatrist in Europe to publish a case of infantile autism (and hence their one and only resident expert at the time), admitted that he'd begun to doubt the existence of autism because there was no mention of it in the European literature for nearly a decade following Kanner's paper. When he finally did encounter an autistic child, he said she was "...as much like those described by Kanner as one raindrop is like another." In the decade following the publication of his paper, Van Krevelen, the expert for an entire continent, saw only ten more cases.[5]

Clearly autism was once highly unusual. It wasn't brought into public awareness in the US until 1988, when Dustin Hoffman portrayed an autistic savant in the movie *Rainman*. Despite impressive abilities in memory and mathematical calculation, the character he played had very rote language, no social skills, and a disabling need for routine. For most people, the savant character in *Rainman* defined autism because they had no other model.

Concern in California

Starting in the mid-1980s, more and more children were being diagnosed. Through the 1990s, rates rose exponentially. The State of California has tracked the numbers of people with autism enrolled in their developmental services program since 1960. In 1969, the Lanterman Act established regional centers to care for people with developmental disabilities throughout the state; in 1973 autism was included in the list of disabilities for which the centers were required to provide services. It's estimated that 75-80% of developmentally disabled children in California are enrolled in this system.[6]

In March 1999, the California Department of Developmental Services (DDS) issued a report entitled "Changes in the Population of Persons with Autism and Pervasive Developmental Disorders in California's Developmental Services System: 1987 through 1998." They reported a 273% increase in DSM-IV full-criteria autism cases enrolled in their program during that decade. Other ASDs increased at an even higher rate—1,965%. Alarmingly, the explosion of cases was from the youngest age groups.

The following graph shows the number of enrolled cases in the California system per birth year between 1960 and 1991. You can see that the rates were fairly flat until the late 1970s when they began to rise:

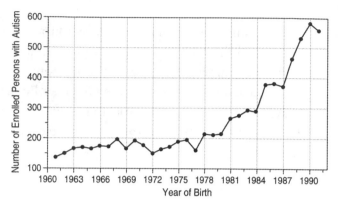

Fig. 1: Distribution of birth rates of regional center eligible persons with autism. Source: DDS Report to the Legislature 3/1/99.

The slope of the rise increased substantially in those children born after 1984.

Figure 2 shows a marked skewing of the population distribution of autism cases in California between 1987 and 1998:

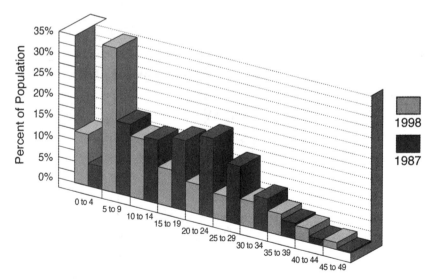

Fig. 2: Age distribution for autistic population in 1987 and 1998. Source: DDS Report to the Legislature 3/1/99.

In 1987, the number of cases was pretty evenly distributed across the age groups, at least between age five and age twenty-nine, after which it dropped off. There is a large percentage increase in 1998 in the five to nine year olds, and two-thirds of the cases were younger than fourteen (up from about 37% in 1987). The rate of general population growth in California between 1987 and 1998 was 20%.

Other disabilities included under the Lanterman Act were also increasing, but not at a rate anywhere close to the rate of autism:

Of all of the children in the California system with developmental disabilities, the percentage of those cases with autism nearly doubled from 4.85 to 9.37%.

What was happening? Why was this previously rare disorder suddenly overwhelming the system? Experts quickly dismissed the idea that these numbers represented a true rise in incidence.[7][8] They reasoned that autism was, after all, a genetic illness, and since there is no such thing as a genetic epidemic, there had to be another explanation. They suggested that changes in the diagnostic criteria had skewed the numbers.[9][10][11][12] Or, that what had been called "mental retardation" was now being called autism.[13][14] Or, that doctors were now more aware of the condition and were better at diagnosing it. Or, that parents were now seeking services for their children with autism instead of keeping them at home, as parents must have done in the past. Or, people with autistic children were moving to California from all over the country to take advantage of better services. Or even that since California was

	1987	1998	Percent Change
Autism (All Combinations)	3,864	11,995	210.43%
Cerebral Palsy (All Combinations)	19,972	28,529	42.84%
Epilepsy (All Combinations)	22,683	29,645	30.69%
Mental Retardation (All Combinations)	72,987	108,563	48.74%
Whole Population	80,483	136,383	69.46%

Table 1: Percent increase in diagnostic populations from 1987 to 1998. Source: DDS Report to the Legislature 3/1/99.

the high-tech capital of the world and since people with autism were particularly adept at computers, these previously undiagnosed adults were now marrying each other and their children were more severely affected.[15][16] Or better yet, autistic males now had a place in the world because of their computer skills and were able to make a lot of money and were, therefore, more attractive to the opposite sex. They were now given the opportunity to procreate when previously they would have been shunned, or relegated to monasteries to spend their days making copies of the Bible.[17] Researchers began diligently looking at the data to see if any of these theories were correct.

The MIND Institute Study

The California Legislature commissioned the University of California's Medical Investigation of Neurodevelopmental Disorders (MIND) Institute in Sacramento to study the possible causes of the rise in the numbers of reported cases of autism in California. The results, "The Epidemiology of Autism in California," were reported to the State Legislature in October 2002. The study included 684 children. Of these, 375 carried a diagnosis of CDER status 1 or 2 autism (equates to full DSM-IV criteria autism). Three hundred nine children were diagnosed with MR (mental retardation) and had no autism diagnosis. Two birth cohorts were compared: children born between the years 1983 and 1985 (cohort #1) and children born between 1993 and 1995 (cohort #2). They used data from the DDS Client Development Evaluation form, the Regional Center records, the Autism Diagnostic Interview-Revised (ADI-R), and their own detailed study questionnaire. The study had several aims:

Aim #1: To investigate whether changes over time in the criteria used to diagnose CDER status 1 autism accounted for a significant proportion of the increased number of cases. In cohort #1, 88% met the current criteria for autism compared to 89% of cohort #2. There was no meaningful change in the CDER or ADI-R criteria over the intervening decade. Their conclusion: "There is no evidence that a loosening in diagnostic criteria has contributed to the increased number of autistic clients served by the Regional Centers."

Aim #2: To investigate whether the past misclassification of some cases of autism as mental retardation had contributed to an apparent increase in the number of children with autism. They found that some children in the mental retardation group did in fact meet DSM-IV criteria for autism. There were 18% in Cohort #1 and 19% in Cohort #2. Since both cohorts had similar numbers, misclassification could not explain the rise. The investigators acknowledged that the numbers might be artificially high because families might have been more likely to enroll in the study if they felt that their MR children also had an autism spectrum disorder (ASD).

Aim #3: To investigate whether children with autism who moved to California for services could account for the increased cases of autism reported to DDS. They found that 87% of cohort #1 was born in California, compared to 93% of cohort #2. Conclusion: "…autistic children in the Regional Center System are largely native to the state and are not coming disproportionately from outside California."

Aim #4: To describe how characteristics of children with autism had changed over time. They reported no significant differences regarding sex, race, parent education, or pregnancy factors between the two groups except that there were more Hispanic children in the younger cohort (28% in cohort #1 vs. 39% in cohort #2). Parents of the older children were more likely to report that their autistic child had mental retardation (41% vs. 21%), and this coincided with Regional Center data (50% in cohort #1 vs. 22% in cohort #2). The older cohort children were also more likely to be reported as having tic disorders, obsessive-compulsive disorder, depression, and bipolar disorder, although that might have been due to an age effect (more likely to be diagnosed as they get older). Parents of the younger cohort were more likely to report improvement of their child's condition over time (93% vs. 81%), gastrointestinal symptoms in the first fifteen months of life, and wheat allergy (12% vs. 4%). There was little difference in the number of children reported to have had a regression of developmental milestones (28% in cohort #1 vs. 34% in cohort #2). The report concluded that none of these differences explained the increased incidence of autism.

Aim #5: To find out what parents of autistic children thought had caused their child's autism, and to determine if perceptions were different between the two cohorts. The most common response in both groups was no response or "don't know" (46% vs. 48%). Other responses included: genetics (31% vs. 27%), immunizations as a contributing factor (18% vs. 33%), birth events (about 15% in both groups), and environmental exposure (11% of combined groups).

Aim #6: To determine if vaccination with MMR vaccine was associated with an increase in the rate of autism recurrence in subsequent siblings. Avoidance or delay of at least one vaccine for the child with autism was reported at 8% for cohort #1 and 22% for cohort #2. There were similar numbers for avoidance of vaccines in younger siblings (10% vs. 21%). The authors acknowledged that they would have needed approximately 7,000 participants in order to answer the question posed by this study aim, far in excess of the 684 enrolled.

Their final conclusion was: "Without evidence for an artificial increase in autism cases, we conclude that some, if not all, of the observed increase represents a true increase in cases of autism in California, and the number of cases presenting to the Regional Center system is not an overestimation of the number of children with autism in California."[18]

Diagnostic Substitution?

Other researchers began looking at the California numbers. Croen reviewed the data collected from the regional centers on children with autism who were born in eight successive birth years, between 1987 and 1994. The prevalence rate increased from 5.8 to 14.9 per 10,000 over the study period, with an absolute change of 9.1 per 10,000. Rates of the diagnosis of mental retardation without autism over the same time period decreased from 28.8 to 19.5, for an absolute change of 9.3 per 10,000. Since the absolute increase in autism was nearly equal to the absolute decrease in MR, she concluded that the rising incidence of autism was a result of substituting the one diagnosis for the other.[19]

Blaxill et al., DSM III-R and DSM IV Criteria for Autism reanalyzed Croen's data and detected several flaws. When looking over the entire eight-year period, the diagnostic trends seemed to offset, but when the period was broken into two- or three-year subgroups, the pattern no longer matched. One period had a large decline in MR and only a short increase in autism, one had a large increase in autism and a very small decrease in MR, and one had a large decrease in MR and a small decrease in autism. If diagnostic substitution were the answer, the trends within each time period should also have correlated.

Blaxill also showed that ascertainment bias within Croen's study probably invalidated the results. Because children with autism were often not diagnosed until after they were four years old, it was likely that Croen underestimated the prevalence in the youngest (1994) cohort, which had just turned four. Using statistical estimation methods to correct for this bias, the true prevalence in the younger kids was more likely to be 21.3- 29.8 and the rate of change closer to 14-24 per 10,000, rather than 9.1. A similar effect was demonstrated in the MR group, in which the diagnosis is often delayed until puberty. It's likely that the true incidence of MR was also increasing slowly during that time period.[20] In a reply to Blaxill's commentary, Croen acknowledged that these points were valid.[21]

What about the Rest of the Country?

Is California an anomaly, or has the incidence of autism been increasing in other states as well? Because of the quality of the California data, many researchers use those numbers for studies. Most other states didn't start tracking autism until the early 1990s, when the Federal Department of Education mandated it as part of the IDEA law. Since then, we have data from every state, but because some children with autism don't go to public school, and because the diagnoses made by the school districts have not always been validated, we can't use these school-based numbers for true prevalence studies; nonetheless, the trend in all states is consistent and unequivocal.

Figure 3 shows the rising prevalence of autism in all of the US; it's apparent that the rates in California are no more than average. There have only been a few prevalence studies of autism in the US published in the medical literature. The three studies done before 1993 all showed rates between three and four per ten thousand.[22][23][24]

In 2001, Bertrand et al. published a study in the journal *Pediatrics*. It was done in response to concern over an apparent high rate of autism in the community of Brick Township, New Jersey. In 1998 they searched for all cases of autism in children between three and ten years old in that community, using several methods for active case-finding, including reviewing school and physicians' records, canvassing community parent groups, and sponsoring a local marketing campaign. They confirmed

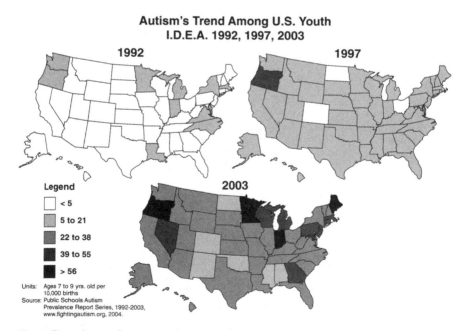

Fig. 3: Prevalence of autism in the public school system of 7 to 9 year-olds per 10,000 births. Source: Public Schools Autism Prevalence Report Series, 1992-2002, www. FightingAutism.org, 2004

the diagnoses with clinical assessment in the majority of cases. They found an alarming prevalence of forty per ten thousand (1 in 250) for full-spectrum autism and sixty-seven per ten thousand (1 in 149) for other ASDs.[25]

A similar study in the metropolitan Atlanta area (published in 2003 in *JAMA*) yielded numbers lower than Brick Township (34 per 10,000 for all ASDs in children between three and ten years old in 1996), but this rate was still much higher than previous US studies and showed higher numbers in the younger age groups.[26] The lower rates were more likely a result of less rigorous case-finding efforts rather than a truly lower prevalence compared to Brick Township.

Finally, in 2004, the CDC published an autism "ALARM," acknowledging that the current rate of ASD in the US was one in 166. They also noted that a developmental disability and/or behavior problem was being diagnosed in one child out of every six.[27]

What about Other Countries?

Other developed countries have reported similar surges in prevalence concurrent with the rising US numbers. Gillberg and Wing showed very low rates in children born in Sweden before 1970: two to five per ten thousand. The rates were at least double in children born between 1990 and 1995 (ten per ten thousand).[28]

A study published in 2001 found a prevalence of 62.6 per ten thousand (16.8 for autism and 45.8 for other PDDs) in preschool-aged children in Staffordshire, England.[29] Many other studies in England confirmed increasing rates.[30][31][32][33][34] A startling 2006 report from England found the rate of ASDs in nine and ten year olds in the South Thames region (out of 57,000 children) to be 116.1 per 10,000 (38.9 for autism, 77.2 for other ASDs).[35] *This is one in eighty-six children.* Other countries have also reported a rise, including Iceland,[36] Sweden,[37][38][39] Finland,[40] Denmark,[41][42][43][44] Canada,[45][46][47] Australia,[48] and Japan.[49][50]

Changes in the Diagnostic Criteria

The rising numbers are undeniable. Many still believe, however, that it's due to changes in the diagnostic criteria. The MIND study refuted this explanation. But the definition has changed slightly over time, so is it possible?

Since Kanner first described it, autism has been defined by its collection of behavioral symptoms. In 1956, Kanner and Eisenberg suggested that the only two defining symptoms were a profound lack of affective contact and repetitive, ritualistic, elaborate behavior. For decades after, the definition remained imprecise, and autism wasn't even included as a separate disorder in the first two Diagnostic Manuals of the American Psychiatry Association.

In 1980, the DSM-III (Diagnostic and Statistical Manual of Mental Disorders, third edition) created a new category called "pervasive developmental disorders," which included "infantile autism." The criteria for infantile autism were as follows: (A) Onset before thirty months of age; (B) Pervasive lack of responsiveness to other people; (C) Gross deficits in language development; (D) If speech is present, peculiar speech patterns such as immediate and delayed echolalia, metaphorical language, pronoun reversal; (E) Absence of delusions, hallucinations, loosening of associations, and incoherence, as in schizophrenia.

This 1980 definition was eventually found to be too restrictive. It didn't allow for the variations commonly seen in individuals thought to be on the spectrum. When the DSM-III was revised in 1987 (DSM III-R), the diagnostic criteria were modified (see appendix). Now there were three primary features: abnormal social interaction, abnormal communication, and narrowed interests or activities. The three features included sixteen separate criteria (each with specific examples), of which a certain number from each category were required for the diagnosis. DSM III-R also specified an onset during infancy or early childhood, and mentioned for the first time the possibility of other symptoms such as sensory disturbances and uneven acquisition of skills.

The other pervasive developmental disorders described in the previous DSM edition were now grouped together as Pervasive Developmental Disorder-Not Otherwise Specified (PDD-NOS). Critics of the new criteria, who had once thought the definition too narrow, now considered the parameters too broad, and felt that many children who previously would not have been considered to have the disorder were now being misclassified.[51]

When the DSM-IV was published in 1994, the criteria for autism were modified yet again (appendix). The defining characteristics were decreased from sixteen to twelve, and the language in some of the criteria was changed. The intent was to narrow the DSM-III-R definition, thus increasing the specificity of the diagnosis. Also, the concept of a spectrum of pervasive developmental disorders was reintroduced and similar syndromes (Asperger's syndrome, Pervasive Developmental Disorder-Not Otherwise Specified, Rett's Disorder, and Childhood Disintegrative Disorder) were now included as separate but related disorders. These defining criteria have remained unchanged and generally accepted since 1994.[52 53]

The argument that the introduction of the DSM-III-R criteria caused an increase in numbers after 1987 doesn't bear scrutiny; the rise would have leveled off over a couple of years as people became familiar with the new diagnostic criteria. In addition, we would expect to see a drop in the rate of new diagnoses after 1994 when DSM-IV standards were narrowed. Certainly, if this most recent change in criteria were responsible for a statistical rise, the curve would have flattened long before now (thirteen years later, at this writing).

Other Explanations?

Are there any other valid theories? It would be irresponsible not to consider them all fairly. One is that the rise in numbers occurred because doctors are now much better at diagnosing autism. Studies have shown (and my own clinical experience confirms) that the vast majority of children are not diagnosed by their primary care physicians.[54] Most are referred from school districts. Most parents report that doctors disregarded their early concerns, often giving a number of other explanations for the child's delayed development including "boys talk later," "his older siblings are talking for him," or even "Einstein didn't talk until he was four years old." Parents often report needing to ask repeatedly for referrals, or having to visit several doctors before their concerns are acknowledged.

This trend could be changing. Because of growing awareness of effective early educational interventions, some doctors are beginning to refer patients to specialists for diagnostic evaluations at a younger age. The average age of diagnosis in California, for example, has dropped from age five to just before four.[55] But earlier diagnosis cannot explain the rising incidence (number of cases per birth year); it only increases the numbers reported in the youngest age group.

The diagnosis of autism requires nothing more than a good history and physical exam. There simply are no other diagnostic tests or technological advances used to make the diagnosis. It's unreasonable to think that doctors today are better at taking a history and performing a physical exam than doctors were twenty years ago. In fact, physicians today rely less on history-taking and exam skills and much more on technology to make diagnoses in general.[56] Full-criteria autism is not a subtle disorder. There is no reason to believe that physicians wouldn't have noticed this degree of abnormality in their patients twenty or thirty years ago.

What about the theory that more parents are suddenly seeking services? Autism is a disabling disease, not only for the patients, but for the entire family. The care needed by an autistic child never ends. It's expensive, difficult, and frequently disheartening. Is it reasonable to think that twenty years ago parents of autistic children would not have gone to their doctors or school districts to seek help for their child? In California alone, three thousand cases are being diagnosed a year. Is it possible that year after year three thousand more California families kept their autistic children hidden at home? It's an illogical conclusion—it defies common sense.

The Hidden Horde Theory Refuted

In spite of overwhelming evidence to the contrary, some experts still deny that an autism epidemic exists.[57] They argue that the rising numbers are no more than a statistical aberration. If the apparent increase reflects more accurate diagnosis and case finding, then there must be "a hidden horde" of undiagnosed autistic adults in the population. Since autism is disabling, undiagnosed individuals would end up where society deposits the mentally ill: outpatient psychiatric clinics, mental institutions, homeless shelters, or prisons.

In fact, studies have been done looking for this large group of autistic adults. Burd et al. did a prevalence study of all autistic children born in North Dakota between the years 1967 and 1983 and found a rate of 3.4 per 10,000.[58] A follow up study on the same cohort done twelve years later showed that the original study detected 98% of the cases of autism (they missed only one individual).[59]

Nylander and Gillberg screened adults at outpatient psychiatric facilities in Sweden, looking for undiagnosed cases of autism.[60] They presumed they'd find people who had never been evaluated for autism in the past, at least using modern criteria. They did find nineteen people who met autism criteria who'd previously been undiagnosed as such, but that brought their prevalence rate to only 2.7 per ten thousand, similar to the other population rates quoted before 1980. Others have tried, but no high-quality study has been done that can validate the hidden horde hypothesis.[61 62] (And if there were such a horde, it would be damning to a medical community that could allow a potentially enormous number of disabled individuals to go undiagnosed and untreated.[63])

California Update

So what has happened to the numbers in California since the original 1998 report? The California DDS published a 2003 update of the autism trends within the state. In December 2002, the number of cases of full-criteria autism being serviced by the system had risen to 20,377 (about double):

	Dec. 1987	Dec. 1998	Dec. 2002
Total Population with CDERs	80,389	129,169	163,791
Persons with Autism (Codes 1 & 2)	2,778	10,360	20,377
Percent of Total Population with Autism	3.46%	8.02%	12.44%

Table 2: Number of persons with autism (codes 1 & 2) in 1987, 1998, and 2002. Source: DDS "Changes in the CA Caseload. 1999-2002.

The prevalence rate for the 1997 birth year rose to thirty-one per ten thousand:

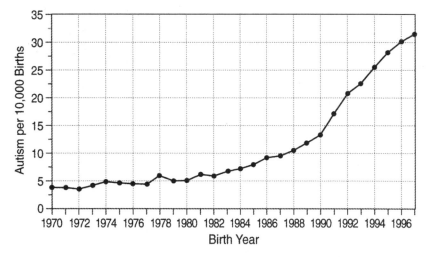

Fig 4: Uncorrected birth year prevalence rates from 1970-1997 for the 2002 population of persons with autism. Source: DDS "Changes in the CA Caseload. 1999-2002.

The preceding graph shows the relative change in prevalence per age group over the five years between 1997 and 2002. The increasingly steep slopes among the younger age cohorts indicate a rapid rise in the number of young children being diagnosed with autism.

The rates of autism continue to rise alarmingly above other developmental disorders, as in figure 6 on the following page.

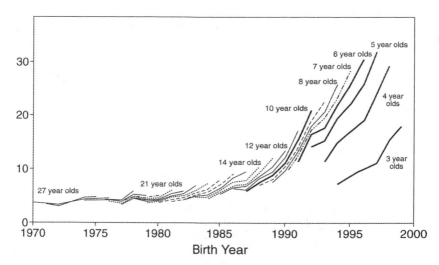

Fig. 5: Rates in CA over six years: 12/9712/02. Prevalence rate by age cohort (cases per 10,000). Source: Blaxill, M. The Question of Time Trends in Autism. Autism One Conference. 5/28/06.

Through the 1970's, autism accounted for roughly 3% of the new cases entering California's developmental services system. By 2003, that number had increased to 40%, but by the third quarter of 2006, autism accounted for 76% of all new intakes entering the system.

Age at first diagnosis continues to decrease. The following graph shows the age at which people with autism and other disabilities first accessed the DDS system. You can see that the most common age for diagnosing autism is now two to three. For other disorders, including mental retardation, there is a spike at birth, and then again as they enter the school system, which continues through their teenage years. This is exactly what Blaxill predicted in his rebuttal to Croen's diagnostic substitution paper.[64]

The age distribution of all cases in the system continued to skew toward a younger population, which also indicates a rising incidence. The next graph shows that in 2002, the percentage of the autism population under age fourteen increased to 70%, up from 66% in 1998 and 35.5% in 1987, as in figure 7.

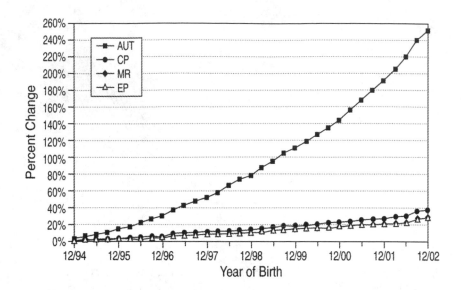

Fig. 6: Percent change in all disabilities from 1994 through 2002. Source: DDS "Changes in the CA Caseload." 1999-2002.

Remember that these numbers and graphs represent people with full-criteria autism only, not PDD or other ASDs. As of September 2006, the number of people receiving services in California has reached 31,853.

The Autism Crisis

It is no longer possible to deny that autism is rampant. It represents a major social and medical crisis. A recent Harvard School of Public Health study by Dr. Michael Ganz estimates that the direct and indirect costs of caring for an individual with autism are as much as $3.2 million over his or her lifetime.[65] Even if, starting today, no more autistic children were born, long-term care for those already living will cost trillions of dollars and will conceivably completely absorb, and then bankrupt, the federal social services budget. Ignoring this problem is no longer an option.

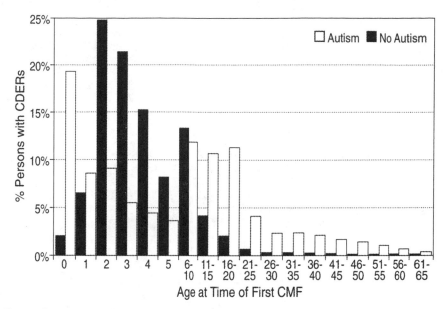

Fig. 7: Comparison of age at time of first request for services between persons with autism (codes 1 & 2) and persons without autism. Source: DDS "Changes in the CA Caseload. 1999-2002.

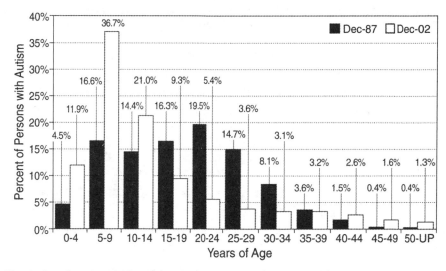

Fig. 8: Age distribution for all persons with autism (codes 1 & 2) in 1987 and 2002. Source: DDS "Changes in the CA Caseload. 1999-2002. *www.dds.ca.gov/autism/pdf/ AutismReport2003.pdf.*

chapter five

AUTISM IS A DISEASE, NOT A DISABILITY

Autism: An Environmental Illness

WHY IS ANSWERING THE QUESTION ABOUT THE RISING INCIDENCE of autism important? *Because there is no such thing as a genetic epidemic.* If the increase in numbers is real, and available evidence suggests that it is, it strongly implicates an environmental component to this disease. There is no other explanation. This reality must force a complete shift in the way that we view autism, the way we fund research, and the way we approach treatment.

Autism can no longer be viewed as a purely genetic illness with the outcome written in the chromosomes. If we can determine which environmental factors are triggering the epidemic, we can potentially prevent it and even find a cure. Although logical, this represents a major shift in thinking for the medical community and the government agencies that fund medical research.

To date, relative to far less common disorders, autism research has been poorly funded. If autism is truly an epidemic, it should be considered as high a priority as other threatening world-wide epidemics such as bird flu, West Nile Virus, and HIV. This is especially true since it is a chronic, disabling condition with lifetime care the usual expectation if untreated.

Incidence vs. Private Funding

- Leukemia: Affects 1 in 25,000 / Funding: $310 million
- Muscular Dystrophy: Affects 1 in 20,000 / Funding: $175 million
- Pediatric AIDS: Affects 1 in 8,000 / Funding: $394 million
- Juvenile Diabetes: Affects 1 in 500 / Funding: $130 million
- Autism: Affects 1 in 150 / Funding: $15 million

National Institutes of Health Funds Allocation

- Total 2005 NIH budget: $29 billion
- Of this, only $100 million goes towards autism research. This represents 0.3% of total NIH funding.

Table 1: Source: Autism Speaks *www.autismspeaks.org*

If understanding the role of the environment will lead to prevention or treatment, the funding balance should now be shifted so that the majority is directed toward environmental causes and interactions. Unfortunately, altering medical dogma is like turning an aircraft carrier. In spite of obvious misdirection, it takes time to change course. The history of medicine is full of examples of new ideas that were rejected by the medical community only to be widely recognized decades later as undisputed fact.

Disease, Not Disability

Independent researchers and physicians have been adding pieces to the complex biochemical puzzle of autism. Many of them are the parents or grandparents of autistic children. Others were moved by the compelling stories of grief and frustration told them by parents. As the parent of an autistic child myself, I feel indebted to each of these dedicated people. They have persisted in their efforts to add to our understanding, often in the face of strong institutional and political pressures. While there's bound to be controversy in any paradigm shift, it can be particularly heated when major environmental causes might be to blame, and governments, politics, and business lobbies are involved.

In the chapters that follow, I'll describe the current accumulated research on the metabolic abnormalities of autism. Each piece of information adds clarity to the emerging scientific picture. Autism is among the most complex diseases that I have ever encountered, in the scope of its physical effects on the human body.

Currently the definition of autism is a collection of behavioral symptoms, and it's classified as a developmental disability or disorder. This oversimplification does not account for the many differences in the neurological presentation of children within the autism spectrum, and certainly doesn't account for the symptoms in the other organ systems. Whatever the root cause, autism affects a fundamental and critical part of metabolism. Calling it a developmental disorder is like calling a brain tumor a headache. "Autism" is merely one symptom of an underlying disease process that affects the immunological system, the gastrointestinal system, and the toxicological system, as well as the neurological system.

It's certainly possible that we're dealing with more than one cause and more than one disease, manifesting with similar overlapping neurological syndromes. Anyone who has treated many autistic patients will tell you they are not all alike, neither in their symptoms nor in their response to treatment. Ultimately, sorting out the subgroups will be important to determine the most effective treatment strategy.

We need to redefine autism as a multi-organ metabolic disease that should be removed from the DSM-IV, placed in the medical textbooks instead, and routinely taught in medical schools and residencies.

The Multiple Hit Hypothesis

The most likely scenario for the development of this disease involves a series of negative responses to the environment in a baby who is at risk genetically. As in most diseases, coupling genetic predisposition with environmental factors raises the risk. For example, a positive family history of heart disease is a significant risk factor, but when you add environmental insults such as smoking, obesity, poor diet, etc., the cardiac risk rises substantially. I believe autism works in a similar way. Evidence shows a higher rate of autoimmune disease in the families of autistic children.[1,2] This suggests a genetic predisposition in the immune system of children with ASD (autism spectrum disorders). As discussed in later chapters, children with autism have abnormal detoxification systems, which also increase their risk of damage from environmental insults.

Almost immediately after conception, the growing fetus is exposed to a variety of toxins and foreign substances. Many studies have documented increasing levels of placental toxins.[3,4,5,6,7] These come from the food the mother is eating, the air she is breathing, the medications she is taking, and the vaccinations she might have received. These substances pass through her blood, through the placenta, and into the fetal tissue. Because the baby has a weak detoxification capacity, the toxins can accumulate rather than be excreted.

After birth, more toxins and chemicals are introduced. These could start with the medications given to the mother during delivery, in prophylactic medications given to the baby as part of hospital routine, and hepatitis B vaccinations given within hours of birth (since the early 1990s).

Over the next year of the baby's life, he or she is introduced daily to potentially millions of other new exposures, including breast milk, formula, baby food, other foods, chemicals in the air, soaps, clothes, vaccines, medications like acetaminophen or ibuprofen, and, all too often, antibiotics. Most children seem to tolerate these exposures without obvious ill effects, but if a child has an abnormal immunological or toxicological system because of genetic factors, risk of injury will be much higher.

As environmental toxins accumulate, a critical point is reached when the struggling immune system can no longer deal with them appropriately, and damage occurs. I refer to this as the toxic tipping point. Once this toxic tipping point is exceeded, a series of reactions is likely to happen. First the toxin will damage tissues directly, setting off an inflammatory reaction. The inflammation itself creates more damage, triggering further inflammation, forming a vicious cycle. The immune system then loses its ability to deal with incoming exposures and begins to misinterpret "self" for "non-self." This results in an autoimmune reaction, i.e., the body defends itself against itself. With this impaired regulation of the immune system, the body becomes vulnerable—more susceptible to even graver injury from both new and ongoing exposures—until it can no longer compensate and a disease state is manifest. In the case of autism, this often correlates with a neurological regression, after what appeared to be normal early development (chapter 7).

Can the multiple-hit theory explain an epidemic? We know an epidemic must arise from either exposure to a new toxin or infectious agent, or an increased exposure of a previously known toxin(s) that is capable of causing the immune system damage described above. Another possibility is that the general toxic load in the environment has risen to a point where so many of us have reached our genetically-determined toxic tipping point that the human species has now edged into a state we might call herd vulnerability.

chapter six

BASICS OF THE IMMUNE SYSTEM

FROM AN EVOLUTIONARY PERSPECTIVE, THE PURPOSE OF EVERY LIVING thing is to survive long enough to pass on its genes, so each species has developed an elaborate defense system to ensure this end. The human body is a perfect breeding ground for many microorganisms; unfortunately for us, some of these have no interest in preserving their host after they've replicated, causing us damage, disease, and sometimes death. To combat these invaders, our bodies have developed an intricate defense—the immune system.

This system has many layers and barriers. Within each redundant layer there's a network of cells and chemicals designed to communicate with each other, providing maximum protection to the body as a coordinated unit. A perfectly functioning immune system will quickly identify a foreign invader (antigen), destroy it, remove the remains, and clean up any damage—all done with the least amount of injury to the host tissues. An effective immune system will also learn from past experience and become more efficient at killing particular invaders should they attack again in the future.[1][2][3]

Although well designed, our immune system doesn't always work as planned. The result is disease, either from the persistence of harmful microorganisms, or excessive damage to the host (meaning us) during the defense process, or misinterpretation and assault on our own tissues (autoimmunity). In the sections that follow, I'll describe how the immune system is designed to work. This crash course in immunology might seem like a lot of information to process, but it should fall into place in the next chapter, which explains what goes wrong in autism.

The First Line of Defense

The first objective of any good defense is to prevent the need for a battle. The body does this with physical barriers that prevent invading organisms from reaching our internal structures. The most obvious of these is our skin, which is the largest human organ. It performs a variety of functions including excreting toxins or waste products, absorbing some nutrients and sunlight, maintaining our core body temperature, and protecting more delicate underlying tissues from damage due to physical contact. Most importantly, it prevents microbes from accessing internal tissues. The major risk of death to burn victims, for example, is from secondary infections because of the loss of this protective barrier.

Another access point for microorganisms is the gastrointestinal tract, which is essentially a hollow tube that goes from mouth to anus. Everything within the GI tube is, by definition, outside the body, even though we think of it as our "insides." (Only when something trespasses the lining of the GI tract is it actually inside us.) Like the skin, the mucosal lining of the GI tract is designed to absorb what we need and to exclude everything else. It's also a source of toxin and waste product excretion.

The lining of the gut has very tight junctions between cells; this is how the cells control what gets in and out. Think of gut-lining cells as a border patrol, with an impenetrable fence between gates. These cells also produce mucus, which provides a protective layer between the microbe and the cell wall and further discourages the invader.4 Because of this mucous layer, most microorganisms are demobilized and excreted, never having made true contact with the cell lining.

The respiratory tract is the third inlet for invading organisms. Nose hair acts as a filter, trapping organisms until they can be expelled. Our bronchial tubes also have microscopic hairs that perform the same task, called cilia. (Cilia are often destroyed by cigarette smoking—one reason why smokers have a higher risk for pulmonary infections.) Like the gut, the respiratory lining produces mucus to discourage microorganisms from attaching.

The Non-Specific or Innate Immune Response

When microbes do manage to gain access to our internal tissues, the immune system kicks in and starts fighting. And just like a nation's military, it has a hierarchy of specialization. The first level, called the innate immune response, carries out its actions in a non-specific way, reacting to invaders indiscriminately. Innate immune cells patrol the blood and the body tissues, reacting immediately when they locate something foreign, and at the same time signaling other types of immune cells to migrate to the area to help out. Cytokines (chemical messengers) recruit more specialized components of the immune system to join in the battle. The result is inflammation at the point of origin.

Innate immune cells kill invaders in different ways. One is by direct phagocytosis, meaning they engulf and internalize the microorganism and then kill it—in effect devouring it. Another method is to activate something called the complement system. The complement cascade starts a series of reactions, damaging the organism directly by making its cell membrane rupture. Cells in the innate immune system include neutrophils and macrophages.

The Antigen-Specific or Adaptive Immune Response

Compared to the innate immune system, the adaptive immune response is more intricate; it has the advantage of targeting antigens (invaders) in a specific and refined way that allows it to kill more efficiently, and with less body damage. It's also the mechanism by which the body creates immune memory, so that on re-exposure to the same antigen the killing process is quicker and even more targeted. The adaptive immune system is composed primarily of three types of cells: antigen-presenting cells, T-cells, and B-cells. Since each has a part to play, and each plays a different role in the new ASD paradigm, I'll describe them separately.

Antigen-Presenting Cells (APCs)

These are the sentinel cells of the immune system. They're responsible for detecting antigens, internalizing them, processing them, and then presenting the remains on their surface so that the other cells in the adaptive immune system can see and identify them. APCs also send out cytokine messengers (primarily IL-1) that tell the naïve (undifferentiated) T-cells that they need to activate and specialize. Macrophages, which also operate in the less-sophisticated innate immune system, can function as APCs.

Dendritic cells are another kind of APCs, and they are more efficient than macrophages. They're usually found in the structure of lymphoid organs (the spleen, the thymus, and lymph nodes), but can circulate in the bloodstream. It's believed that they capture antigens and then bring them to the lymphoid organs where an immune response is initiated. The HIV virus, for example, is found in large amounts within the dendritic cells. This virus disables the killing mechanism of the cell and uses it as a reservoir, until it is transmitted to other cells during a re-activation event. In chapter 8, I'll discuss this potentially important observation with regard to immune activation and viral issues in autism.

T-Cells

The majority of cells that function within the adaptive immune system are called lymphocytes, and are divided into two classes based on function: T-lymphocytes and B-lymphocytes. T-cells are responsible for cell-mediated immunity, meaning that they engage in face-to-face combat with the targeted microorganism. There are three basic T-cells: T-helper (Th) cells (also called CD4 cells), cytotoxic (killer) T-cells (CD8), and T-suppressor cells.

The T-helper cells receive the signal from the APC cell, activate, and then stimulate the rest of the adaptive immune system. First, they send out a cytokine called IL-2, which stimulates production of more Th cells. Then, they send out another cytokine called IL-4, which stimulates B-cell production. And they send other cytokines (IL-5, IL-6, IL-10, IL-13, gamma interferon, and lymphotoxin) that activate other parts of the immune response, such as cytotoxic T-cells, macrophages, and natural killer cells.

When activated, cytotoxic T-cells (Tc) bind to foreign organisms and make holes in their cell membranes, causing them to lyse, or rupture. When the body has recovered, either T suppressor cells (Ts) or T-regulatory (Tr) cells shut down the immune response; they stop production of Th and Tc cells, using regulatory cytokines, IL-10 and TNF-β, so that unnecessary tissue damage doesn't occur.

B-Cells

B-cells form antibodies (immunoglobulins), which are proteins that bind to specific antigens and signal the other parts of the immune system to react. This is called humoral (or antibody-mediated) immunity, and it's how the body creates immune memory. Th cells use the cytokine IL-4 to stimulate B-cells during the primary immune response. Once stimulated, naïve B-cells mature to become either plasma cells or memory B-cells. Plasma cells can produce a large amount of antibodies in a very short period, but have a life span of only about a week. Memory

B-cells remain partially activated, but when re-exposed to the particular antigen can work quickly in activating the humoral immune system and forming new plasma cells (secondary immune response). They can persist on stand-by in the blood for years or even a lifetime; on re-exposure to a particular antigen, they rapidly differentiate to plasma cells and produce large amounts of antibodies. This allows the body to remove microorganisms within a matter of days when re-exposed, compared to possibly several weeks with the first exposure.

Several kinds of antibodies, i.e., immunoglobulins (Ig), are produced in our bodies, each with a different structure and a different function:

IgG: the predominant type of antibody in our system, comprising about 80% of the total. It can diffuse out of the blood stream and is commonly found in extravascular tissue spaces. Its concentration increases rapidly in particular areas during inflammation and is particularly effective in neutralizing extracellular bacterial toxins and viruses. It also crosses the placental barrier, providing passive immunity from the mother to the fetus and newborn baby. A baby generally has the full complement of its mother's IgG antibodies; they circulate for about six months after birth, giving the baby partial immune protection while its own immune system is developing.

IgM: this antibody type protects against blood-borne pathogens. Located mainly in the bloodstream, it comprises 10% of circulating antibodies. It functions early in the immune response, and its multiple binding sites can cause clumping or aggregation of the specific antigens, allowing the innate immune cells to more easily engulf the antigens by phagocytosis.

IgA: primarily produced in gut-associated lymphoid tissues, it's secreted in the mucous surfaces. It accounts for about 15% of total antibody production. The predominant antibody found in GI fluids, nasal secretions, saliva, tears, and other mucous secretions, it plays a key part in protecting these mucosal layers and neutralizing the bacterial toxins that are secreted in an effort to break down the mucosal barrier. IgA is transferred in breast milk, especially in colostrum, and provides passive immunity to the infant from the first few days after birth to about six months.

IgE: is found in small amounts (only 0.002% of total) and is produced especially by the plasma cells in the respiratory and intestinal linings. It's firmly bound to receptors on mast cells, which are responsible for histamine release. When activated, the result is immediate inflammation and activation of the immune system. IgE is responsible for immediate hypersensitivity reactions like hives, bronchospasm (asthma), hay fever, etc. Some of these symptoms are atopic, i.e., they take place in a part of the body not in direct contact with the allergen.

IgD: is a lesser-known antibody that appears to function as an immunoregulator for control of B-cell activation and suppression.

In addition to signaling the other parts of the immune system, antibodies can directly defend the body against organisms. When bound by antibodies, foreign organisms are more easily engulfed by phagocytic cells and are less able to attach to other cell membranes. Antibodies can neutralize bacterial toxins and also stimulate the complement cascade that results in organism death.

Th1 Vs. Th2 Response

T-helper cells play a central role in controlling the adaptive immune pathway by encouraging the development of other cell lines. In addition, there appears to be a differentiation within Th cells that makes them more prone to stimulating either the B-cells (humoral response) through IL-4, or the cytotoxic T-cells, NK cells, and macrophages (cellular response) through IL-12 and IFN-γ. The type of immune response that's stimulated changes the relative effectiveness of the immune system against certain microorganisms.

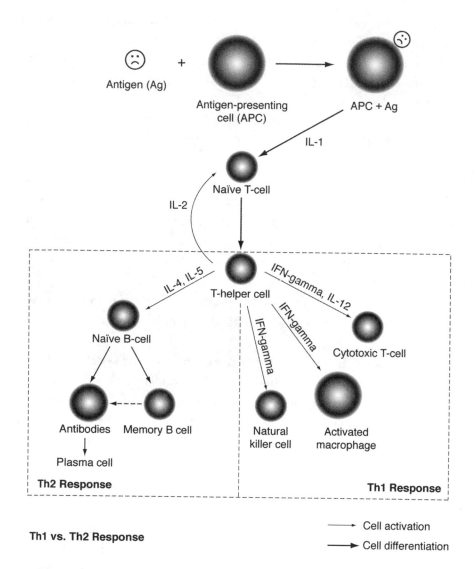

Th1 vs. Th2 Response

⟶ Cell activation

⟶ Cell differentiation

Th1 cells stimulate the cell-mediated response, which is more effective at targeting intracellular organisms such as viruses and some bacteria. Th2 cells stimulate the humoral immune response by creating antibodies, which are more effective against extracellular pathogens. If the antigen can escape inside the cell before it's recognized and stopped by the immune system, it's no longer accessible to be bound with an antibody. The balance between Th1 and Th2 is normally tightly controlled by feedback mechanisms between the two systems, and also by other cells in the immune system such as APCs. If this balance is disrupted, a shift toward Th2 means the individual will be more prone to forming antibodies and allergies, but less able to fight off viruses; there is also a tendency to develop systemic autoimmune disease. If shifted toward Th1, more organ-specific autoimmunity results.[5]

Other Immune Cells

Macrophages. Macrophages can take many forms, including phago-cytic cells and antigen-presenting cells. They can be activated by IFN-γ (a cytokine produced by Th cells). When activated, they have an increased ability to destroy intracellular pathogens such as viruses and certain bacteria. They're also good at recognizing and destroying tumor cells.

Natural killer cells. NK cells are a type of lymphocyte found in blood and the lymphoid tissues. Unlike Tc cells, they don't require cell-sur-face antigen activation to become cytotoxic, but are activated by cyto-kine signals sent from Th cells, including IL-2 and IFN-γ.

chapter seven

THE PROBLEM OF IMMUNE DYSREGULATION

THE WEAPONS OF THE IMMUNE SYSTEM, WHILE MEANT TO PROTECT us, have the potential to cause unintended harm to the surrounding tissues. An effective immune response is a quick attack, with minimal surrounding damage, that can easily be repaired after the battle is over. Shutting down the immune response is as critical to the defense and repair process as turning it on. Many of the symptoms that we feel when we are infected, including swelling, redness, pain, and warmth at the site of the infection, are the results of the activities of our own immune system on the tissues of our body rather than from the organism itself.

Disease results when the immune system can't immediately get rid of infection and there is damage to local tissues from the organism, or from the immune response trying to kill it. Often, invading organisms develop their own protective mechanisms that weaken the immune system, preventing it from doing its job. The infection then becomes disease, and the disease becomes chronic or even fatal. (The HIV virus is a good example.)

Chronic disease can also result from abnormalities within the system's communication network that prevent effective regulation of the inflammatory response. This can lead to ineffective or imbalanced cell differentiation in the adaptive immune system as a result of abnormal chemical signals telling the T-helper (Th) cells whether to favor a Th1 response (cell-mediated) or a Th2 response (antibody-mediated). Instead of choosing the path that is most needed based on the type of organism that's being fought, a dysregulated immune system always favors one particular pathway. This is called Th1 or Th2 shifting, or imbalance.

If the immune system is shifted away from Th1 towards a Th2 response, it will be less protective against viruses, which might then persist in a chronic state, hidden inside cells. (Remember that the Th1 response is better at killing intracellular organisms such as viruses and some bacteria.) With Th2 predominance, antibody formation is also more likely, often to an abnormal degree, so that it induces allergies and systemic (widespread) autoimmune reactions. Th1 predominance leaves a person vulnerable to recurrent infections since the antibody memory is weak, and prone to the kind of autoimmune reactions that attack specific organs.

Another abnormal immune response results from an imbalance of the cytokines that activate the inflammatory response (such as IL-1, IL-2, IL-4, IL-5, IL-6, IFN-γ, and TNF-α), and those that turn it off (IL-10 and TNF-β). If the anti-inflammatory cytokines don't do their job, the inflammatory cycle continues, and can lead to tissue damage even after the original microorganism has been eliminated.

Finally, one of the major tasks of the immune system is to recognize which cells are foreign and which cells are "self." It should attack "nonself" and leave "self" alone. Since the foreign cells often mimic our own cells, the task can be difficult, and mistakes are often made. When the immune system accidentally attacks "self" cells, it is called an autoimmune *reaction*. The immune system has checks and balances to prevent this type of reaction, but if they aren't working properly, the ongoing damage will result in autoimmune *disease*.

Do Individuals with Autism Have Immune Dysregulation?

Paul Ashwood, an immunologist at the MIND Institute in California, published a review of the immune response in autism in 2006.[1] By referencing almost two hundred studies, he builds a strong argument for the disease's immunological basis. There's a great body of evidence in the literature documenting immune dysregulation in autistic children leaving them prone to infection, chronic inflammation, and autoimmune reactions; it can affect any organ system, but the brain and the GI tract seem to be the worst hit.

These immune system issues haven't been traced to a single underlying abnormality, and aren't always consistent among children on the autism spectrum. Just as there are subgroups based on behavioral characteristics, there appear to be subgroups within the autism spectrum related to the type and severity of immune abnormalities.

The research shows that both the quantity and function of immune cells are abnormal in children with autism. Many reports have documented decreased numbers of lymphocytes, including naïve T-cells, T-helper cells, cytotoxic T-cells, and B-cells.[2,3,4,5,6,7,8] Natural killer cell numbers are reduced.[9,10] Other cells in the immune system, including monocytes and eosinophils, show abnormal patterns.[11,12] There is a skewing of the balance of serum immunoglobulin subtypes, with low total IgM, IgG, and IgA, and elevated total IgE and IgG subtypes (IgG2 and IgG4).[13,14,15,16,17] Platelets are often elevated, reflecting a non-specific inflammatory response.[18]

Studies have documented decreased responsiveness or abnormal function in both T-cells and natural killer cells.[19,20,21,22,23,24] Apoptosis, the body's method for removing unwanted or disabled cells, is found to be dysregulated in these children.[25] Researchers have found an imbalance of the Th1/Th2 response in autistic patients with an overall tendency toward a Th2 response.[26,27,28,29] Abnormal cytokine profiles and responses have been demonstrated, with elevation of proinflammatory cytokines and reduction of regulatory cytokines.[30,31,32,33,34,35,36,37,38]

Excessive Inflammation

While abnormal GI tract inflammation in children with autism is well documented (chapter 9), standard brain images such as MRI scans or standard analysis of CSF (cerebrospinal fluid) do not typically reveal brain inflammation in autism. Until a 2005 study out of Johns Hopkins by Vargas et al. laid the question to rest, many people believed it didn't exist. They analyzed brain tissue samples from autistic patients who had died from other causes such as drowning, comparing them to controls. They also compared CSF (using cytokine protein arrays) from living patients with autism to controls. They found a significant activation of the innate immune system within specific regions of the brain (particularly the cerebellum), indicated by activation of astroglial cells, macrophages, and monocytes (all cells that are part of the nonspecific immune response). The brain's astroglia and microglia act like macrophages by detecting pathogens and starting the immune response through cytokine signaling. Vargas found abnormal levels of proinflammatory signals (such as IL-6, MCP-1, and TARC), anti-inflammatory signals (TNF-β), growth/differentiation factors (IGFBP-1), and complement activation. This type of immune activation is similar to what happens in other chronic brain conditions like Parkinson's, Alzheimer's, amyotrophic lateral sclerosis (ALS) and HIV-related dementia.

Interestingly, there was no evidence that the adaptive immune system was activated, and consequently no lymphocyte proliferation or antibody production, although many of the cytokines found were from lymphocytic origins. This suggests that the primary target of the immune activation might not be located in the brain at all. Rather, a source outside of the brain might be causing a system-wide activation of the innate immune response due to circulating cytokines.

The authors stated that their study provides evidence that the neurological disease in autism does not stem from a single in utero event, but is a disease of ongoing, postnatal inflammation. They hypothesized that the neuroimmune abnormality could be genetically based or that it could be induced by environmental factors, either before or after birth.[39][40]

Autoimmune Reactions

I've mentioned the increased prevalence of autoimmune illness in families with autistic children.[41][42] This suggests an inherited tendency of the immune system to develop autoantibodies. In fact, many research studies have documented the existence of autoantibodies in people with autism (30-70%).[43][44][45][46] Autoantibodies against many regions and structures of the brain have been detected, including myelin basic protein,[47] serotonin receptors,[48] caudate nucleus,[49][50] prefrontal cortex,[51] cingulate gyri,[52] putamen,[53] neuron axon filament protein,[54] cerebellum[55][56] nerve growth factor, alpha-2-adrenergic binding sites, endothelial cell proteins,[57] and an as-yet-unidentified brain protein.[58][59][60][61]

In spite of the many anti-brain antibodies found in the blood, Vargas et al. were unable to detect lymphocytes when examining brain tissue. This could indicate that although antibodies are being formed, they're not actively proliferating and causing tissue destruction. An antigen-antibody complex should trigger an inflammatory response with ongoing production of antibody-producing B-lymphocytes (plasma cells). This would typically lead to the kind of tissue destruction we see in myelin in multiple sclerosis or pancreatic cells in type 1 diabetes. In spite of elevated anti-brain antibodies, studies have failed to document active autoimmune destruction in the brains of autistic patients;[62] nonetheless it's possible that antibody-mediated inflammation occurred early in the disease process but does not persist as a chronic state. Autoimmune destruction of the epithelial membrane in the GI mucosa in autism has been documented.[63]

Antibodies from maternal blood have the potential to damage the fetus by passing through the placenta.[64] A study done by Dalton et al. showed that when serum from the mother of a child with autism was injected into pregnant mice, it induced altered exploration, motor coordination difficulties, and structural changes in the cerebellum in the mouse offspring. When serum from mothers with NT (neurotypical, i.e., developmentally normal) children was injected into a control group of mice, no such changes were noted.[65] Others have reported increased antibody production against fetal brain tissue (from rats) in the blood from mothers of autistic children but not in control mothers,[66] and in another study, mothers produced abnormal antibodies to their own children's lymphocytes.[67] It's possible that an abnormal prenatal immune response in the mother could cause damage to her fetus, leading to the development of autism.[68]

Food Reactions

Parents have reported for years that their autistic child improved when foods containing gluten and casein were removed. Gluten is a protein found in wheat, barley, rye, oats, spelt, and some other grains. Casein is a protein from cow's milk. Sections of these proteins (called peptides) have a structure similar to opiates like morphine or heroin. It's theorized that these peptides affect autistic children by attaching to opiate receptors in the brain and acting as false neurotransmitters (chapter 13). Many of these children self-limit their diet to foods containing gluten and casein peptides; they even act as if they are addicted, complete with withdrawal and binging behaviors. Another possibility is that these (and other) foods could stimulate an immune response that contributes to the general inflammatory burden in the GI tract and in the brain.

Research has found evidence of food allergies in autism. Lucarelli et al. detected much higher level of antibodies to casein and other milk proteins in children with autism compared to controls, and saw a marked improvement in behavior after an elimination diet challenge.[69] Jyonouchi et al. showed that when challenged with food proteins from gluten, casein, and soy, children with autism produced a markedly higher amount of proinflammatory cytokines, compared with normal controls. Their immune response was in most cases equal to or higher than non-autistic children with known symptomatic food allergies. Interestingly, the NT siblings of autistic children had an immune response somewhere in between the controls and the autistic and food-intolerant children.

The Jyonouchi report also noted that the addition of an endotoxin similar to one produced by a common species of abnormal gut bacteria heightened the inflammatory response against these food proteins.[70] The same investigators also showed that this endotoxin-stimulated altered immune response was limited to autistic children with GI symptoms, suggesting a possible link between gut, immune, and behavioral response.[71 72]

Jyonouchi's suggestion is consistent with the 2006 report from Campbell et al. identifying a common variant of the MET gene as a risk factor for autism; the MET gene is known to be involved in brain development, regulation of the immune system, and repair of the gastrointestinal system.[73]

Vojdani et al. measured the antibody response against nine common brain proteins, as well as proteins from milk, from Group A streptococcus bacteria, and from Chlamydia pneumoniae (a common cause of pneumonia and bronchitis). They chose these particular species because they are known to cross-react to the brain proteins they were studying. They found that compared to controls, the autistic cases had highly significant increases against all of the measured proteins in each of the immunoglobulin subtypes tested (IgG, IgM, and IgA):

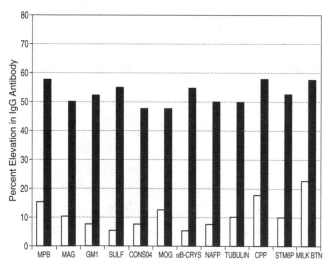

Fig 1. Percent elevation in IgG antibody against neurologic antigens and their cross-reactive peptides in healthy control subjects and patients with autism at a cut-off point of 0.30 O.D. Source: Vojdani et al. Antibodies to neuron-specific antigens. Journal of Neuroimmunology p. 170.

Vojdani hypothesized that the overreaction of the immune system to common brain proteins might reflect an incompetent blood-brain barrier, which normally excludes these antibodies from the brain. They also hypothesized that the antibodies against the cross-reacting proteins from dietary and infectious sources could be a triggering event for autoimmune reactions in the brain.[74]

In a follow up study, the same authors showed that antibodies against casein and gluten (as well as streptokinase and ethylmercury) cross-react to lymphocytes containing specific surface markers called CD26 and CD69. CD26 is a receptor protein also expressed on a digestive enzyme called DPP-IV, used to digest gluten and casein peptides. It also plays a part in T-cell regulation and in adenosine metabolism—two other areas that are abnormal in autistic patients.[75]

Abnormal Response to Infections

Many cases of autism have been caused by exposure to particular infectious agents. Congenital CMV (cytomegalovirus), Borna disease virus, congenital rubella virus, herpes simplex, and measles virus are all known causes.[76 77 78 79 80 81 82] It's thought that these pathogens induce an immune response, resulting in neuroinflammation, autoimmune reactions, and brain injury. This makes sense, considering the evidence of immune dysregulation in autistic patients. Because of a shift towards a Th2 reactivity, for example, viruses are more capable of hiding inside cells for long periods and then intermittently inducing an immune response during replication cycles; this could result in a chronic pattern of inflammatory disease.

There is strong evidence that viruses might be the triggering event for many other autoimmune diseases, including myositis and type-1 diabetes.[83] Th2 predominance also creates a tendency to overreact to common environmental stimuli, resulting in the swelling of the mucosal tissues and histamine-type allergic reactions (e.g., seasonal allergies). Chronic nasal and sinus congestion can lead to secondary eustachian tube dysfunction, and can predispose autistic children to otitis media (ear infections). Physicians commonly prescribe repeated courses of antibiotics to treat conditions such as sinusitis, otitis media, and bronchitis. These are often the result of allergic or viral-mediated phenomena, and so show little or no response to antibiotics. Studies show that autistic children have many more ear infections, a higher frequency of allergies (respiratory, skin, and food), more pediatrician visits, more courses of antibiotics, and more hospitalizations than control children.[84][85][86][87][88]

Among the consequences of repeated antibiotic use are the unfortunate proliferation of antibiotic-resistant organisms and the loss of beneficial bacterial flora in the gastrointestinal tract. This can then lead to secondary GI mucosal damage from abnormal bacteria, increasing immunological response to food proteins and further susceptibility to infections.

chapter eight

MEASLES AND THE MMR CONTROVERSY

IN 1998, A TEAM LED BY ANDREW WAKEFIELD FROM THE Department of Medicine at the Royal Free Hospital in London published a research study that created a very large stir in medical circles and, ultimately, a public outcry. The team examined twelve consecutive children referred to their clinic for chronic gastrointestinal symptoms (e.g., abdominal pain, diarrhea, abdominal bloating, and food intolerance) and developmental disorders (nine with autism, one with disintegrative psychosis, and two with possible post-viral or vaccinal encephalitis). The parents of eight of these children reported that their child's neurological regression coincided with their MMR (measles-mumps-rubella) vaccination. The work-ups included a colonoscopy with biopsy, an EEG, an MRI, a lumbar puncture, a basic metabolic workup to rule out other neurological or bowel diseases, and a barium small-bowel follow-through radiography where possible.

Review of medical records confirmed that all twelve children had a period of normal development followed by a neurological regression. In the cases of the eight children whose regression was believed by the parents to be related to the MMR vaccine, adverse symptoms were reported within fourteen days of vaccination, either by the parents themselves or by their clinicians. Adverse symptoms included a rash, fever, delirium, and, in three cases, convulsions. The average interval from the time of vaccination to the onset of the first symptom was 6.3 days.

The tests revealed that not only did all twelve children have bowel disease, but the way it manifested was quite different from the IBDs (inflammatory bowel diseases) the team was accustomed to seeing, such as Crohn's disease and ulcerative colitis. The most striking abnormality was ileal LNH (lymphonodular hyperplasia), a swelling of the lymph nodes at the final portion of the small bowel (the terminal ileum). LNH was found in eleven of the twelve children studied; the doctors were unable to access that portion of the bowel in the twelfth. LNH wasn't found in any of the seven control children, all of whom had other known bowel diseases.

Other GI findings included patchy mucosal erythema (redness), aphthoid ulcerations (canker-like sores), loss of vascular (blood vessel) pattern, granularity, and the telltale red halo pattern that's an early indication of Crohn's disease. Biopsies showed a chronic patchy inflammation in the colon in all cases, and acute inflammation in five cases. Other explanations for bowel disease or metabolic disorders were ruled out. MRIs, EEGs, and lumbar punctures were all unremarkable.

The authors hypothesized that the GI pathology and the behavior regression might be linked. They suggested it was biologically plausible that the MMR vaccine could be causally associated with regression based on historical evidence of viral-induced autism, the association of measles virus with other bowel disorders, and the fact that other investigators had reported an apparent temporal association of autistic regression with MMR vaccinations. Whatever their suspicions, the team clearly stated in their concluding remarks, "We did not prove an association between measles, mumps, and rubella vaccine and the syndrome described. Virological studies are underway that could help to resolve this issue...further investigations are needed to examine this syndrome and its possible relation to this vaccine."[1]

The Epidemiology Wars

News of this study, with its implication of a possible association between autism and a government-mandated childhood vaccine, spread rapidly through the press and ruffled the mainstream medical community. There was general concern that the results of the study would undermine public confidence in the MMR vaccine and could affect the entire UK immunization program. Some people feared there would be a decline in vaccine uptake followed by an epidemic re-emergence of vaccine-preventable infectious diseases. Not surprisingly, soon after Wakefield's 1998 *Lancet* paper appeared, a number of studies were published which attempted to discredit his theory. Unfortunately, in the years that followed, what should have been a matter of scientific enquiry too often devolved into personal attacks on some of the researchers.

In 1999, the *Lancet* published an article by Taylor et al. entitled "Autism and measles, mumps, rubella vaccine: no epidemiological evidence for a causal association." The authors did a chart review of cases of autism diagnosed in a defined region in England, in children born between 1979 and 1992. They identified 498 cases of ASDs in the population, of which only 293 could be confirmed according to ICD-10 criteria. They analyzed the data in three different ways to test the hypothesis that autism was related to the MMR vaccination. First, they examined whether or not there had been a sudden step-up in autism diagnoses in children (born in 1987 or later) who received the MMR vaccine after it was introduced in England in 1988. They found that the prevalence rates of autism began an exponential rise starting with children born a couple of years before the introduction of the MMR vaccine, and that there had been no sudden step-up after 1988 (figure 1). They concluded that this refuted a temporal relationship.

Their second aim was to determine if the age of diagnosis was different in children given MMR before the age of eighteen months, compared to those who received it after eighteen months. They reasoned that if autism were temporally related to MMR, more children should be diagnosed soon after the vaccine was given. They

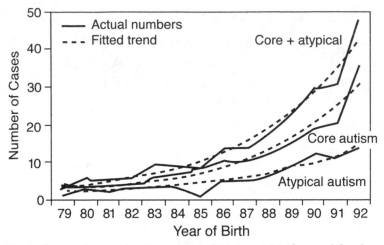

Fig. 1: Core and atypical autism cases under 60 months of age and fitted trends by year of birth 1979-92. Source: Taylor, The Lancet, June 1999.

found no difference. The third analysis examined whether or not there was a clustering of the diagnoses associated with either a reported developmental regression or with the timing of the first reported parental concern in any time period up to two years after vaccination. They found a clustering for first-reported parental concern at six months after vaccination, but dismissed it as a statistical artifact based on the probability that, unable to recall the exact age of initial concern, parents arbitrarily chose eighteen months. Their final conclusion, as stated in the study title, was that there was no epidemiological evidence for a causal association between MMR vaccine and autism.[2]

Many have been critical of this study's methodology.[3 4 5 6] Stott et al. challenged their "no step-up after 1988" argument by pointing out that a substantial number of older children (those in the pre-1987 cohort who were born between the years 1984 and 1986) participated in a "catch-up program" in which they also received the MMR vaccine. When this is accounted for, a temporal relationship between the introduction of the vaccine and the rising incidence of autism is evident. Reevaluating the graph as presented above shows that there is, in fact, a step-up between the 1985 and 1986 birth cohort. And, if you analyze the pre-1985 group compared to the post-1985 group, the slope of the incidence line has risen dramatically.

There are several other methodological problems with this study. First, it's a retrospective chart review attempting to evaluate data such as age of developmental regression and onset of first parental concern. Parents of children with autism typically complain that their pediatrician initially ignored their concerns,[7] so it's unlikely that this information was systematically recorded in all of the patient charts. In those cases in which it is recorded, there is no way to verify the accuracy of the records (i.e., recall bias). The authors argue this point themselves when trying to explain away the temporal clustering they found at six months after MMR. The concern about the quality of the records is indeed appropriate when you consider that they couldn't even confirm the accuracy of the diagnosis in 41% of the cases.

Second, the number of affected children in the younger age groups in this cohort is likely to be underestimated due to ascertainment bias. The median age of diagnosis that they reported from their data is thirty-seven months for autism, forty-two months for atypical autism, and seventy-three months for Asperger's syndrome. They included all children who were age five or older in their data set. But many children in the five-to-seven year age group were not likely to have received a diagnosis yet; in all probability this would affect their results. They didn't even include the Asperger's children in their vaccination analysis, stating that the number was too small to be useful—despite the fact that it made up 10% of their study population.

A third criticism concerns the use of the ages of diagnosis, regression, and parental concern in relation to MMR vaccination. Note that the age of diagnosis and the age of symptom onset are not equivalent. Taylor et al.'s own data show that the average age of diagnosis is between three and seven years old. Age of diagnosis merely reflects the quality of their diagnostic system—it has nothing to do with any true temporal relationship between symptom onset and MMR vaccination.

Finally, in their discussion, the authors make their goals for this study very clear. They state, "We *hope that our results will reassure parents* and others who have been concerned about the possibility that MMR is likely to cause autism and that they *will help to restore confidence* in the MMR vaccine [italics added]." The bias of the authors is hardly surprising, since several of them were members of the UK Immunization Division of the Public Health Department, as reported on the front page of the study.

In 2002, Madsen et al. published a population study in the *New England Journal of Medicine* refuting an association between MMR and autism.[8] Using the Danish National Civil Register database (the record of all available information on Danish residents), they looked at all children born between 1991 and 1998. Information on autism diagnoses was obtained from the Danish Psychiatric Central Register. (Virtually all autistic children in Denmark are diagnosed by pediatric psychiatrists, who then report to this database.)

The authors used national vaccination data to determine if there was an increased incidence of autism in those children who received the MMR vaccine compared to those who did not. They found that although there did appear to be a continual rise in the diagnosis rates in the 1990s, it didn't appear to correlate with the introduction of MMR in Denmark in 1987, nor with vaccine uptake rates. They did not find any difference in the autism prevalence rates in vaccinated versus unvaccinated children. They also were unable to detect a temporal clustering of cases at any time after immunization. This study was the first population-based study (data captured from an entire national population) that looked at the association between the vaccine and cases of autism, so it was highly anticipated at the time it was published.

But not everyone agreed that this study was bulletproof. Goldman and Yazbak criticized the methodology of the Madsen study for several reasons.[9] They suggested that the rising incidence of autism in the 1990s could likely be explained by "greater diagnostic awareness." Several changes in diagnostic practices occurred in the 1990s that could have affected Madsen's data. In 1995, the Denmark registry began including data from children diagnosed with autism as outpatients (prior to that, only inpatient records were included). Also, in 1993-1994, Denmark began using the new ICD-10 definition of autism instead of ICD-8. Goldman et al. reviewed the Danish database carefully, and presented a graph showing the marked difference in diagnostic rates after 1995:

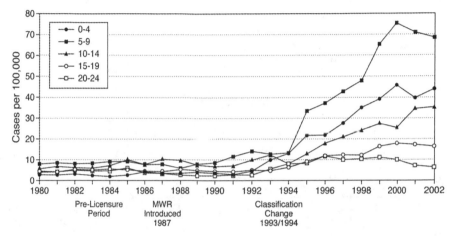

Fig. 2: Prevalence of autism in Denmark by age group and year, 1980 to 2002. Source: Goldman. *Journal of American Physicians & Surgeons*, 2004.

Lauritsen et al., presented a similar graph (fig. 3), also derived from the Danish Psychiatric Registry, which showed a sudden increase in incidence rates starting in 1990[10].

Goldman also points out a strong ascertainment bias in the Madsen study because of substantial under-reporting both of cases of autism and of frequency of MMR vaccination in the younger age group. Five was the average age of diagnosis reported in the Madsen study. Since the study period included children born as late as December 1998 and the data was collected at the end of 1999, a substantial portion of their study population was not yet old enough to have been diagnosed, and many of these had not yet received their MMR vaccine. Children born in 1997 and 1998 alone represent 39% of the observation years. Madsen

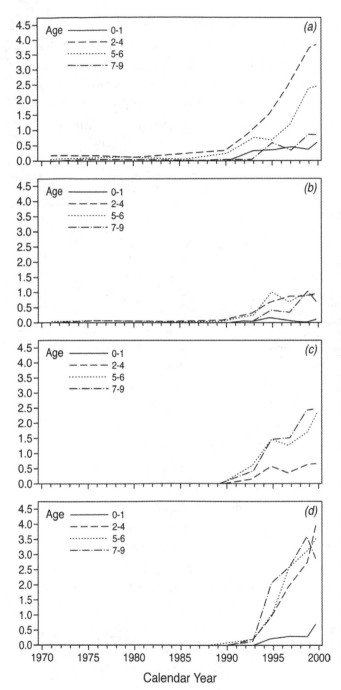

Fig. 3: Incidence of Childhood (a), atypical autism (b), Asperger's Disorder (c) and PDD-NOS (d) by age and calendar year. The incidence measures the number of new cases observed per 10,000 children per year. Each calendar year estimate of incidence was based on an average background population of 127,000, 194,000, 132,000, and 202,000 children aged 0-1, 2-4, 5-6, and 7-9 years respectively. Source: Lauritsen, *Psychological Medicine*, 2004.

argued that they accounted for this confounder with an "age-adjust-ment" factor, but the reliability of their study conclusion rests entirely on the accuracy of their adjustment. Without the age adjustment from Madsen, there is a statistically significant 45% increase in the risk of autism associated with the introduction of MMR. There was another group of children who had received the MMR shot but were not yet old enough to be diagnosed with autism. These were included in the MMR/no autism group although the outcome of the study could have been substantially affected if a percentage of those children later devel-oped autism.

In a response sent to the *New England Journal of Medicine* (which they declined to publish), Suissa from the Department of Epidemiology and Statistics at McGill University argued that the Madsen data actu-ally shows an association between MMR and autism when the calcula-tion is based on autism rates in relation to time after vaccination; a more accurate way to present the data would have been to base it on the birth year of affected children rather than on the age of diagnosis.

Stott's group showed steady prevalence rates between 1982 and 1987 (the year that MMR was introduced) and a sharp increase thereafter, consistent with the steady increase in uptake of the MMR in the Dan-ish population (fig. 4).

SafeMinds, an autism advocacy group in the US, has also published a critique of the Madsen article on their website (*www.safeminds. org*). They point out that the rates of autism in Denmark are much lower than in other reported populations such as the US and the UK, although virtually the same diagnostic criteria are used. This suggests either an underlying difference in the genetics of the Danish popula-tion (which is fairly homogenous), or a potential difference in other environmental factors that might work synergistically with MMR to increase the risk of autism (like thimerosal, for example—see chapter 11). They also argue that the Madsen data cannot rule out the possibil-ity that a subgroup of children regressed into autism after MMR, as per Wakefield's original hypothesis. Madsen failed to account for a positive

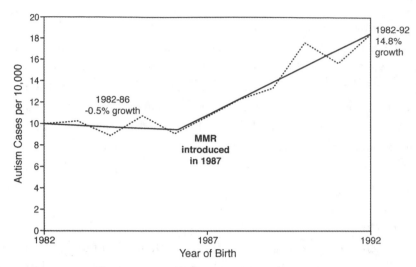

Fig. 4: Autism prevalence in Denmark by year of birth, 1982-1992. Lines of best fit are shown for birth years 1982 to 1986, and from 1986 to 1992. Children born in 1986 were first to receive MMR in Denmark. The annual growth before MMR was -0.5% [trend= -0.15; 95% Cl, (-1.06) – (-0.76), ns], compared with 14.8% after MMR introduction (t – 6.94, p<0.001; trend 1.54, 95% Cl, 0.97 – 2.11). Source: Stott, et al. *Journal of American Physicians & Surgeons*. 2004.

family history of autism or autoimmune disease, which might be a factor in a parent's decision not to vaccinate their child, thereby affecting the unvaccinated risk pool. Finally, it must be noted that, similar to the Taylor study, three of the Madsen study authors worked for the Statens Serum Institut, the largest vaccine manufacturer in Denmark.

Other investigators have examined the MMR-autism debate.[11] Several studies compared rising prevalence of reported autism and coverage rates of MMR and found no correlation.[12 13 14 15 16] Others have failed to find a temporal association of the timing of administration of the MMR vaccination and a clustering of autism diagnoses.[17 18 19 20 21 22] Several studies looked for a relationship between developmental regression, GI symptoms, and MMR vaccine, and were unable to detect an association.[23 24 25 26] But each of these studies has been widely criticized in the literature for incomplete case ascertainment, methodological flaws, and inherent biases.[27 28 29 30 31 32 33 34 35]

A couple of Japanese studies have looked at the relationship between autism and MMR. Japan is unusual in that it's one of the only developed nations that do not currently use MMR as the primary source of measles prevention. They began using MMR in 1989, but discontinued it in 1993 because of case reports of meningitis associated with the Urabe mumps strain in the vaccine. After the initial 70% uptake of MMR in Japanese children born in 1988, the percentage of children receiving the vaccine decreased rapidly until 1993, when it was withdrawn from the market. Honda et al. hypothesized that if autism were caused by MMR, there should be an initial increase after the introduction of MMR followed by a decline in the autism incidence after it was withdrawn.[36] They looked at an area in Japan where there were clear diagnostic practices and good services for developmental delays. The results of their study are presented in figure 5.

The black bars indicate the percentage of uptake of the MMR vaccine, which declined over a four-year period. The shaded areas on the graph represent the incidence rates of autism and other PDDs. There is a small peak in 1990, followed by a decline, and then a second, larger peak reaching its highest point in 1994. The authors suggest that since

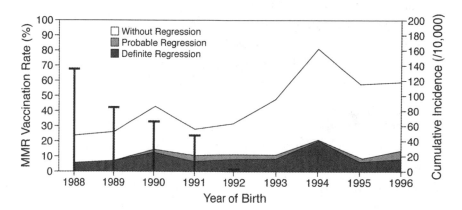

Fig. 5: Yokohama City MMR vaccination rates by birth year (1988-1992), and annual trends in cumulative incidences of ASD with and without developmental regression up to seven years in the birth cohort in the catchment area. Source: Honda, *Journal of Child Psychology and Psychiatry*. June 2005.

autism clearly continued to increase after the removal of MMR, it could in no way be to blame for the rising numbers.

In a rebuttal to this study, Wakefield pointed out that the prevalence of autism in Japan in 1987 (the birth year before MMR was introduced) was less than 25 per 10,000 (not shown in Honda's graph). In the years that followed, the incidence rose to 85.9 per 10,000. There was a subsequent decline in cases corresponding to the declining uptake of the MMR vaccine, and then, a second rise peaking in 1994. The study region was redistricted in 1994 and although the authors claimed no effect on the study results, the widening confidence intervals of the statistics in the study would suggest otherwise.

The second peak in autism incidence might in fact support Wakefield's hypothesis. In Japan, the substitute for the MMR vaccine was monovalent measles, mumps, and rubella, spaced four weeks apart. Dr. Wakefield's initial concern about MMR was based on the exposure to three live-virus vaccines within a short time period. Whether multiple exposures are in the same shot, the same day, or within a few weeks of each other could be irrelevant. Other studies on the synergistic effects of viral-related immune suppression suggest that exposure within several months, or even up to a year, during critical points of development might still be close enough to cause synergistic harm.[37] It is likely that what we see in figure 5 is a decrease in autism cases when MMR uptake declined, followed by an increase when it was replaced with the virtual biological equivalent.

It's interesting that this incidence curve has a very different appearance from those of the US and the UK, which show steady, exponential rises. The curve in Japan is bimodal, which might very well document a challenge/re-challenge effect for measles, mumps, and rubella given within close temporal proximity to each other.[38] Another study team in Japan compared diagnosis rates for autism in children receiving MMR versus measles monovalent vaccines, and did not find an increased risk in the MMR group, but the same criticisms involving synergistic risk as those of the Honda study would also apply.[39]

A study by Geier and Geier found a positive epidemiological association between MMR and autism.[40] They reviewed the VAERS (Vaccine Adverse Event Reporting System) data maintained by the CDC (Centers for Disease Control and Prevention) in the United States. This is a mandatory reporting system for any adverse event that is temporally associated with any vaccine. The Geier study compared serious neurological events occurring within thirty days of the receipt of MMR to those reported from the DTP vaccine between 1994 and 2000. The neurological events they evaluated included autism, cerebellar ataxia, mental retardation, and permanent brain damage. Tables 1 and 2 show the results of their comparison.

The results suggest that although the reports of immediate neurological events are quite low, they are significantly more frequent with the MMR vaccine compared to the DTP vaccine. This is interesting, because due to the high risk of neurological events associated with DTP vaccine, it was pulled from the market in 2001 and replaced with DTaP (diphtheria, typhoid, acellular pertussis).

There are several criticisms of this study, chief of which is the use of the VAERS database. Critics have suggested that the use of this database grossly underestimates the real incidence of adverse vaccine

Table 1 - A summary of serious neurologic reactions following MMR vaccination

Type of Reaction	Number of Male Reaction Reports	Number of Female Reaction Reports	Mean Age (Years)	Mean Onset (Days)	Incidence per Million MMR Vaccines
Cerebellar Ataxia	23	21	1.4 ± 0.66	4.9 ± 4.7	1.8
Autism	29	8	1.8 ± 1.1	6.5 ± 7.2	1.5
Mental Retardation	23	12	1.9 ± 2.0	5.5 ± 6.0	1.4
Permanent Brain Damage	8	9	1.9 ± 1.2	9.7 ± 8.4	0.69

Table 2 - A comparison of serious neurologic reactions following MMR vaccination in comparison to DTwcP vaccination

Type of Reaction	Relative Risk	Attributable Risk	Percent Association	Statistical Significance	95% Relative Risk Confidence Interval
Cerebellar Ataxia	8.2	7.2	89	$p < 0.0001$	4.4 to 15
Autism	5.2	4.2	84	$p < 0.0001$	3.0 to 9.2
Mental Retardation	1.7	0.7	63	$p < 0.05$	1.1 to 2.6
Permanent Brain Damage	2.3	1.3	70	$p < 0.05$	1.2 to 4.4

reactions because it relies on busy clinicians to report an event, and only a small proportion of the adverse reactions get reported.[41] In addition, this study can't detect any subacute or delayed vaccine reactions that might not manifest within thirty days after the vaccination (note that in the case of SSPE (subacute sclerosing panencephalitis), reactions to measles exposure typically manifest between two and ten years later).

Richler et al. published a study in 2006 attempting to determine if there is a subgroup of children with regressive autism and GI symptoms whose onset of developmental symptoms is closely related in time to MMR vaccination.[42] Through the use of a telephone interview with the parents, confirmed with review of the original ADI-R (interview given at the time of initial diagnosis), they found a group of children who had experienced a loss of developmental skills (the regression group). They compared these with age-matched autistic children without regression. They found some interesting differences between the groups. To begin with, most of the children with defined regression showed evidence of atypical development in several areas before their regression, suggesting a pre-existing slowing of development. In addition, they found that the regressive children had lower verbal IQ scores and more severe social impairment than the non-regressive group. Furthermore the regressive group had a significantly higher amount of GI symptoms. The data presented by Richler's group also show that the group of children most representative of Wakefield's hypothesized phenotype (children with behavior regression and GI symptoms) received their MMR at an earlier age (14.3 months vs. 17.7 months) and had a later age of onset of symptoms (19 months vs. 14.5 months) compared to the other ASD cases.

They did not find a significantly shorter interval between the MMR vaccine and the onset of autistic symptoms (although a trend in this direction is evident in their graphs). The authors suggest that this "definitively" proves that MMR is not related to autistic regression. But this conclusion is not clear from their data. Assuming that their retrospective data related to the onset of autistic symptoms are correct, the only accurate statement that can be made is that the onset of autistic symptoms might not be immediate after the MMR vaccine. In fact, the data suggest that the receipt of the MMR vaccine at an earlier age is more likely to result in GI symptoms and a post-vaccine onset of autistic symptoms. Since we know measles virus can produce devastating effects on the brain months (or even years—eight years on average for SSPE[43]) after the primary infection, a time correlate within a couple of months is not necessary to establish causation.[44]

The more relevant question regarding the Wakefield hypothesis is the timing of the GI symptoms in connection to the MMR vaccine. Wakefield's theory is that the measles virus creates an abnormal immune response resulting in immune dysregulation that allows persistence of the measles virus in a subacute or chronic state. The gut inflammation would allow the entrance of toxins from a variety of sources (e.g., food, flora) into the blood, which can ultimately cause secondary brain injury resulting in autistic behaviors.[45][46] This hypothesized process might take longer than a couple of weeks to manifest as recognizable autistic behaviors. Measles virus might also cause damage to the brain indirectly through immune suppression, resulting in secondary infections from other organisms; evidence suggests that this immunosuppression can last for up to a year after the primary viral infection.[47]

The only accurate conclusion from the Richler study would be that they did not see evidence of immediate behavior regression related to the MMR vaccine, but this is by no means definitive evidence against Wakefield's theory.

In spite of many studies evaluating the MMR connection to autism, we still do not have a conclusive answer. None of the epidemiological studies to date have adequately addressed this fundamental question: does the attenuated measles virus found in the MMR vaccine contribute to the pathology and consequent disability of a sub-group of children with autism?

Biological Plausibility

What do we know about the measles virus? Could it in fact induce the changes documented in the children studied by Wakefield et al. in 1998? Dr. Wakefield published a review of the history of the measles virus and the development of attenuated live measles virus vaccines.[48] Prior to the vaccination era, measles virus was a common childhood disease worldwide; it remains a significant cause of illness and death in developing nations today. Rarely, measles infection can cause both acute and persistent central nervous system disease, sometimes not manifesting for many years, including acute encephalitis (brain inflammation) and SSPE.[49][50] It can cause diseases of the GI system, including acute gastroenteritis, mesenteric adenitis, inflammatory bowel disease, and acute appendicitis.[51][52] The virus also has profound immunosuppressive effects. Just like wild measles, the live but attenuated (weakened) virus strain in monovalent measles vaccine and MMR has been known to cause complications (beyond the common rash and fever many children experience right after vaccination), including acute gastroenteritis, IBD (such as Crohn's and ulcerative colitis), arthritis, seizures, ITP (idiopathic thrombocytic purpura), meningitis, and encephalitis.[53][54][55] These sequelae were all well-known long before Wakefield's interest in the virus.

High titer monovalent measles vaccine was administered to babies less than one year of age in several developing nations and resulted in a significant increase in death, especially from diarrheal illness. There was also a large increase in delayed effects such as wasting and growth delay.[56] All of this eventually led the World Health Organization (WHO) to withdraw this vaccine.

The pre-licensure safety studies on the various forms of MMR were grossly inadequate in terms of methodology, presence of a good control group, and duration of active follow-up (all follow-ups were less than twenty-eight days; the latent period of the virus is known to last up to twenty-one days). Many of the side effects were reported as part of a post-licensure passive surveillance system requiring doctors to self-report adverse reactions—a system that is known to severely underestimate the true incidence of reactions. All of the adverse reactions were either dismissed by authorities as coincidental or accepted as an unavoidable element of an overall risk/benefit analysis, a ratio that has never been adequately established through appropriate research studies.

The safety of combining three live viruses, each of which is independently associated with autism, is open to question. Evidence shows that when natural exposure to measles and other neurologically active viruses (including mumps, chicken pox, and enterovirus) are closely linked in time, the risk of long-term neurological sequelae (like SSPE) and inflammatory bowel disease increases.[57] Measles is a strong suppressor of the cell-mediated immune response, predisposing the body to more damage from attack by a secondary virus. At one time, some versions of MMR included a particular strain of the mumps virus (Urabe strain) that caused many cases of mumps encephalitis; it was eventually pulled from the market, but not before millions of children were exposed.[58][59]

The importance of including mumps and rubella in early childhood vaccine programs is debatable. Although measles causes significant worldwide disease, mumps is relatively benign, rarely causing death or chronic disability in children. It can result in a viral meningitis syndrome that's almost always transient and well tolerated. Mumps is a potential cause of sterility in pubertal males, but the mumps vaccine doesn't guarantee immunity for more than a few years. Rubella can cause developmental disability (congenital rubella syndrome) if a woman is infected during pregnancy (incidence in the US was about twenty cases per year before introduction of rubella vaccination policy). As a childhood disease, rubella is typically mild. It would make more sense to target susceptible risk groups, i.e., immediately pre-pubertal males for mumps and pubertal females for rubella, rather than requiring all toddlers to receive a vaccine with viral-viral interactions that are not yet clearly established, and that provide them with time-limited protection at the time in their lives when they least need it.

Confirmation

Once Wakefield et al. proposed the association between MMR and autism in 1998, they and several other research groups began looking for further evidence of measles virus in children with autism. Wakefield's group expanded their original study population to ninety-one patients, taking biopsies of enlarged ileal lymph nodes. Using a technique called TaqMan RT-PCR, they isolated measles virus RNA sequences in seventy-five out of ninety-one children with autism, but in only five out of the seventy controls (p value < 0.0001). Interestingly, the measles virus was mostly located within the dendritic cells of the lymphoid follicle. (Remember from chapter 6 that the job of the dendritic cells is to capture and present viral antigens on their own cell membranes and then use cytokine signaling to initiate an immune response, leading to the death of the cells containing the virus. This cytokine signaling should also lead to an antibody response that will prevent more of the virus from entering the cells.) It appears that the measles virus might be acting as an immunological trigger to recruit lymphocytes to these lymph nodes, but the virus is not destroyed, due to its immunosuppressive properties, and so the cells become chronically infected. (This is not unlike the effects of the HIV virus on the immune system in general, and on the gut specifically).[60]

Ashwood et al. used a different method, confirming measles-virus antigen in 87.5% of ileal biopsy specimens from ten autistic children, compared to none of the samples from the eighteen controls. They tested for but were unable to detect the presence of other viruses, including rubella, mumps, adenovirus, herpes simplex types 1 and 2, and HIV and the bacteria *Pneumocystis carinii* (common in AIDS patients). The Ashwood group speculated that the immunosuppressive effects of the virus might be responsible for systemic immune dysregulation, and, further, that the secondary gut inflammation allowed absorption into the bloodstream of potentially neurotoxic substances, eventually leading to the encephalopathy (brain disease) seen in autistic children.[61]

The remaining question was whether the measles virus antigen found in the bowels of autistic children was from an atypical wild measles strain or from the cultivated strain in the MMR vaccine. A group from Japan was able to isolate measles virus from the blood samples of a small group of autistic children. They found that in every case the RNA sequence was consistent with the vaccine strain.[62]

A recent study from Montreal (D'Souza) also detected a high level of measles viral RNA in the blood of autistic children using a PCR technique reported by Uhlmann.[63] However, using their own PCR assay, all of these positive reactions went away. This led them to suggest that the findings of Uhlmann and others were false positives for measles.

In the United States, Walker et al., using a variety of techniques (including the Uhlmann primers), have found measles virus in a high percentage of biopsy tissues from autistic children with enterocolitis. They confirmed positive samples with specific RNA sequencing, which eliminates false-positive PCRs (which refutes D'Souza's argument). They found the Uhlmann technique actually yielded very few false positives from bowel tissues, and the RNA sequences are consistent with vaccine strain measles.[64] Since the samples in this study were from bowel biopsies in autistic children with known autistic enterocolitis rather than blood from a group of children both with and without gastrointestinal symptoms (as in the D'Souza study), Walker's results should be more definitive in evaluating Wakefield's initial theory.

In 2006, Wakefield et al. published a study that further suggests a causal association between the MMR vaccine and autism in children with gastrointestinal abnormalities and developmental regression. In a review of evidence concerning the strength of the association between MMR and autism, the IOM (Institute of Medicine) suggested that a study documenting an effect from a "challenge/re-challenge would constitute strong evidence of an association."[65] Wakefield and colleagues compared two groups of autistic children with developmental regression and gastrointestinal abnormalities. The first group had received only one MMR vaccine and the second group had received two (initial shot and booster). They found that the 69% of the children in the second group had new onset or worsening of GI symptoms after the booster. On endoscopy and biopsy, the double-exposure group had a more severe degree of lymph node hyperplasia and acute inflammation, indicating an apparent worsening of the bowel disease after repeat exposure. This study is highly suggestive of a causative role of the MMR vaccine in the bowel disease of these children.[66]

An abnormal immune response to the measles vaccine in autistic children has been associated with other problems as well. Dr. Vijendra Singh published a series of studies evaluating the antibody response to measles virus in relation to anti-brain autoantibodies. In the first study, he documented an association between elevated antibodies to measles and HHV-6 (human herpes virus-6) and autoantibodies against two brain proteins, MBP (myelin basic protein) and NAFP (neuron-axon filament protein). As the level of viral antibody titers (the number of antibodies present in the blood) increased, the likelihood of finding brain autoantibodies also increased. These antibodies against brain tissue were not found in the neurotypical controls. He concluded that this strong association might indicate a viral trigger to an autoimmune reaction affecting the brain in autistic children.[67]

In another study, Singh looked for antibodies against the MMR vaccine and found high levels in 60% of samples from autistic children and none from the controls. Based on molecular weight, he determined that the antibody was specifically targeting the measles component of the vaccine. Of the autistic children that had an MMR antibody, 90% were also positive for antibodies against their own MBP. This suggests an inappropriate immune response against MMR that might be triggering an anti-brain autoimmune reaction. Antibodies against this particular brain protein might be clinically meaningful because of the critical part that myelin plays in the nervous system. Myelin is a substance that forms an insulating sheath around the long axons of nerve cells, protecting them from damage and speeding the transmission of the electrical impulse from one end of the cell to the other. If myelin is damaged, the processing time of the nerve will be delayed and the nerve cell will be vulnerable to injury. This is the primary mechanism for the neurological injury in patients with multiple sclerosis.[68]

Singh also tested specifically for serum antibody titers to each of the viruses in the MMR vaccine (measles, mumps, and rubella). He compared titers in autistic children to normal controls and to siblings of autistic children. He found much higher measles titers in the children with autism compared with controls ($p = 0.003$), and with the siblings ($p<0.0001$). There was no real difference in the antibody levels against rubella or mumps virus. When he tested the antibody using an immunoblotting technique and compared it to vaccine-strain measles from MMR, he found that it was exactly the same weight and size. This particular vaccine-strain measles antibody was not detected in the blood of normal children or siblings. He again hypothesized that the vaccinestrain measles virus from MMR is inducing an autoimmune response in autistic children that might be contributing to their neurological disease.[69]

Bradstreet et al. tested CSF (cerebral spinal fluid) from three children who had previously been evaluated and found to have measles virus in their bowel biopsies. They found measles virus gene in all three cases. None of the control samples were positive for the virus. All three autistic children had serum antibodies against MBP, and antibodies were present in the CSF in two out of the three. IgG measles antibody titers were high in the serum and present in the CSF in two of the three autistic children. This confirms that in these children, evidence of the measles virus was not localized to the bowels. Additionally, the fact that measles virus antibodies persist in the CSF of these patients is suggestive of ongoing viral replication, since the CSF volume is replaced several times a day.[70]

In a larger follow-up study, 68% of 28 autistic children with developmental regression tested positive for measles-virus antigen in their CSF. All but one of the control samples were negative for the virus (a child with Burkett's lymphoma and leukemia). Bradstreet's group tested for the vaccine-strain viral sequence in a subset of the cases with autism; it was positive in 100% of the samples. They also detected measles virus in bowel tissue and blood cells in a subset of the children with autism in which tissue samples were available.[71] These two studies are highly suggestive of an etiological association between the vaccine-strain measles virus and the encephalopathy found in a subset of children with regressive autism.

It has been suggested that the vaccine-strain measles virus might be a causative factor in a subgroup of autistic children with developmental regression and GI symptoms. Most epidemiological studies have refuted the association, but all had methodological flaws and were unable to adequately answer the fundamental question of an association between MMR and a subset of autism. This hypothesis of an association is entirely plausible when we consider the precedents of other known risks associated with both naturally occurring measles virus and MMR vaccination, and now several published studies have confirmed the presence of vaccine-strain measles virus in the bowel tissues, the blood, and the CSF of children with autism and gastrointestinal disorders. As there is also evidence of a concomitant antibody response to measles and antibrain antibodies in children with autism, this area of investigation cannot be dismissed. Further research is mandatory, both to further define the connection between measles virus and autism and to investigate effective treatment.

chapter nine

IS AUTISM A GUT DISEASE?

THROUGHOUT ITS HISTORY, AUTISM HAS BEEN CONSIDERED A psychiatric disorder. Because of this model, many of the physical symptoms common in patients with autism have gone largely unrecognized, or even ignored. This error was compounded by the fact that most people with autism have trouble communicating, so getting an accurate history has always been challenging.

The medical establishment's failure to take note of coinciding GI symptoms in autistic children is but one example of the system's inability to look beyond the psychiatric model. Recall from chapter 2 how Kanner himself recorded GI abnormalities, only to sweep them aside, in the earliest description of this disease.

More recent medical literature clearly shows that gut symptoms are common in autism: in a prospective study by Fombonne and colleagues, GI symptoms were present in 80% of their autistic population studied in Montreal.[1] Valicenti-McDermott reports 70% of autistic children had GI symptoms compared with 28% of neurotypical controls;[2] and Melmed,[3] Levy,[4] and Horvath[5] reported similar rates in various studies of American children with autism.

In several retrospective reports, mostly chart reviews of medical records, an increased frequency of GI disease in children with autism was refuted. These records have minimal documentation of GI disease, but also fail to document its absence. [6][7][8][9] This is a discrepancy that underscores the importance of using prospective study design when evaluating symptoms in autism, especially when considering symptoms not previously assigned to the disease complex. (A prospective study establishes a hypothesis and then tracks the development of outcomes such as the onset of symptoms or side effects during the study period. A retrospective study looks back at accumulated information to see if it fits a given hypothesis. The quality of a retrospective study relies solely on the quality of note-taking, record-keeping, and personal recall, so errors due to confounding and bias are much more common.)

It's unlikely, in light of the high rates of GI disease documented in prospective studies, that the low incidence of these symptoms in the chart reviews is an accurate reflection of the true incidence. It's much more likely that the treating physicians failed to ask the right questions or didn't document symptoms they considered irrelevant to the presenting disease. Symptoms such as unexplained irritability, aggressive behavior, mood changes, discomfort, and nighttime awakenings could easily be dismissed or misinterpreted as neurological or "behavioral" rather than manifestations of gastrointestinal discomfort in a child who could not clearly express how he was feeling.

Diagnostic Confirmation of Upper GI Disease

Even when acknowledging GI symptoms in autistic children, some physicians continue to believe that the symptoms are the result instead of the cause of the behavior. They might think that the constipation, the reflux, and the abdominal pain occur because of unusual eating habits only. To find out if the GI symptoms reflected underlying gut pathology in autistic children, Horvath et al. did endoscopic evaluations of the upper GI tract of thirty-six children with autism and GI symptoms, including abdominal pain (n=25), chronic diarrhea (n=21), gaseousness/bloating (n=21), nighttime awakening (n=15), and unexplained irritability (n=18). Many of these children also had symptomatic food allergies.

An EGD (esophagogastroduodenoscopy—i.e., an upper endoscopy) was performed on each child; the researchers measured small intestine and pancreatic digestive enzymes, and took biopsy samples and bacterial and fungal cultures. They found reflux esophagitis in 69.4% of the children, (88% of whom had symptoms including nighttime awakening with irritability, abdominal discomfort, and pushing on the abdomen). There was chronic stomach inflammation in 42% and in the duodenum (small intestine) in 67%. They also found abnormal carbohydrate digestive enzyme activity in 58% of the patients (all of whom had loose stools and/or gaseousness).

In addition, the children had an unusual hypersecretory response to the injection of secretin, a gut hormone used to stimulate pancreatic fluid secretion; all of the children with this response had improvement in diarrhea that either lasted for several weeks or was sustained indefinitely. They also found an unusually large number of Paneth cells in the duodenum, similar to the numbers that have been documented in other chronic IBDs such as Crohn's disease. Paneth cells produce substances that are important for local immune defense, providing protection against pathogenic bacteria and *Candida albicans*, a common yeast that causes infections.[10]

Abnormal Stools

It's frequently observed that children with autism do not have normal stools. Constipation and/or diarrhea are common. Constipation is defined as either (a) the passage of hard, painful stools, regardless of how often they are passed, (b) the passage of infrequent stools, regardless of the degree of hardness of the stool, or (c) the difficult passage of stool, regardless of the other factors. It's rare to see hard, painful stools from children with autism, in spite of days between bowel movements.

This by itself suggests an abnormality of the colonic mucosa, which should have absorbed most of the water from the stool if it was sitting in the colon for days.

Children with autism are more likely to meet the criteria for constipation defined by (b) or (c) above. Stools are infrequent or difficult to pass, but are generally loose or diarrheal in consistency and often described as mushy or pudding-like. It's common for the stool to contain undigested food and be especially malodorous.[11] Diarrhea was the most common stool pattern reported to a large gastroenterology referral center, present in 78% of the children. Abdominal pain was reported in 59% and constipation in 36%.[12]

Afzal et al. studied 103 autistic children presenting to their GI clinic; abdominal X-rays revealed that 36% met radiological criteria for moderate to severe constipation. Moderate to severe rectosigmoid loading or acquired megarectum (stretching of the rectum from chronic fecal impaction) were present in 54%.[13] The researchers were unable to predict which children would have abnormal X-rays based on clinical symptoms alone. Milk consumption was the strongest predictor of constipation. In spite of stool retention evident on radiography, these children had a fairly normal number of bowel movements per week without evidence of a true impaction. Their symptoms were manifest by avoidance posturing (hunching forward on the toilet while defecating or defecating while standing) and soiling.

Autistic Enterocolitis

In 1998, Wakefield and colleagues at the Royal Free Hospital in London performed ileocolonoscopic examinations on twelve children with autism or related developmental disorders, and GI symptoms. They described a new variant of inflammatory bowel disease that they named autistic enterocolitis. The salient features were chronic patchy inflammation and lymphonodular hyperplasia (LNH), typically located in the terminal ileum (the last part of the small intestine), and to a lesser extent in the colon. This pattern was unique to the twelve chil-

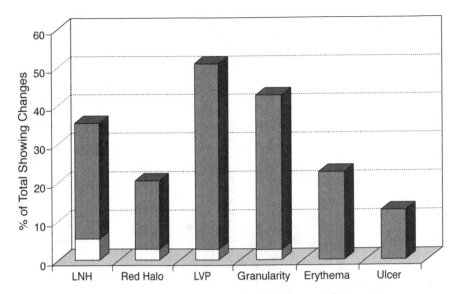

Fig. 1: Colonoscopic features in affected children (dark gray) and non-inflammatory bowel disease controls (light gray). Colonoscopies were scored for either the presence or absence of LNH, red halo sign, loss of vascular pattern (LVP), mucosal granularity, mucosal erythema, and ulceration. All of the features except ulceration were statistically significantly more common in affected children than in controls (p < 0.01). Source: Wakefield, *American Journal of Gastroenterology*. 2000.

dren with ASD when compared to the control children in the report who had bowel disease but no developmental disorder, and also when compared to other children that had been seen previously at the Royal Free GI clinic.[14]

Since then, many studies have confirmed and further defined these original findings. The first was a follow-up by Wakefield et al. on sixty children with ASD.[15] Ileal LNH was found in 93% of the autistic children, compared to 14% of the controls (thirty-seven developmentally normal children undergoing investigation for possible IBD); they also compared biopsies from twenty histologically normal samples and twenty samples with ulcerative colitis. Colonic LNH was found in 30% of the study group and 5.4% of the controls. Other common findings included "red halo" signs (pre-ulcerative erythema around lymphoid

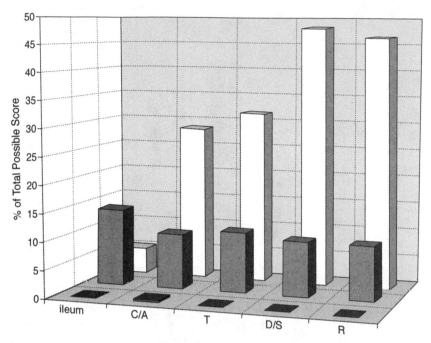

Fig. 2: Severity of histopathological changes in the ileum and colon (C/A=cecum / ascending, T= transverse, D/S=descending/sigmoid, and R=rectum) of affected children (gray w/lines) compared with controls whose biopsies were reported as normal (non-IBD controls (plain light gray)), and children with ulcerative colitis (white). The differences between both affected children and those with ulcerative colitis, and non-IBD controls, for severity of histological change at each site are significant (p < 0.001). Ulcerative colitis biopsies showed statistically significantly more severe change at each site, except the ileum, compared with those from affected children (p < 0.001). Source: Wakefield, *American Journal of Gastroenterology*. 2000.

nodules), loss of vascular pattern, mucosal granularity, mucosal erythema, and ulceration. These abnormal symptoms were all much more frequent in autistic children than in controls, with the exception of ulceration, which was uncommon in both groups.

The biopsies from the autistic children showed reactive follicular hyperplasia (enlargement of the lymph node follicles) in 88.5% compared with only 29% of children with ulcerative colitis, and none in the control children without IBD. In many cases they also saw infiltration of inflammatory cells (like neutrophils and lymphocytes) in the epithelium (the most superficial layer) of the bowel mucosa. Active neutrophilic inflammation in the ileum was present in 8% of the autistic children and in none of the controls. Chronic lymphocytic inflammation in the colon was present in 88% of the autistic cases, 4% of the controls, and 100% of the ulcerative colitis cases. Frequency and severity of inflammation were higher in both the autism and the ulcerative colitis cases than in the controls. The severity of inflammation in the autistic cases was generally milder than in the ulcerative colitis cases.

In 2005 the same group published a report on endoscopic evaluations of 148 autistic children confirming the findings of their earlier, smaller studies. Table 1 shows the frequency of GI symptoms in autistic children compared to controls (developmentally normal children with GI symptoms).

The Wakefield team found ileal LNH in 90% and colonic LNH in 59% of the autistic children compared with 30% and 23% of the controls, respectively. The LNH severity was significantly higher in the autistic children; less than 3% of the entire sample had isolated LNH (without evidence of other colon inflammation). This strongly suggests that LNH is neither a benign nor a normal condition (as has been suggested by some), but is strongly associated with mucosal pathology. It was also pointed out that many biopsy-proven cases of follicular hyper-

Symptoms	ASD ($n = 148$)	Developmentally normal controls ($n = 30$)
Constipation	75 (51)	4 (13)
Diarrhoea/loose stool	45 (30)	8 (27)
Abdominal pain/diarrhoea/ constipation	19 (13)	0 (0)
Abdominal pain	6 (4)	14 (47)
Rectal bleeding	0 (0)	4 (13)
Other	3 (2)	0 (0)

n = number of cases in symptom group (%).

Table 1: Symptoms in the ASD and the control groups. Source: Wakefield, *European Journal of Gastroenterology & Hepatology.* 2005.

plasia were not apparent by visual inspection of the mucosa, indicating the importance of biopsy for accurate diagnosis of the condition.[16] These studies from Wakefield and colleagues have been duplicated in the United States,[17 18] in Italy,[19 20] and in Venezuela.[21]

In Italy, Balzola et al. reported the first-time use of wireless endoscopy ("pillcam") in an autistic patient. The new technology enabled them to see the entire small intestine—impossible with traditional endoscopy. They found evidence of patchy erythema, mucosal erosions, and ulcers in the jejunum and the ileum.[22] This shows that, as in Crohn's disease, the bowel inflammation in autism is patchy, and is panenteric, i.e., it can exist anywhere along the GI tract.

The research group from the Royal Free Hospital further refined the characterization of the immunohistological abnormalities seen in autistic enterocolitis, recorded in a series of studies. In each of these, biopsies from children with autism were compared to developmentally normal children with bowel disease as well as to normal, non-diseased controls. The first study reported a degree of chronic inflammation in the colons of autistic patients that was intermediate in severity between subjects with classic IBD and normal subjects, results that were similar to the Wakefield study in 2000.

However, when doing an immunohistochemistry assessment (a different staining technique from routine histology, allowing specific identification of immune cell types) of the biopsies, they showed a marked infiltration of T-cells (particularly CD-8 cells and gamma-delta T-cells) and plasma cells (B-cell derived) of the gut mucosa. This inflammatory response was worse than was evident from the routine histological exams, and was different from both the other IBDs and the normal controls. The inflammation was more localized to the epithelium and basement membranes (superficial layers) of the gut mucosa than is commonly seen in classic IBD.[23]

Torrente et al. used similar techniques to evaluate biopsies from the duodenum (upper part of the small intestine) obtained with EGD.[24] They found a similar pattern of immunological abnormalities as the above-mentioned studies, with increased lymphocytic infiltration of the superficial layers of the gut lining and invasion into the crypt cells (cells that secrete digestive enzymes). Another striking abnormality was the deposition on the basolateral membrane of the gut epithelium of IgG antibodies, and complement immune activation (chapter 6). This strongly suggests that an autoimmune process is attacking this layer of the gut lining, and could be one explanation for the increased intestinal permeability reported by D'Eufemia et al. (see "Leaky Gut" syndrome, below).

The same research group found a similar immunohistochemical profile in biopsies taken from stomachs of children with autism, again with characteristic infiltration of primarily CD8+ T lymphocytes and immune deposition along the basement membrane of the stomach epithelium.[25]

Ashwood and colleagues added further evidence of the presence of GI inflammation in autistic children by looking at cytokine profiles in intestinal biopsies and in the blood, finding a dysregulated pattern that favors a pro-inflammatory response. This is represented by excess levels of TNF-α, IFN-γ, IL-4, and IL-5 (proinflammatory), and a marked reduction of IL-10 (regulatory) cytokines[26] (chapter 6).

Leaky Gut Syndrome

Wakefield et al. hypothesized that part of the neurological disability in children with autism results from absorption of neurotoxic molecules across a gut membrane damaged by inflammation.[27] D'Eufemia et al. used the lactulose-mannitol test to determine the gut permeability level in autistic children. Their study group comprised forty autistic children without apparent GI complaints and a group of controls; they documented an abnormal level of intestinal permeability in 43%, compared to 0% of the control group.[28]

Horvath et al. did the same test on twenty-five autistic children with GI symptoms and found that 76% had abnormal intestinal permeability.[29]

Dr. Rosemary Waring did a series of studies on children with autism that could partly explain the mechanism for a leaky gut. The GI mucosa forms a barrier against the contents of the gut, normally exerting tight control over what is allowed to enter the bloodstream (chapter 6). The lining of the gut is composed of cells with absorptive surfaces (the brush border) that interact with the contents of the lumen. Between these cells are gates called tight junctions that prevent substances from entering the blood stream without passing directly through the cells. In certain situations, these gates can open to allow substances to enter between the cells (paracellular transport). The locks to these gates are made of sulfate bonds. Dr. Waring and colleagues showed that children with autism have decreased levels of sulfate, which might predispose them to leaky gut syndrome.[30] Inadequate calcium in the blood could be another mechanism that triggers these gates to open, in which case calcium deficiency would be another predisposing factor for a leaky gut.[31]

A leaky gut means that molecules that wouldn't normally gain access can enter the bloodstream. This can lead to immune activation and tissue damage and effects on the brain, including damage to brain tissue. Over the years many parents have reported that their child's behavior improved measurably after gluten and casein were removed from the diet. Gluten is a protein found in grains and casein is a protein found primarily in cow's milk. These proteins have been shown to be highly immune-reactive in children with autism, particularly those with GI symptoms (chapter 7). There is also strong evidence that parts of these protein molecules act directly on the opiate receptors in the brain.

Goodwin et al. were among the first to document an abnormal brain response to gluten from food in autistic children with GI symptoms.[32] Starting in the mid 1980s, several researchers found an elevation of molecules consistent with gliadomorphine (derived from gluten) and casomorphine (derived from casein) peptides in the urine of autistic subjects; these are substances that attach to the opiate receptors in the brain. They also showed that children who maintained a gluten- and casein-free diet did much better neurologically (improved cognition, language, etc.) than those who did not. [33 34 35 36 37 38 39 40]

They hypothesized that these opioid (opiate-like) peptides disrupt normal neurotransmitter function in the brain, creating or contributing to behaviors such as decreased socialization, decreased response to pain, abnormal language, and self-abusive or repetitive behaviors. They also proposed direct effects on the neuronal structure of the brain tissue and on the immune system. They suggested that people with autism are more likely exposed to these opioids because of abnormal digestive enzyme activity, most probably genetically influenced. The enzyme diaminopeptidase IV (DPP-IV) is thought to be involved because it is part of a family of enzymes called adenosine deaminase binding proteins, which are known to be abnormal in some cases of autism.[41]

Intestinal Dysbiosis

Trillions of bacteria populate the human bowel. In fact, there are ten-fold more of them than there are human cells in the entire body. Most of them are beneficial to us, producing or making certain vitamins available, helping us digest food, and protecting the bowel lining. However, dozens of species of pathogenic (harmful) bacteria and yeasts are living in the bowel that, if allowed to overgrow, can cause disease. A good example of a pathogenic bacteria is *Clostridium difficile*. It's a common cause of severe colitis when broad-spectrum oral antibiotics have killed the beneficial gut bacteria and allowed this antibiotic-resistant, opportunistic organism to overgrow and cause inflammation.

In addition to causing damaging local effects on gut tissue, abnormal bacteria have been shown to affect the brain. For example, patients with chronic liver failure can develop a brain disease called hepatic encephalopathy. Because of liver pathology, the toxins that are produced by the harmful bacteria in the gut aren't adequately metabolized. These toxins, ammonia among them, can build up in the brain by way of the bloodstream, resulting in confusion, delirium, and even coma. One treatment for this condition is to rid the bowel of the harmful bacteria, which allows toxin levels to drop.

Probably because of GI inflammation and abnormal immune function, children with autism have abnormal levels of harmful bowel organisms. Frequent antibiotic use in the first years of life can contribute to the chronic imbalance referred to as intestinal dysbiosis. Several investigators have found evidence of this imbalance in autistic patients. In particular, a variety of clostridia (known for their production of neurotoxins) are found in higher amounts in children with autism compared to controls.[42][43][44][45][46] In one study, treatment with an antibiotic known to be effective against clostridia (oral vancomycin) improved autistic behaviors. Unfortunately, the behaviors returned shortly after discontinuing the medicine, presumably from reversion to a dysbiotic state.[47]

Dr. William Shaw has also suggested an association between autistic symptoms and yeast overgrowth in the bowel. Evaluation of urine organic acids in children with autism indicated elevated levels of chemicals (e.g. arabinose and tartaric acid) that are unknown in human metabolism, but are commonly found in yeast. Yeast species are known producers of chemicals that have neurological effects (e.g., alcohol).[48] Children with autism could be vulnerable either because of larger-than-normal yeast populations or an impaired capacity to detoxify the yeast metabolites.

I know of no other studies documenting yeast overgrowth in stool cultures or gut biopsies, but many parents and treating physicians report meaningful improvement in both GI and behavioral symptoms in autistic children with the use of antifungals, which kill yeast.[49][50] It's possible that the antifungals work via a different mechanism to produce clinical improvement rather than by killing the yeast. As of this writing, I'm not aware of any controlled studies on the use of antifungals for children with autism.

A great deal of evidence establishes that children with autism have a high incidence of bowel pathology that includes abnormal stool consistency, diminished digestive enzyme activity, intestinal permeability, intestinal dysbiosis, and a painful, unique inflammatory disease called autistic enterocolitis. Whether the GI disease is a primary event or is secondary to an underlying immune system abnormality is less clear. In light of the known gut-brain connection as established in other diseases (such as celiac disease and hepatic encephalopathy), it's possible that the neurological effect could be secondary to a widespread immune activation that started in the gut, or that there is injury from neurotoxic compounds derived from food substances or abnormal bowel microflora. Whatever the reason, almost all physicians who regularly care for the medical needs of autistic children agree that treating the GI disease results in significant improvement in core autistic behaviors.

chapter ten

WHY CAN'T THEY DETOXIFY?

THE EXPLOSION OF CASES OF AUTISM STARTING IN THE MID-1980s implicates a strong environmental role in this disorder, but a definite cause is still unknown. Is there some new toxin introduced in the last thirty years that makes babies develop autism? Or has the general toxic load increased in the environment to the point that children with limited detoxification capacities are neurologically affected? We should be able to find the answers to these questions by examining both the toxic exposures we now live with and the detox capacities of autistic children.

Detoxification 101

We're constantly exposed to substances that can cause damage to our tissues. Toxins are in the air we breathe, the water we drink, and the food we eat. To prevent injury from these substances, we have a multilayered and complex system for detoxification.

The liver is the main organ of detoxification; it's the first stop for harmful substances absorbed from the gut into the bloodstream. It processes most toxins before they can reach and damage the other organs—this is called *first-pass metabolism*. The liver uses different metabolic pathways to safely excrete harmful substances via the urine or the stool. The main detoxification pathways are called glucuronidation and trans-sulfuration. Depending on their structure, toxins are usually metabolized more effectively by one or the other.

But the liver can't completely detoxify every harmful substance, and because of this inevitable exposure, each cell in the body has its own mini-detoxification system.

The brain is particularly sensitive to damage from toxins, so it has an additional level of protection, the blood-brain barrier, which prevents many harmful substances from gaining access. But because the brain is exquisitely dependent on the blood supply for glucose and oxygen, certain small toxic molecules are able to slip through.

Many substances that are initially innocuous become toxic during normal metabolism. Some of these metabolic by-products are known as free radicals, and are produced by a process called oxidation. A counter-process, reduction, converts free radicals back into a harmless form. Imbalance between oxidation and reduction (redox) creates oxidative stress, which can result in tissue injury; anti-oxidants, including sulfate, cysteine, glutathione (GSH), and several vitamins and minerals (particularly vitamin C, vitamin E, vitamin B6, zinc, and selenium) combat this problem.

The Methylation Cycle

A number of researchers independently began looking at detox dysfunction in children with autism. They found abnormalities in the methylation cycle, a critical metabolic pathway that among other things produces precursor molecules for detoxification and anti-oxidation. Although this is complicated biochemistry, I am going to go through it in detail because it plays such an important part in so many of the pathways that appear to be disrupted in autism.

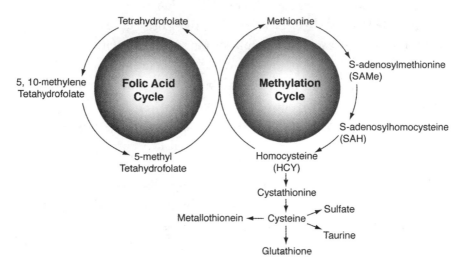

The diagram above gives an overview of the cycle, along with its interaction with two other metabolic pathways, the folic acid cycle and the transsulfuration pathway.

If we think of the methylation cycle as a central bank, the currency would be an organic molecule called a methyl group (-CH3). When a larger biochemical is "methylated," its structure and function change.

For example, a methyl group released from a chemical reaction with SAMe can attach to specific DNA sequences in our genetic code. If methylated, gene expression of that particular DNA strand is turned off. If the methyl group is removed, the gene is turned on. Methylation therefore controls which genes are active and which are repressed. The methylation patterns are established during embryogenesis (early development of the embryo) and are inherited in a tissue-specific manner. This allows cells to differentiate or specialize, accomplishing different tasks in different tissues, and it helps stabilize the chromosome structure, resulting in fewer mutations. It allows the body to inactivate genes (like the extra X chromosome in females) and to activate the inherited genes that give us the characteristics of our family tree. It's also used to suppress the expression of DNA sequences inserted by foreign invaders like viruses.[1]

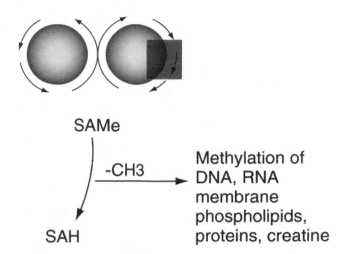

SAMe

$-CH_3$ → Methylation of DNA, RNA membrane phospholipids, proteins, creatine

SAH

SAMe, the body's primary methyl donor, also methylates neurotransmitters (like norepinephrine and serotonin), neurohormones (like melatonin), proteins, membrane phospholipids (form the cell membrane), myelin (the protective layer around nerve cells) and creatine (used in energy transfer). It's used to make precursors to carnitine (used in fatty acid metabolism) and to inactive histamine (modulates allergic responses). If methylation is impaired, then neurotransmitter function, protein and cell membrane structure and function, fatty acid metabolism, allergic responses, myelination, and cellular energy transfer are all adversely affected.

Currency has to flow both ways in banking, and this is so for the methylation cycle as well. As methyl groups are dispensed via SAMe, they must be added to another part of the cycle. Since methylation plays such a big role in cellular function, the body has several sources for regaining methyl groups to ensure that the cycle is continuous.

The first is methionine, an amino acid we mostly get from food. If it is lacking in the diet or absorption is impaired, the methylation cycle can create methionine from homocysteine by accepting a methyl group from the folic acid cycle. (5-methyl-tetrahydrofolate becomes tetrahydrofolate, and the methyl group is added to homocysteine via methyl-B12 to become methionine.) An enzyme called methionine synthase

(MS) drives this process. A parallel pathway can also transfer a methyl group from betaine (trimethylglycine, i.e., TMG) to homocysteine to make methionine; this one is catalyzed by betaine-homocysteine methyltransferase (BHMT). The existence of this backup pathway underscores the critical importance of maintaining adequate methionine (and SAMe) for the essential methylation reactions.

The methylation cycle requires a constant supply of folic acid, which is converted in a series of steps to 5-methylTHF (donates methyl group to homocysteine). The contribution from the folic acid cycle can be diminished for several reasons, not the least of which is a deficiency of folic acid in the diet.

Yet another cause of disruption in methionine recycling is inadequate methylcobalamin, a form of vitamin B-12 that's converted from B12 in the diet. Methylcobalamin is the most important cofactor for normal function of the methionine synthase (MS) enzyme that converts homocysteine back into methionine.[2] If methylcobalamin is deficient, methylation will be impaired. Oxidative stress can also inhibit the function of methionine synthase; it shunts homocysteine to the detoxification pathway rather than recycling it to methionine for methylation.

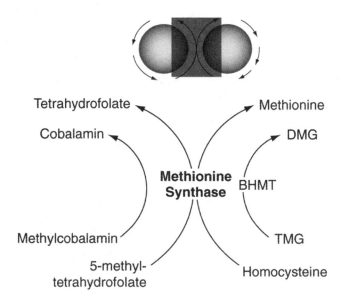

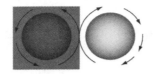

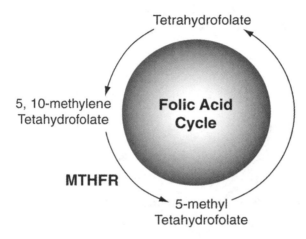

Tetrahydrofolate

5, 10-methylene Tetahydrofolate

Folic Acid Cycle

MTHFR

5-methyl Tetahydrofolate

Certain toxins such as thimerosal, mercury, and antimony are known to disrupt MS function.[3]

Another function of the methylation cycle is to produce or re-circulate the structural basis for cellular energy transfer, adenosine monophosphate (AMP), through the metabolism of S-adenosylhomocysteine (SAH). When adenosine starts to build up, the conversion of SAMe to SAH production slows down until the extra adenosine is removed. This negative feedback loop prevents recycling of methyl groups and inhibits the essential methylation reactions of SAMe.

The final key molecule in the methylation pathway is homocysteine. When exposed to either oxidative stress or a heavy toxic burden, the body considers protection from damage more essential than methylation, so homocysteine is shunted towards the detoxification/antioxidant pathway rather than recycling back to methionine for methylation. The enzyme that controls this decision process is called cystathione beta-synthase (CBS). This metabolic decision pathway is dependent on pyridoxl-5-phosphate (P5P, the active form of vitamin B6) and zinc. P5P

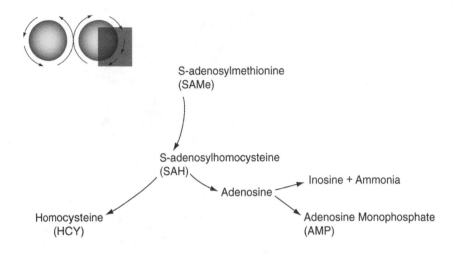

functions as a cofactor (assisting the primary enzyme) for CBS, in moving the reactions from one step to the next.

When homocysteine is diverted to this transsulfuration pathway, it's converted into a molecule called cystathionine, which becomes cysteine. Cysteine plays a central part in many body processes. It can become taurine, an amino acid used to produce the bile salts that help the bowel break down fats. It is also a source of sulfate, which is used extensively for detoxification by bonding with heavy metals and other toxic substances, preventing their absorption and facilitating excretion. Sulfate also forms the joints in the tight junctions between the cells lining the gut's absorptive surface, preventing unwanted molecules from leaking into the bloodstream.

In yet another process, cysteine is used to build metallothioneins (MTs), a family of proteins that are important regulatory molecules in gene expression, cellular metabolism of metals, and cellular adaptation to stress. They are especially active in maintaining normal intracellular balance of copper and zinc, and thereby influencing zinc-dependent biological processes (chapter 16). MTs also reduce the toxic effects of heavy metals on the cells (chapter 11) and can protect brain cells against glutamate-induced toxicity (chapter 20).[4]

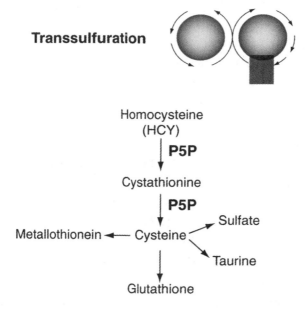

Note that brain cells don't produce the enzyme that breaks down cystathionine to cysteine, so all of the cysteine needed by the brain must be imported from liver stores.[5]

Cysteine is also the immediate precursor and the rate-limiting step in the production of GSH, the most important antioxidant and detoxification molecule.

The Importance of Glutathione

I remember reading about glutathione (GSH) in my biochemistry course in medical school, but I didn't really grasp its importance until I was a practicing emergency medicine physician. In the Emergency Department, we frequently treat patients who have overdosed on over-the-counter medications; one of the most common is acetaminophen (Tylenol). Acetaminophen has an excellent safety profile at the appropriate dose, but in overdose it can be deadly. Normally it's metabolized in the liver through the transsulfuration pathway, and GSH converts it to a non-toxic metabolite. In overdoses, the available GSH stores are used up and a toxic metabolite of acetaminophen accumulates, causing damage directly to the liver cells. Overdose patients can die shortly thereafter from liver failure.

Fortunately, there's an antidote for acetaminophen poisoning, N-acetylcysteine (Mucomyst) that almost always prevents liver damage when given early enough. This medication becomes cysteine, the immediate precursor of GSH. Cells don't generally absorb intact GSH across their cell wall; it's first broken apart into its three amino acid components: cysteine, glutamate and glycine. The cysteine is then taken up by the cell membrane and GSH is reassembled from the other components inside the cell. The N-acetyl cysteine given in the antidote is actually a better supplier of intracellular GSH than GSH itself, because it's better absorbed and skips a step in the intracellular transfer. In either case, GSH stores are replenished, the extra acetaminophen is detoxified, and the patient survives.

GSH performs a lot of vital intracellular functions.[6] It is the main anti-oxidant, both intracellular and extracellular, preventing free radical-induced cellular damage from oxidative stress. It maintains mitochondrial integrity and ATP production (necessary for cellular energy production). It works in the immune system to maintain normal T-cell subsets and to protect cells against intracellular viruses.[7] It is essential for the function and structural integrity of the gut; mucosal GSH depletion is associated with inflammatory bowel disease.[8][9] It is the foremost means for detoxifying and eliminating heavy metals and other environmental toxins, and it maintains vitamin C and vitamin E in their active forms. Without adequate levels of GSH, our bodies are compromised on many levels.

Impaired Methylation in Autism

In her work on children with Down syndrome (many of whom had autistic features), Dr. Jill James, a Ph.D. biochemist at the University of Arkansas, learned that they had abnormal methionine metabolism. She has since done similar studies on children with ASDs.[10][11] By measuring the components of the methylation cycle and comparing results to

	Control[a] (n=73)	Autistic[a] (n=80)	P-value
Methionine (μmol/L)	28.0 ± 6.5	20.6 ± 5.2	<0.0001
SAM (μmol/L)	93.8 ± 18	84.3 ± 11	<0.0001
SAH (μmol/L)	18.8 ± 4.5	23.3 ± 7.9	<0.0001
SAM/SAH ratio	5.5 ± 2.8	4.0 ± 1.7	<0.0001
Adenosine (μmol/L)	0.19 ± 0.13	0.28 ± 0.13	0.001
Homocysteine (μmol/L)	6.0 ± 1.3	5.7 ± 1.2	0.03
Cystathionine (μmol/L)	0.19 ± 0.1	0.24 ± 0.1	<0.0001
Cysteine (μmol/L)	207 ± 22	165 ± 14	<0.0001
Cysteinylglycine (μmol/L)	39.4 ± 7.3	38.9 ± 11	0.78
Total GSH (μmol/L)	7.53 ± 1.7	5.1 ± 1.2	<0.0001
Free GSH (μmol/L)	2.2 ± 0.9	1.4 ± 0.5	<0.0001
GSSG (μmol/L)	0.24 ± 0.1	0.40 ± 0.2	<0.0001
Total GSH/GSSG ratio	28.2 ± 7.0	14.7 ± 6.2	<0.0001
Free GSH/GSSG ratio	7.9 ± 3.5	4.9 ± 2.2	<0.0001

SAM, S-adenosvlmethioninie; SAH, S-adenosylhomocysteine; GSH, glutathione; GSSG, glutathione disulfide.
[a]**Means ± SD.**

Table 1: Transmethylation and transsulfuration metabolites in autistic cases and controls. Source: James, *American Journal of Medical Genetics*, 2006.

neurotypical controls, she demonstrated an abnormal pattern of methylation and transsulfuration in the autistic children. The results of her study are shown in table 1.

All of the methylation and transsulfuration markers in the autism group were much lower than in the controls with the exception of SAH and adenosine, which were significantly elevated in a subset of the children. This suggests an abnormality in adenosine metabolism that's causing an accumulation of this molecule in some autistic children, inhibiting the rest of the negative feedback loop described earlier. This finding is of special interest because there are rare genetic disorders that are known to cause autism, and these disorders affect adenosine metabolism.[12] The enzyme that's used to break down adenosine is called adenosine deaminase and it's bound to a molecule called DPP-IV, the enzyme in the gut that digests gluten and casein. Abnormalities in this enzyme might explain why children with autism have both gluten and casein peptide sensitivity and abnormalities in their methylation cycle. It has recently been found that DPP-IV also has immunomodulatory properties through cleaving numerous chemokines and cytokines and influencing their effect. It's also a surface marker that controls production of certain cells called thymocytes, which are active in the immune system.

The autistic children in Dr. James' study also had low levels of the molecules in the transsulfuration pathway including cystathionine, cysteine, and GSH. In addition, they had an abnormal ratio of oxidized GSSG to reduced GSH, a very sensitive marker of oxidative stress.

Dr. James tested a two-part intervention in a smaller trial.[13] First, she supplemented eight children with autism with betaine (TMG) and folinic acid, both of which add methyl groups to the methylation bank. She found that the methylation cycle values all improved measurably with these two dietary manipulations.

Next she added methylcobalamin injections, and levels of cysteine and GSH essentially returned to normal. Although preliminary, this study has great meaning because it demonstrates that a significant abnormality in a critical metabolic pathway in children with autism can be returned to near-normal standards using nutritional supplementation. It was mentioned that the clinician who conducted the study saw a simultaneous improvement in the children's behavior, but the improvement was not adequately quantified and therefore not reported. This study is now being repeated with a larger number of children, and behavioral observations are part of the study design.

Recent evidence suggests that some of the genetic susceptibility in autism could be related to the methylation pathway as well. Several polymorphisms (small variations in the genes) have been identified at critical points in the folic acid and methionine cycles that can decrease the activity of the enzymes and the overall efficiency of methylation and oxidative metabolism. These polymorphisms are common in the general population, but are found at much higher rates in children with autism; they've been shown to be independent predictors of autism risk. (The polymorphisms that carry the highest risk include: MTHFR (methylene tetrahydrofolate reductase—creates 5-methyltetrahydrofolate to act as a methyl donor to homocysteine); RFC (reduced folate carrier—modulates the delivery of folate to the cells); TCN2 (transcobalamin 2—the major transport carrier required for B12 uptake into the cells); COMT (catecholamine O-methyltransferase—methylates and inactivates the neurotransmitter dopamine in the brain); and GST (GSH-S-transferase—conjugates toxins to reduced GSH to be excreted from the body).[14][15]

Many of the metabolic abnormalities and susceptibilities that we commonly see in autism can be explained after examining the effects of acquired or inherited abnormalities in methylation and detoxification pathways. It's interesting to note that nutritional supplements associated with an improvement in autistic symptoms, either anecdotally[16] or in the medical literature,[17][18] happen to support normal function of these pathways. These include folinic acid, DMG, TMG, methylcobalamin, zinc, vitamin B6 (or P5P), digestive enzymes containing DPP-IV, GSH, cysteine (as N-acetyl cysteine), sulfate, and metallothionein-promoting amino acids.

Much is left to discover, and research will yield new information that will not come too late for many of these children if we enable promising and appropriate studies to move ahead.

chapter eleven

DOES MERCURY CAUSE AUTISM?

THE SEARCH FOR A UNIFYING ENVIRONMENTAL CAUSE OF AUTISM has led many to consider the highly toxic heavy metal, mercury. I want to make it clear that I do not believe that mercury is *the* cause of autism. I don't believe there is a single cause. I believe that autism comes about in children who are born with a genetically vulnerable immune system that sustains damage from multiple environmental exposures acting cumulatively and synergistically. The environmental exposures are likely to be different in different children, which could explain the range of symptoms and the differing ages of onset. Nonetheless, I am writing a chapter about mercury because it's a good example of a toxin with a wide spectrum of negative biological effects, many of which are evident in autistic children. Learning more about mercury and how it affects children with autism will undoubtedly help us to better understand the impacts from other environmental toxins, and so to find more effective treatments. For an excellent review on the issue of the environmental toxicity and the neurodevelopment of our children, I refer you to an article by Dr. Philippe Grandjean out of Harvard that was published in *The Lancet* in December 2006.[1]

The Mercury Cycle

As part of the earth's crust, mercury is ubiquitous in the environment. It's found in the air, the soil, the water, and in living organisms. Natural sources include volcanoes and deep mines, but the majority of atmospheric mercury (70%) is from coal-burning power plant emissions and refining waste. Once mercury is released into the environment, it's there indefinitely. Over the last hundred years, atmospheric mercury has increased three-fold from industrial emissions. From there it enters our waters as rainfall, and is then converted to an organic form (methylmercury) by aquatic bacteria. Because living organisms can't effectively excrete methylmercury, it accumulates in the tissues of sea life and is transferred up the food chain; we absorb it when we eat seafood. Other sources of exposure include mercury vapor from dental amalgams (metallic fillings) and contaminated air. It's also been used as a preservative in medical products and vaccines (thimerosal). Some cultures still use mercury in their traditional medicines (in the form of cinnabar or calomel) because they believe it has magical or healing properties.[2]

The Toxicity of Mercury

The first reported cases of mercury poisoning were in 23-79 AD in miners, in what is now Spain. Shakespeare wrote about murder with quicksilver (liquid mercury) in *Hamlet.* The Mad Hatter from *Alice in Wonderland* is actually mercury toxic; in the nineteenth century, hat makers were exposed to vapor from the mercurous nitrate used to cure felt, causing a syndrome characterized by the onset of bizarre behavior (including excessive shyness or rages and aggression, depression, anxiety), loss of coordination, slurred speech, tremors, and gingivitis. The phrase "mad as a hatter" became popular not from Lewis Carroll's story, but because the mental instability of hat makers was once so well known.

An example of mercury poisoning in more recent history is pink disease (acrodynia). In the nineteenth and continuing through the first half of the twentieth century, some babies mysteriously developed symptoms of irritability, photophobia, pain and redness of the hands and feet, hypertension, depression, and GI and other symptoms; about 7% died. It was eventually determined that calomel-based teething powders and worm powders caused these symptoms. The disease all but disappeared once mercury was removed from these powders in 1960.[3]

In recent decades, there has been much in the medical literature about the toxicity of the biologically active form of organic mercury, methylmercury (MeHg). High doses of MeHg have been shown to be extremely harmful and often fatal (for an excellent review of MeHg toxicity, read Sanfeliu's "Neurotoxicity of organomercurial compounds"[4]). Classically, patients present with paresthesias, dysarthria, sensory deficits, deafness, cerebellar ataxia, and progressive constriction of the visual fields. This collection of symptoms is referred to as Hunter-Russell syndrome. The neurological impairments can progress to paralysis, coma, and death.

In the 1950s, neurological illness and death resulted from the contamination of Minamata Bay in Japan by mercury-containing waste. Over eighteen thousand people reported symptoms and over nine hundred died from what became known as Minamata Disease. The symptoms were much the same as Hunter-Russell syndrome. Those with lower exposures had less severe sensory disturbances. There was a wide variation in the severity and onset of symptoms (from weeks to months after exposure), depending on the amount and duration of exposure and on individual susceptibility. There is a chronic form of Minamata Disease in which symptoms manifest years after exposure; there is also Congenital Minamata in babies born to mothers who were exposed, indicative of the far reach of the effects.

A similar incident occurred in Iraq in the early 1970s—the accidental consumption of seed grain contaminated with organic mercury used as a fungicide resulted in the hospitalization of over 6,500 people and 439 deaths. It's estimated that as many as forty to fifty thousand people were affected.

In both the Japanese and the Iraqi exposures, the neuropathological consequences of acute MeHg toxicity in exposed adults included a significant loss of granule cells in the cerebellum with focal atrophy (wasting), and less severe effects in other brain regions. Asymptomatic mothers produced babies born with neurological impairments and even more widespread cellular damage than was seen in symptomatic adults. Misorganization of the brain cells was a common feature in the children's brains.

In Iraq, prenatal exposures caused symptoms of mental retardation with associated language delay and impaired sensory, motor, and autonomic functions. This indicates a particular sensitivity in developing brains, with unique pathophysiological consequences at lower levels of exposure, compared to adults.[5]

Two large studies looked at the neurological effects of prenatal methylmercury exposure from maternal fish consumption, one study in the Faroe Islands and one in the Republic of Seychelles. The patterns of fish consumption differed somewhat between the two regions. Mothers from Seychelles ate regular daily amounts of ocean fish with relatively low concentrations of mercury. The women in the Faroe Islands had episodic intake of large amounts of pilot whale meat, which has much larger concentrations of mercury (and also PCBs, or pesticides).

Long term follow-up of the neurodevelopmental outcomes of children whose mothers had high mercury levels in their hair showed different results between the two studies. The Seychelles children showed a mild abnormality on only one of forty-six endpoints tested (time to complete a pegboard task)—the mercury effects were minimal.[6 7] The Faroes study in contrast reported an adverse relationship between mercury exposure and memory, attention, language, and visual-spatial perception in children at seven years of age.[8] The differences in exposures between the two populations might account for the difference in their study results. It's certainly possible that bolus (high intermittent) doses of mercury differ from daily low doses in their effect. In a review of these and other studies, the EPA set the "safe" limit of daily methylmercury exposure at 0.1 mcg/kg/day.[9] [Note: A 2006 study on the prevalence of ASDs from the Faroe Islands shows an overall rate of 56/10,000 (1 in 178) in children born between 1985 and 1994 who were still living in the region.[10] The authors suggest that this is equal to rates published by other epidemiological studies, but in fact that's only true for prevalence rates in children much younger than this cohort. Prevalence rates in similar age groups are much lower, especially in nearby regions such as Finland, Iceland, and Denmark (chapter 4).]

Perhaps the most important observation to be drawn from these reports is that there is wide variation in the onset and in the manifestations of mercury toxicity in individuals, in spite of equivalent exposures. For example, only one in 500-1,000 infants exposed to mercury in teething powders developed acrodynia. Note that in many cases, symptoms of toxicity didn't become apparent for months or even years after the exposure.[11]

The EPA Reports Concern about Mercury

Because of ever-increasing levels of environmental mercury, the EPA has placed it on their watch list of toxins of highest concern. The following information about the potential risk of mercury to developing brains is reported on the EPA website (italics added):

"For fetuses, infants, and children, the primary health effect of methylmercury is *impaired neurological development*... Impacts on cognitive thinking, memory, attention, language, and fine motor and visual spatial skills have been seen in children exposed to methylmercury in the womb."

"Outbreaks of methylmercury poisonings have made it clear that adults, children, and developing fetuses are at risk from ingestion exposure to methylmercury. During these poisoning outbreaks some mothers with no symptoms of nervous system damage gave birth to infants with severe disabilities, it became clear that the *developing nervous system of the fetus might be more vulnerable* to methylmercury than is the adult nervous system."

"The Environmental Protection Agency believes that about 630,000 of the roughly 4 million babies born annually in the United States—twice as many as previously thought—may be exposed to dangerous levels of mercury in the womb...The EPA's analysis reflects a new understanding among scientists in the US and Japan that umbilical cord blood has higher mercury concentrations than a mother's blood..."

"Given the new finding that umbilical cord blood has higher concentrations of mercury, the EPA believes that the safe level for mercury in mothers' blood is 3.5 parts per billion. About 15% *of women of childbearing age* had blood levels that high, according to the CDC study."

Noting the EPA's "15% *of women of childbearing age*," perhaps it isn't coincidental that the CDC has recently reported that 15% of American children are currently being diagnosed with a neurodevelopmental disorder (including autism and ADHD).[12]

Mercury and Autism

In 1999, a group of parents of autistic children got together because they were concerned that mercury was possibly the cause of their children's neurological disease. An exhaustive search of symptoms related to mercury poisoning in the medical literature revealed some haunting similarities to symptoms of autism.

Sallie Bernard et al. published a study of their findings in *Medical Hypotheses* in 2001.[13] The table on pages 118 and 119 depicts neurological characteristics common to the two diseases.

The tables on pages 120 and 121 show the similarities of biological disturbances.

The Bernard paper hypothesized that autism is a previously unrecognized manifestation of mercury toxicity and that the likely culprit is thimerosal, the mercury-based preservative in childhood vaccines. It noted that the first cases of autism were described in 1943 in children born in the early 1930s, shortly after the introduction of thimerosal in 1930. The paper stated that as the mercury dose increased through the addition of more TCVs (thimerosal-containing vaccines) to the pediatric schedule, so did the prevalence of autism.

Summary comparison of traits of autism and mercury poisoning

Psychiatric disturbances

Social deficits, shyness, social withdrawal

Repetitive, perseverative, stereotypic behaviors; obsessive-compulsive tendencies

Depression/depressive traits, mood swings, flat affect; impaired face recognition

Anxiety; schizoid tendencies; irrational fears

Irritability, aggression, temper-tantrums

Lacks eye contact; impaired visualfixation (HgP)/problems in joint attention (ASD)

Speech and language deficits

Loss of speech, delayed language, failure to develop speech

Dysarthria; articulation problems

Speech comprehension deficits

Verbalizing and word retrieval problems (HgP); echolalia, word use and pragmatic errors (ASD)

Sensory abnormalities

Abnormal sensation in mouth and extremities

Sound sensitivity; mild to profound hearing loss

Abnormal touch sensations; touch aversion

Over-sensitivity to light; blurred vision

Motor disorders

Flapping, myoclonal jerks, choreiform movements, circling, rocking, toe walking, unusual postures

Deficits in eye-hand coordination; limb apraxia; intention tremors (HgP)/ problems with intentional movement or imitation (ASD)

Abnormal gait and posture, clumsiness and incoordination; difficulties sitting, lying, crawling, and walking; problem on one side of body

Summary comparison of traits of autism and mercury poisoning, continued

Cognitive impairments

Borderline intelligence, mental retardation – some cases reversible

Poor concentration, attention, response inhibition (HgP)/ shifting attention (ASD)

Uneven performance on IQ subtests; verbal IQ higher than performance IQ

Poor short term, verbal, and auditory memory

Poor visual and perceptual motor skills; impairment in simple reaction time (HgP)/ lower performance on timed tests (ASD)

Deficits in understanding abstract ideas & symbolism; degeneration of higher mental powers (HgP)/sequencing, planning & organizing

(ASD); difficulty carrying out complex commands

Unusual behaviors

Self injurious behavior, e.g. head banging

ADHD traits

Agitation, unprovoked crying, grimacing, staring spells

Sleep difficulties

Physical disturbances

Hyper- or hypotonia; abnormal reflexes; decreased muscle strength, especially upper body; incontinence; problems chewing, swallowing

Rashes, dermatitis, eczema, itching

Diarrhea; abdominal pain/discomfort, constipation, "colitis"

Anorexia; nausea (HgP)/ vomiting (ASD); poor appetite (HgP)/restricted diet (ASD)

Lesions of ileum and colon; increased gut permeability

Mercury exposure

Biochemistry

Binds · SH groups; blocks sulfate transporter in
Intestines, kidneys

Reduces glutathione availability, inhibits enzymes of glutathione
metabolism; glutathione needed in neurons, cells, and liver
to detoxify heavy metals; reduces glutathione peroxidase and
reductase

Disrupts purine and pyrimidine metabolism

Disrupts mitochondrial activities, especially in brain

Immune system

Senstitive individuals more likely to have allergies, asthma,
autoimmune-like symptoms, especially rheumatoid-like ones

Can produce an immune response in CNS, causes brain/MBP
autoantibodies

Causes overproduction of Th2 subset; kills/inhibits lymphocytes,
T-cells, and monocytes; decreases NK T-cell activity; induces or
suppresses IGNg & IL-2

CNS structure

Selectively targets brain areas unable to detoxify or reduce
Hg-induced oxidative stress

Accummulates in amygdala, hippocampus, basal ganglia, cerebral
cortex; damages Purkinje and granule cells in cerebellum;
brain stem defects in some cases

Causes abnormal neuronal cytoarchitecture; disrupts neuronal
migration, microtubules, and cell division; reduces NCAMs

Progressive microcephaly

Neuro-chemistry

Prevents presynaptic serotonin release and inhibits serotonin
transport; causes calcium disruptions

Alters dopamine systems; peroxidine deficiency in rats resembles
mercurialism in humans

Elevates epinephrine and norepinephrine levels by blocking
enzyme that degrades epinephrine

Elevates glutamate

Leads to cortical acetylcholine deficiency; increases muscarinic
receptor density in hippocampus and cerebellum

Causes demyelinating neuropathy

Neurophysiology

Causes abnormal EEGs, epileptiform activity, variable patterns,
e.g., subtle, low amplitude seizure activities

Causes abnormal vestibular nystagmus responses; loss of sense
of position in space

Results in autonomic distrubance: excessive sweating, poor
circulation, elevated heart rate

Autism

Biochemistry
Low sulfate levels

Low levels of glutathione; decreased ability of liver to detoxify xenobiotics; abnormal glutathione peroxidase activity in erythrocytes

Purine and pyrimidine metabolism errors lead to autistic features

Mitochondrial dysfunction, especially in brain

Immune system
More likely to have allergies and asthma; familial presence of autoimmune diseases, especially rheumatoid arthritis; IgA deficiencies

On-going immune response in CNS; brain/MBP autoantibodies present

Skewed immune-cell subset in the Th2 direction; decreased response to T-cells mitogens; reduced NK T-cell function; increased IFNg & IL-12

CNS structure
Specific areas of brain pathology; many functions spared (36)

Pathology in amygdala, hippocampus, basal ganglia, cerebral cortex; damage to Purkinje and granule cells in cerebellum; brain stem defects in some cases

Nauronal disorganization; increased nauronal cell replication, increased glial cells; depressed expression of NCAMs

Progressive microcephaly and macrocephaly

Neuro-chemistry

Decreased serotonin syntheses in children; abnormal calcium metabolism

Either high or low dopamine levels; positive response to peroxidine, which lowers dopamine levels

Elevated norepinephrine and epinphrine

Elevated glutamate and asparate

Cortical acetylcholine deficiency; reduced muscarinic receptor binding in hippocampus

Demyelination in brain

Neurophysiology

Abnormal EEGs, epileptiform activity, variable patterns, including subtle, low amplitude seizure activities

Abnormal vestibular nystagmus responses; loss of sense of position in space

Autonomic disturbance: unusual sweating, poor circulation, elevated heart rate

This set off a heated, politically charged debate between autism advocacy groups and government health regulatory organizations such as the CDC, the FDA, and the American Academy of Pediatrics. In 1999, the FDA published a review of exposure to mercury in medicinal products, finding that children who received all of the routine vaccines on schedule were being injected with 187.5 mcg of mercury by the age of six months and 237.5 mcg by age two. (This does not include the children who were exposed to thimerosal through influenza vaccines or pre-natal Rho(D) immunoglobulin shots, such as RhoGAM.)[14] At routine check-ups, infants were usually given more than one hundred fifty times the EPA's safe daily standard for methylmercury for an adult (there are no safety standards for ethylmercury). In other words, to be within the government-approved "safe" level, a two-month-old baby would have to weigh 1,375 lbs, assuming that ethylmercury is as toxic as methylmercury.

In an effort to lower overall mercury exposure in children, the FDA recommended that vaccine manufacturers find an alternate preservative for childhood vaccines. They did not ask for a recall of products that were already on the shelves, nor did they acknowledge publicly that the level of mercury exposure that they'd been implicitly endorsing might cause harm to children. Production of thimerosal-free vaccines didn't begin until two years later, in 2001, and the new vaccines slowly replaced the existing supply of TCVs over the course of the next few years.

But even today, not all vaccines that children and pregnant women receive are thimerosal-free. Many forms of Rho(D) shots and the most common forms of flu vaccines contain thimerosal. Flu vaccine (without stipulating preference for thimerosal-free versions) is promoted for pregnant women, and it's recommended that starting at six months old, babies get two doses in the first year followed by single doses in subsequent years. TCVs are still the primary vaccines shipped to developing countries. The question of thimerosal safety is still therefore both relevant and immediate.

What Is Thimerosal?

Thimerosal is used in the manufacturing process of vaccines and as a preservative in multi-dose vaccine vials, as well as in other medical products. It's bacteriostatic (discourages the growth of bacteria), which reduces the chance of bacterial contamination from repeated punctures of the seal on the multi-dose vial. This allows manufacturers to package vaccines more cost-effectively. It costs ten cents per dose to produce a multi-dose vial, compared to twenty-five cents for a single-dose vial.

Thimerosal consists of two principal compounds: ethylmercury (49.6% of the compound) and thiosalicylate. First manufactured by Eli Lilly and Company in 1930, the original safety studies were done on twenty-two patients with meningococcal meningitis. Most died within a few days. Lilly concluded that since they died from meningitis, thimerosal was safe, and brought it to market.[15] The FDA didn't become powerful enough to mandate safety testing of medical products until 1938; by that time thimerosal was "grandfathered" in and no further safety studies were done. Until recently, there were few studies done regarding ethylmercury, and the pharmacodynamics (drug metabolism) of the compound were not well understood. Many studies have documented toxic or allergic effects to the skin, ear, and conjunctival tissues from this product, either through vaccination or ear and eye drops. In the late 1990s, it was removed from most contact lens solutions because of the high rate of sensitivity in the population.

Before the FDA's 1999 announcement, almost nothing had been published looking at developmental issues, neurotoxicity, or immune suppression related to ethylmercury. A 1977 Russian report described a group of adults still suffering from neuropathology several years after exposure to ethylmercury. It's startling that these adults were debilitated by far lower concentrations than American children were to receive in vaccines in the 1990s.[16]

Information obtained through the Freedom of Information Act (FOIA) reveals that since 1947, scientists concerned about the toxicity of thimerosal have sent Lilly half a dozen reports delineating their reasons for alarm about its continued use and manufacture.[17] Even as far back as 1935, Lilly received a letter from the director of biological services at Pittman-Moore (an animal vaccine manufacturer) warning that their own assessment of thimerosal's safety did not agree with Lilly's; 50% of the dogs in the study who received an injection containing thimerosal became ill. Pittman-Moore pronounced it "unsatisfactory as a preservative for serum intended for use on dogs."[18] In 1950, an article was published in the *Annals of the New York Academy of Sciences* stating that mercurials are toxic when injected.[19] In 1967, a study in *Applied Microbiology* found that thimerosal killed mice when added to injected vaccines.[20]

In 1971, Lilly did their own study, determining that thimerosal was "toxic to tissue cells," but they blithely continued to promote their product as non-toxic and even started using it in their topical disinfectants.[21] As a result, in 1977 ten newborn babies died at a Toronto hospital when an antiseptic containing thimerosal was applied to their umbilical cords. In 1982, an FDA panel determined that thimerosal was toxic to cells and unsafe for over-the-counter products.[22] In 1991, thimerosal was banned from use in animal vaccines.[23] Yet the FDA was oddly content to leave it in the early childhood vaccines. Not only was it left in, US children were subjected to higher doses.

When the Haemophilus influenza B (Hib) (1990) and the hepatitis B vaccines (1991) were added to the recommended schedule, thimerosal exposure increased by 150%. Previously, children received eleven vaccines in the first six months—now they received twenty-eight. In 1999 Dr. Peter Patriarca, director of the Division of Viral Products at the FDA, wrote the head of the CDC complaining that no one had done the simple math required to determine that the mercury levels in the new vaccine schedule were unsafe. He went on to write, "I am not sure if there will be an easy way out of the potential perception that the FDA, CDC, and immunization policy bodies may have been 'asleep at the switch' regarding thimerosal until now."[24]

Thimerosal Studies

After the Bernard paper was published and after the FDA announcement, there was understandable alarm among parents. Vaccine manufacturers and vaccine regulatory agencies such as the CDC were also alarmed; perhaps for different reasons. Was it possible that vaccines were responsible for the epidemic of autism? Could autism be an iatrogenic illness (induced inadvertently by physicians)? If so, this would be one of the biggest medical and political catastrophes in history—a government-mandated program ruining the lives of thousands of children with autism, and the lives of their families as well. The credibility of the vaccine program, many high-powered jobs, and large sums of money in potential lawsuits and lost revenues were at stake. The trust of the Third World countries in the US government might be threatened, and with cause. There was an immediate flurry of press releases and news stories, mostly engineered by government agencies, to reassure doctors and the general public that vaccines were safe and that there was no evidence that thimerosal was the cause of neurological injury.

Danish Epidemiological Studies

Not long after the thimerosal-autism link was suggested publicly, several related epidemiology studies were published. Madsen, who had published an MMR/autism study a couple of years before (2002), reviewed data to see if there was a connection between the autism rise and the thimerosal content in pediatric vaccines.[25] He and his colleagues looked at Danish children between two and ten years old diagnosed with autism during the period from 1971-2000. Thimerosal was removed from pediatric vaccines in Denmark in 1992. Since (according to their analysis) the diagnosis rate of autism continued to rise after the discontinuation of thimerosal from pediatric vaccines, they concluded that thimerosal was not related to autism.

However, Mark Blaxill from SafeMinds (an autism advocacy group) points out flaws in the Madsen study design that make it impossible to draw accurate conclusions from the data.[26] There were changes made in the practices of the Danish Registry during the 1990s. One was the 1995 addition of outpatient cases. In Madsen's previous study using the same database, the ratio of outpatients to inpatients was 13.5 to one, and the total number of outpatients represented over 93% of the total cases, but the effect of this large confounder was deemed unimportant by the authors. (A confounder is an unknown or unaccounted for factor in a research study.) In fact, addition of outpatients can account for the entire increase in cases of autism in Denmark after 1994.

Another potential confounder was the addition of cases from a large clinic in Copenhagen in 1992, which accounted for 20% of the total Danish caseload. Also serving to inflate the apparent incidence after 1992, the Danish psychiatry registry changed their diagnostic criteria in 1993 from ICD-8 psychosis proto-infantalis (an unusual inpatient classification that has never been used in autism surveys outside of Denmark) to the more appropriate ICD-10 childhood autism. The use of psychosis proto-infantalis as a diagnostic code is unusual—and even puzzling—because ICD-8 includes a clearly more suitable code, infantile autism. In addition, Madsen reported the incidence of autism based on year of entrance into the system rather than year of birth, although these data were available to him. Many of the outpatients entered the system after 1995, even though they were in the seven-to-nine-year-old age group, artificially weighting the post-thimerosal numbers. The reason that Madsen reports the numbers this way isn't made clear.

A closer look at these incidence rates reveals something else that's highly unusual. The reported rate of autism in Denmark before 1990 was less than one in ten thousand—lower than in any previous autism study in the world. This could either reflect a population that is at much lower risk for autism than the rest of the developed world, or an underreporting of cases in the early years of the study. The rate of two to five per ten thousand in the more recent years is still much lower than reported rates in the US and elsewhere (more than thirty per ten thousand at the time).

It's highly pertinent that there are differences in thimerosal exposure in vaccinated Danish children compared to American children. The only thimerosal-containing vaccine used in Denmark between 1970 and 1992 was the whole-cell pertussis vaccine, but this exposure was later and less frequent than in the recommended US schedule. In Denmark the total thimerosal exposure by six months of age was 125 mcg compared to 187.5 mcg in the US. Their reported thimerosal content of 50 mcg per shot is unusually high, twice as much as the vaccines from any manufacturer in any other country (25 mcg).

Danish children received vaccines against fewer illnesses than US and UK children—a key point because of the possibility that vaccines interact synergistically. And thimerosal-containing Rho(D) injections were not given to pregnant women in Denmark. Because of these exposure and population differences, whatever the Madsen study might tell us about Danes, it simply cannot rule out the possibility of an association between thimerosal and childhood vaccines in a US population. Madsen et al. appear to hand-select data to justify vaccine safety—not surprising, given the affiliation of several of the authors with the Statens Serum Institut, Denmark's premier vaccine manufacturer.

Another epidemiology study from Denmark was published by Hviid et al. in *JAMA* in 2003. This time the subjects were children in the Danish Registry born between 1990 and 1996. As mentioned, the only TCV in Denmark was the whole-cell pertussis vaccine phased out in 1992. Children given thimerosal-containing pertussis were compared to those who received thimerosal-free pertussis, in order to find out if there was a higher rate of autism in children exposed to thimerosal. They also looked at children who received thimerosal in only one or two of the vaccine doses, as an intermediate-exposure group. They did not find an elevated risk of autism in children exposed to thimerosal, in any amount.[27]

SafeMinds reviewed a copy of the same Danish database for cases of autism. They discovered that up to a quarter of the cases simply disappeared from the registry over time. In the ten years before 2000, 815 cases of autism were lost from the records in the Danish database—

more than the total number left in the database in 2000. The majority of these were the older children in the cohort. This would skew the results of the Hviid study, since the children who were more likely to be exposed to thimerosal were also those most likely to have been dropped from the database.

SafeMinds compared children five to nine years old in the database who'd been exposed to thimerosal to a group of the same age who had not. After adjusting for the changes in diagnostic practices (detailed above), they found that those who received TCVs were 2.3 times more likely to be diagnosed with autism compared to those who did not. The incidence in the exposed group was one in five hundred, which is similar to rates reported for the same period in the US. The incidence in the unexposed group was one in fifteen hundred. SafeMinds concluded by calling for a published review of the database by investigators unaffiliated with Statens Serum Institut.[28]

The CDC's Epidemiological Study

CDC investigators published a 2003 study using the vaccine data safety records from some health maintenance organizations (HMOs) to see if there was an association between TCVs and neurodevelopmental disorders. The study had two phases: first, they evaluated the risk of a number of neurodevelopmental disorders in children enrolled in two large HMOs, based on increasing levels of exposure to thimerosal at one month, three months, and seven months of age. In the second phase, they took the disorders that had the highest association with thimerosal from phase one and reanalyzed them using a third, smaller HMO. In phase one, they found an increased risk for tics (exposure at three months, relative risk 1.89) at one HMO and language delay (exposure at three and seven months, relative risk 1.13 and 1.07) at the second HMO, but no association with autism or attention deficit disorder in either group. These associations were not duplicated in phase two using the third HMO, so they concluded that there was no consistent neurological abnormality associated with thimerosal exposure in infants.[29]

This was a highly publicized study, widely used to exonerate thimerosal, so it merits a closer look. Through the Freedom of Information Act, SafeMinds secured copies of the earlier versions of this study, uncovering some interesting findings.[30] Between February 2000 and November 2003 (the date it was published), the study underwent four major revisions. The earliest dataset analysis was done in December of 1999; it's referred to by SafeMinds as "generation zero." This analysis used a straightforward methodology comparing disease risk in the highest thimerosal exposure group to the disease risk in the zero-exposure group. What it revealed was striking. It showed a risk of autism, ADD, sleep disorders, and speech/language delays that was consistently at variance between the two groups—on the order of 1.5 to 11 times higher in the group given thimerosal. The CDC looked for an increased risk of other diseases (for control outcomes) and found none. The strongest effect was in the group with the highest mercury exposure at the youngest age.

Each time they reinterpreted the data over the next few years, Verstraeten and colleagues (the CDC) made numerous statistical adjustments to the dataset, gradually diluting the original results. A transcript from a closed-door meeting in June 2000 at Simpsonwood, Georgia between the study investigators and their advisors reveals clear evidence of statistical manipulation. In introducing the discussion, the lead author, Thomas Verstraeten, reported a positive risk of autism with increasing doses of thimerosal; asked for his opinion of this finding, Verstraeten said, "When I saw this and I went back through the literature, I was

	November relative risk (>25 meg at one month)	December relative risk (>25 meg at one month)
Autism	7.62	11.35
ADD	3.76	3.96
Sleep disorders	4.98	4.64

Table 3: SafeMinds. "Generation Zero."

actually stunned by what I saw because I thought, 'It is plausible.'" At another point in the meeting he said, "Personally, I have three hypotheses. The first is that it is parental bias. The children that are more likely to be vaccinated are more likely to be picked up and diagnosed. Second, I don't know. There is a bias that I have not yet recognized, and nobody has yet told me about it. Third hypothesis. It's true. It's thimerosal." He also said they had found "statistically significant relationships" between thimerosal exposure and neurological disorders.[31]

In each of the different generations of the study, the CDC made adjustments to the study population. Phillip Rhodes (of the National Immunization program at the CDC) suggested many of them. He said, "So you can push, I can pull. But there has been substantial movement from this very highly significant result down to a fairly marginal result."[32] The fudging took the form of first combining the zero-exposure group and the low-exposure group. This had the effect of diluting the two extremes of exposure, making it less likely that a measurable effect would emerge. They excluded all children who had not received at least two polio vaccines—most of these children probably missed many if not all of their vaccines and would have ended up in the zero-exposure group. Their justification for doing this was that these children might not have received all of their primary care through their HMO. They also removed the highest exposure group at age one month, effectively eliminating the children who were exposed to the hepatitis B vaccine at birth. These were the children who were most seriously affected in the zero generation analysis and drove the relative risk of autism higher.[33]

They included data from children who were as young as one year old, although the age of diagnosis of almost all of the primary outcomes was much older than that, so it's likely there was under-ascertainment of their primary diagnostic endpoints, diluting the results even further. (It's important to remember that the average age of autism diagnosis is four to five years old, so many children would later be diagnosed who were still undetected at the time of this study.)

Look at how the data from the California HMO vaccine safety database compares to the autism rates in California in general. It's clear that they're missing cases in their data (fig.1).

In later generations of data analysis, a second phase was added look-

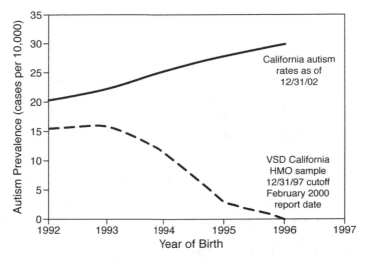

Fig. 1: Ascertainment Bias in Generation 1 Autism Sample Compared to Known California Prevalence Rates. Source: VSD analysis, 2/29/00, California DDS, courtesy SafeMinds.

ing at data from yet another HMO called Harvard Pilgrim. This was an odd choice, since Harvard Pilgrim had recently undergone bankruptcy, and the quality of their record system and the integrity of their database were questionable. This HMO also used a classification system that wasn't based on ICD codes. Very few cases of autism were found in Harvard Pilgrim's records, and because of the results of phase 1, autism was not even included as an endpoint in phase 2. Based on phase 2, any remaining statistically significant risk of neurodevelopmental delays associated with thimerosal was explained away by concluding that since trends differed among the HMOs, they occurred by chance. In my opinion, the differences are more likely a result of poor records, differences in diagnostic practices, and inadequate ascertainment.

The actual increased risk of autism and other developmental delays disappeared from their data as a result of the statistical manipulations. Remember that in generation zero (the earliest version of the data analysis) the relative risks were 11.46 for autism and 3.96 for ADD. Any relative risk above two is considered highly significant for causation, but even with the lower total relative risks, the trend of increased risk with increased exposure remains intact (fig.2).

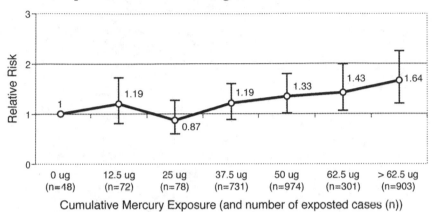

Fig 2: Relative Risk From Mercury Exposure At 3 Months of Age: Neurologic Developmental Disorders (NDD): Generation 2 Findings. Trend (RR per added microgram): 1.007 (1.004, 1.010), p < 0.01. Source: SafeMinds.

The authors acknowledged data weaknesses that could have biased the study toward a null hypothesis (no effect from thimerosal). One was the inherent weakness of using a retrospective computerized records system. They estimated that up to 18% of the children in the database did not have a clear record of receiving their birth dose of hepatitis B vaccine. They acknowledged that the thimerosal content of the vaccines might have been inappropriately labeled in some cases. The diagnostic coding of autism and other disorders was not consistent among the HMOs, which could have resulted in misclassification of cases of autism, or an underreporting of cases. They selected a number of charts to review for verification of the diagnosis and found low reliability, particulary with ADD (28-44% among the three HMOs). Only one of the HMOs had enough cases of autism to use in their statistical analysis, but rather than increasing the size of their dataset they simply excluded autism from the final analysis.

Diagnoses such as "misery disorder" (excluded in later study gen-

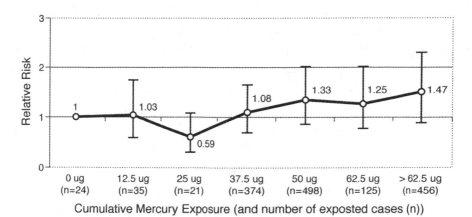

Cumulative Mercury Exposure (and number of exposted cases (n))

Fig. 3: Relative Risk of Speech Delay From Mercury Exposure at Three Months of Age, Generation 2 Findings. Trend (RR per added microgram): 1.008 (1.004, 1.013), p=0.0004. Source: SafeMinds.

erations), speech delay, or language disorder could have in fact been applied to children who were later diagnosed with autism, but the study didn't allow sufficient time for following up these cases. Despite all of the weaknesses in the data, a positive risk was still detected in their early sets of analyses.

In spite of this study's obvious biases, the CDC and the news media announced that it proved thimerosal did not cause autism. After critiques of the study's methodology were published and the transcript from the Simpsonwood meeting revealed, the lead author defended his methodology decisions but acknowledged that the study could not disprove an association, and at best should be described as a neutral study (one that could not prove or disprove an association).[34] Verstraeten later accepted a job at GlaxoSmithKline's vaccine division in Europe.

A Canadian Study

An ecological study from Quebec published in 2006 delineates the changes made in Canadian vaccine policy in relation to the prevalence of ASD in the public school system in children born between 1987 and 1998.[35] It reported an increase in prevalence over the twelve grade-years from 45.7 per 10,000 (Grade 11) to 107.6 per 10,000 (kindergarten).

The vaccine policy in Canada changed over that period as follows: MMR was introduced in 1976 and was recommended for babies at age twelve months; the uptake rate was in the mid-90th percentile throughout the study period. Twenty years later (1996) a booster MMR at eighteen months was recommended. TCVs began in 1985, with increases in cumulative amounts of mercury in 1988, 1992, and 1993, caused by the addition of more HIB doses and a meningococcus vaccine; the highest exposure was 225 mcg. of ethylmercury before age two in 1993. Thimerosal was removed from the vaccine schedule in 1996.

The authors did not detect a significant trend with either MMR exposures or thimerosal exposures that could explain the increase in prevalence in the younger age group. They concluded that there was no relationship between vaccines and autism. But they went on to explain away the increasing prevalence as the result of changing diagnostic practices in Canada over that time period. They acknowledged that their study population was from public schools only, excluding special education schools, and that they did not account for any shift in enrollment in the various school settings. They also acknowledged that many children with autism might have moved into the study region because an autism-specific treatment center in the tertiary care hospital was established, and the local school district received an "Excellence in Autism" rating.

All of these variables would skew their prevalence numbers and make any trend related to vaccine exposure as perceived by the researchers unreliable. It's worth noting that potential negative effects are not exclusive to any one vaccine, and so it's impossible to separate out the possible effects of MMR from those of TCVs. This study serves little purpose, in that it cannot rule out the effect of any vaccine on any subgroup of children with autism.

Positive Epidemiological Evidence

While the researchers linked with the CDC and the vaccine manufacturers were busy presenting their data showing no association between thimerosal and autism, some independent researchers were also busy reviewing databases and reaching very different conclusions. David and Dr. Mark Geier examined the possibility of a connection between thimerosal and autism, publishing several studies. Using the CDC's own Vaccine Adverse Events Reporting System (VAERS) database, they compared reported cases of autism thought to be associated with standard DTaP vaccination (thimerosal-containing diphtheria, tetanus, acellular pertussis) with those cases associated with thimerosal-free DTaP.[36] They found an increased relative risk of 6.0 for autism, 6.1 for mental retardation, and 2.2 for speech disorders. Keep in mind that any relative risk over two can imply causation. To control for reporting bias, they evaluated a variety of other outcomes (deaths, vasculitis, seizures, Emergency Department visits, total adverse reactions, and gastroenteritis) and did not find any association with thimerosal.

In spite of this attempt to control for bias, this study has methodological issues that cannot be overlooked. First is the use of the VAERS database. Although physicians are required to report any adverse vaccine reactions, this system is famously underutilized—only a small percentage of events get reported. The haphazard reporting to this system is a large source of bias in any studies using this data. Since autism hasn't traditionally been considered a vaccine reaction, it's unlikely that most physicians would even think to report it as such.

Parents can report adverse events to this database too. It's possible that after the thimerosal debate became public in 1999, there was a sudden increase in reporting autism to VAERS. The Geiers said that they controlled for this reporting bias by including many years before the controversy began, but they don't present data showing which years account for the most cases of autism. Since the number of autism cases reported to VAERS was quite low (eighteen), any change in the frequency of reporting in later years could have been significant.

As with the other epidemiological studies that I review in this book, it's likely that there is considerable ascertainment bias in this study. The Geiers reported on cases of autism in children receiving vaccines through the year 2000, so many of these children might have been less than two years old, and not yet diagnosed. The thimerosal-free vaccine data was analyzed from 1997 to 2000, so most of those children would have been younger than five years old when the data was analyzed.

Since VAERS is designed for reporting immediate adverse reactions, the system won't capture the children diagnosed in retrospect with vaccine-associated autism. And as we know from the history of mercury poisoning, the effects can be both cumulative and delayed. So even if thimerosal is a cause of autism, it's not likely to ever be highly associated with immediate adverse vaccine reactions.

In 2003, the Geiers published another study using the VAERS database, but this time they compared children receiving thimerosal-containing diphtheria, tetanus, whole-cell pertussis (DTwcP) or DTaP between the years 1992-2000 with those who received thimerosal-free DTaP between 1997-2000. Once again they saw a higher relative risk that rose exponentially with increasing doses of thimerosal. They found a similar association with the risk of speech disorders and cardiac arrest, but not for any of the other control events (febrile seizure, fever, pain, edema, or vomiting). The autism risk was basically the same for DTwcP and thimerosal-containing DTaP, although the other adverse reactions were more common with DTwcP.

Then they evaluated the number of cases of autism in birth-year cohorts ranging from 1984 to 1994 as reported to the US Department of Education (DOE) in 2001, and compared that number with the amount of mercury these children would have received based on the routine vaccination schedule at the time. Again, they found that the cumulative dose of thimerosal correlated with an increasing number of reported cases of autism and speech disorders. This association was not present with the other disorders tracked by the DOE. This study suffers from some of the same inherent biases described above in using the VAERS data; it cannot clearly prove direct causation, but the positive association is interesting.

A third study by the Geiers used just the US DOE data and compared the number of cases of autism in many birth cohorts (mid 1980s until 1996) with the relative thimerosal exposure of each cohort. Since all of the subjects were at least six years old, ascertainment bias caused by the young age of the children in previous studies should not have been a significant factor. They found levels of association similar to their previous studies, leading them to suggest that the similar odds ratios help to validate their earlier VAERS studies (fig.4).

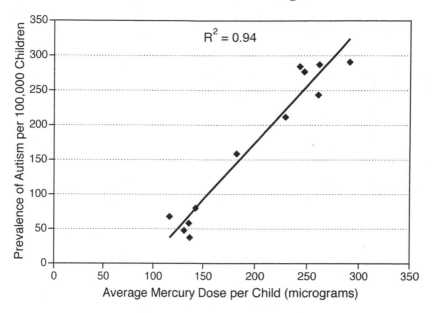

Fig. 4: The prevalence of autism in comparison to the average mercury dose from thimerosal-containing childhood vaccines (birth cohorts: 1981 through 1985 and 1990 through 1996). Geier DA, Geier MR, *Med Sci Monit.* 2004 Mar;10(3): PI33-9.

The Geiers also showed that the highest prevalence rate of autism was found in children born in 1993, correlating with the highest exposure of thimerosal in vaccines; the prevalence rates were lower in subsequent years as thimerosal exposure was also lowered (fig. 5).

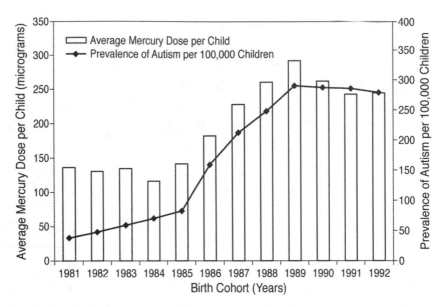

Fig. 5: A birth cohort evaluation of the prevalence of autism in comparison to the average mercury dose from thimerosal-containing childhood vaccines. Geier DA, Geier MR, *Med Sci Monit.* 2004 Mar;10(3):PI33-9.

The validity of the US DOE data for epidemiological studies is questionable because of potential biases introduced by changes in reporting practices or diagnostic criteria; this study did not try to control for either of those factors. Better-controlled data from California have shown increasing prevalence rates beyond 1993, contrary to the numbers reported in the Geier study, adding further question to the validity of the database. But all in all, the Geiers have shown a consistent positive association between thimerosal and autism, using three different methods, each of which demonstrated conclusions contrary to the other epidemiological studies.[37]

We know that mercury is toxic to developing brains. The leading source of early significant mercury exposure to infants has been through childhood vaccines. The possibility that autism could be caused or made worse by a vaccine component has embedded autism in a deep controversy, with much at stake. The politics behind the mercury debate are demonstrative of the power and the problem of big money, which has produced defensive science (trials designed to rule out an uncomfortable theory) rather than real science. By definition, real science would involve an open and aggressive quest to find out what is truly behind the epidemic. Instead, epidemiological studies were done (and touted) to exonerate thimerosal, but suffered from clear bias and weak methodology. More study of this issue was, and is, clearly required.

chapter 12

FURTHER EVIDENCE AGAINST MERCURY

CASES OF ACUTE OVERDOSE ASSOCIATED WITH THIMEROSAL OR ethylmercury (EtHg) have been reported, but few studies have specifically looked at adverse reactions with more typical exposures. In a review of the overdose cases, Magos et al. reports neurological symptoms, including dysarthria (difficulty articulating words), ataxia (inability to coordinate muscle movements), deafness, constricted visual fields, and coma, as well as death. In most cases, the onset of the neurological symptoms occurred weeks to months after the exposure, and in each case the level of exposure was extremely high.[1]

Where Does Ethylmercury Go?

In 2000, Stajich et al. evaluated twenty newborns admitted to a Neonatal Intensive Care Unit immediately after birth.[2] They measured levels of blood mercury after the infants were given the hepatitis B vaccine (contains 12.5 mcg of ethylmercury) and compared fifteen premature/low birth weight (<1000 g) infants to five full-term infants (weights >3500 g). When compared with pre-vaccination levels, there was a significant rise in mercury levels in blood taken forty-eight to seventy-two hours after vaccination in both groups (p<0.05). The level of blood mercury was even higher (p<0.01) in the preterm infants:

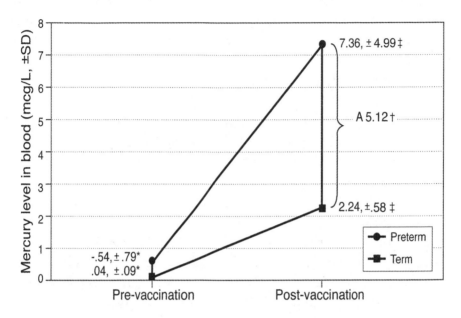

Fig. 1: Difference in mean mercury levels (in micrograms per liter) between preterm and term infants. ++P < .01; +P < .01; *P = .2. Source: Stajich, *Pediatrics*, 2000.

The authors point out that since there is no dose adjustment for birth weight in TCVs (thimerosal-containing vaccines), premature and low birth weight infants have higher relative exposure to a neurotoxic substance—a two-pound baby receives the same burden as a baby weighing nine pounds.

In 2002, Pichichero et al. reported on the excretion patterns of mercury in infants after exposure to TCVs.[3] Samples from 20 two-month-old babies and 20 six-month-old babies with varying degrees of thimerosal exposure were compared to a control group of twenty-one children who received thimerosal-free vaccines. Blood, stool, and urine samples were measured at varied intervals after vaccination. Based on blood mercury levels in the babies, and using a prediction model that they developed from broad assumptions about the distribution of mercury into body tissues, they estimated that the half-life of ethylmercury in the blood was about seven days. They also suggested that most of the thimerosal is rapidly eliminated from the body via the stool, and concluded that thimerosal therefore poses very little risk to full-term infants.[4]

But the methodology in this study is weak and the conclusions premature. There was no control in the timing of sample collection after immunization, and only one sample was obtained per child. A single sample gives only a snapshot of the mercury concentration at a random moment whereas multiple samples reflect the change in concentrations over time per individual. So multiple sample measurements from the same individual is the measure that would be needed to truly assess excretion patterns.

Their prediction model does not account for differences in the detoxification capacity among individuals. In fact, their results confirm a wide variation in individual distribution of mercury. Among the two-month-olds in his study, there was a range of over 400% in the blood concentration (between 5 nmol/L and 20.55 nmol/L) in the first week after receiving the vaccines. Oddly, the child with the highest blood concentration was given only half of the total dose of thimerosal because he didn't get all the vaccinations scheduled for that particular doctor visit.

Pichichero assumes that since there's an increase of mercury in the stool after receiving the vaccine, all of the mercury is being excreted. In fact, if you look closely at Pichichero's numbers, the greater part of the mercury remains unaccounted for. Where did the rest of the mercury go, and how long would it take to actually leave the body—assuming that it does? It cannot be assumed that thimerosal is safe for infants until this pivotal question is answered.

The other crucial question regarding thimerosal is whether there is a population subgroup with genetically weakened detoxification and immune systems, placing them at high risk of injury from even low doses. The prevalence of autism is currently about one in 150 children, and yet Pichichero evaluated only forty infants—so if there is a subgroup, it's statistically unlikely that any of these higher-risk babies would happen to be in the study group. All of the infants in his study were healthy and remained so during the study period; evidence shows that autistic children were frequently ill during the first year of life, so it's possible that higher-risk babies were selected out of the study at inception. This study does not answer pertinent questions such as what happens to the mercury distribution in children who are ill or concurrently being treated with antibiotics or fever-reducing medication?

So, although widely quoted, this study does nothing to answer the question regarding the role of thimerosal in causing or contributing to autism. Suggesting that thimerosal is safe based on this study is nonsensical. It's worth noting that Pichichero did research and consulting work for Eli Lilly, the maker of thimerosal.

A study done on adult squirrel monkeys answers some of the question about where thimerosal ends up.[5] The monkeys were given daily nasal sprays containing low doses of thimerosal. After six months, they sacrificed the animals and did autopsies to determine true tissue concentrations of mercury in various body compartments, finding large accumulations of mercury in the kidney, liver, muscle, and brain (in descending order of highest concentration). Much of the ethylmercury (EtHg) had been converted to inorganic mercury, a form that's particularly difficult to excrete. There was also a wide range of body tissue concentrations among the monkeys in spite of identical exposures, once again confirming that there are differences in individual susceptibility to mercury.

None of the monkeys developed outward signs of mercury toxicity, although the authors point out that it's conceivable that subtle or ongoing changes might have been made apparent with continued exposure or longer observation. Although a study on adult monkeys might not be completely relevant to what's happening in developing human infants (infant brains in any species are more likely to be affected), the results confirm that mercury does indeed accumulate in body tissues from low dose thimerosal exposure.

Is Ethylmercury as Bad as Methylmercury?

In 1985, Magos et al. did a study comparing the relative toxicity of EtHg (ethylmercury/thimerosal) to MeHg (methylmercury) in rats fed high doses of the compounds.[6] They found a few important differences. First, EtHg-treated rats lost much more weight compared with MeHg-treated rats at equivalent doses. The EtHg-treated rats had higher organic mercury concentrations in the blood, but lower concentrations in their kidneys and brains. But the inorganic mercury concentration was higher in the EtHg-exposure organs, and in the kidney especially—this form resulted in more extensive damage.

MeHg resulted in more widespread cerebellar damage in the brain, although the neurotoxic effects on the dorsal root ganglia were quite similar. Magos theorized that because of its larger size, EtHg is less likely to cross the blood-brain barrier than MeHg. He also suggested that because of lower weight and higher metabolic rates, infants should metabolize mercury more rapidly than adults. Based on these assumptions, he surmised that ethylmercury does not reach levels in infants that could cause any harm.[7] But this weight-based calculation does not account for the less effective blood-brain barrier and immature detoxification systems in infants compared to adults. In addition, the undifferentiated neurons in infant brains are more sensitive to toxins than those in an adult brain, even in lower doses or for shorter periods of exposure.

A 2005 study by Burbacher et al. compared the pharmacokinetics (metabolism and distribution) of EtHg and MeHg in infant primates (macaques) at exposures typical of human infants, adjusted for weight and life span. They injected one group of infant monkeys with thimerosal in amounts and frequencies comparable to the CDC's infant vaccination schedule. Another group was fed commensurate oral MeHg solution. Both were compared to a control group not exposed to either form of mercury. Blood samples were taken from each individual on several occasions following exposures, and the primates were sacrificed at different intervals (up to twenty-eight days) after the last mercury exposure, in order to evaluate brain concentrations and to estimate the half-life of brain mercury.

They found some important differences between the two organic forms. EtHg was cleared more rapidly from the bloodstream compared with MeHg (6.9 days vs. 21.5 days). EtHg was also more rapidly cleared from the brain (24.2 days vs. 59.5 days). The elimination kinetics were different, with methylmercury following a simple first-order pattern and ethylmercury following a biphasic pattern. Both forms had high tissue-to-blood concentrations of around twenty to one, i.e., most of it leaves the blood but lingers elsewhere in the body.

There were other striking differences between the two groups—anywhere from 21-86% of the brain mercury in the EtHg group was converted to inorganic mercury, compared with 6-10% in the MeHg group. The much higher concentration of brain inorganic mercury (16 ng/ml for EtHg vs. 0-7 ng/ml for MeHg group) is critical because inorganic mercury is effectively trapped in the brain. It takes years to be excreted, if it ever is in fact removed. The relative concentration of EtHg in the kidneys was also much higher (kidney:blood ratio of 95.1 vs. 5.8).[8]

And consistent with other studies that I have referenced, there was a wide variance (up to two-fold) of mercury concentration in the blood and the brain among the study subjects, even though their initial exposure was exactly the same.

The authors concluded that since the pharmacokinetics of methylmercury and ethylmercury are quite different, methylmercury studies are not appropriate to assess the risk of ethylmercury exposure in infants. The potential for brain accumulation between thimerosal exposures in the routine childhood vaccine schedule is a concern, since inorganic mercury is associated with increased numbers of microglia, decreased numbers of astrocytes, and higher risk of autoimmune reactions. Vargas et al. showed an extensive activation of microglial cells and astrocytes in children with autism and other studies have demonstrated increased numbers of anti-brain antibodies[9] (chapter 7). Could the trapped inorganic mercury derived from thimerosal be driving these adverse reactions?

Burbacher and his colleagues called for increased study of the effects of thimerosal on the developing brain before any conclusions can be reached about the safety of thimerosal in childhood vaccines. Oddly, much of the press about the Burbacher study missed the point entirely, reporting simply that ethylmercury leaves the blood more rapidly than methylmercury. The newspaper articles declared thimerosal safe, with no mention that the mercury cleared the blood only to lodge, perhaps with permanent effects, in the brain.

Cell Death in the Brain and the Immune System

Several other studies looking specifically at the toxic effects of thimerosal on the body have been published since 2001. Baskin et al. showed that neuronal cells (from human cerebral cortex) and fibroblasts (from skin and soft tissues) sustained membrane damage within two hours of exposure to micromolar (a concentration of 1/1,000,000 (one millionth, 10^{-6}) molecular weight per liter (mol/L)) concentrations of thimerosal. By six hours, there was DNA damage and evidence of impending cell death by apoptosis. The severity and speed of injury escalated with increasing concentrations of thimerosal exposure.

Brain cells were more sensitive to the negative effects than skin cells. The authors pointed out that the concentrations used were almost four times higher than what would be assumed from a typical vaccine exposure, but they tested cells for less than twenty-four hours. With longer exposures, damage to cells was noted at much lower concentrations. The authors therefore concluded that further research is warranted to assess potential damage from low-level but chronic exposures, such as would be seen in children routinely receiving TCVs.[10]

A similar study by Makani et al. confirmed the dangerous effects of thimerosal on T-lymphocytes; it induced glutathione depletion, increased oxidative stress, and apoptosis (cellular suicide).[11]

Thimerosal Inhibits Glutamate Transport

Mutkus et al. studied thimerosal's effects on glutamate receptors in the brain. Glutamate, an excitatory neurotransmitter, becomes excitotoxic if it accumulates in extracellular brain tissue, so glutamate transport systems manage it by pulling it back into the cells; astrocytes are brain cells that are agents of this balance. These authors found that micromolar concentrations of thimerosal inhibit the glutamate transporters present on astrocytes after several hours, with the effect of increased extracellular glutamate (chapter 13). They suggested that it's probably a direct effect of the ethylmercury binding to the sulfate found in the cell membrane receptor's cysteine structure.[12]

Thimerosal Affects Nerve Differentiation

A study by Parran et al. found that even at low nanomolar (10^{-9}) concentrations, thimerosal disrupted several signaling mechanisms essential for neuronal differentiation, a critical process in normal brain development. Thimerosal was also responsible for nerve cell death both by apoptosis and necrosis, depending on the concentration. In each case, as the concentration of thimerosal and the duration of exposure increased (from twenty-four to forty-eight hours), the damage was more severe. Much of the damage to nerve cells was evident at lower concentrations of thimerosal than with comparative doses of methylmercury in earlier studies.[13]

Can You Be Genetically at Risk for Thimerosal Injury?

A Columbia University study by Mady Hornig and colleagues examined postnatal thimerosal exposure in mice, approximating the weight- and age-based exposure from routine childhood vaccines based on the 2001 vaccination schedule. Some of the mice strains were genetically predisposed to autoimmunity, and others were not. They found significant negative effects from thimerosal in the autoimmune-susceptible mice, effects that were not found in the other mice strains, including growth delay, reduced locomotion, exaggerated response to novelty, and abnormal neuronal structure in certain regions of the brain. In the hippocampus, there were an increased number of neurons that were densely packed together, with abnormal glutamate receptors and transporters.

These structural abnormalities are analogous to those found in the brains of autistic children, which have been shown to be hypertrophic (overgrown) in certain regions, with an abundance of cells that normally would be weeded out during the neuronal maturation process (chapter 13). Hornig found this structural brain abnormality correlated with abnormal behaviors in the mice. This study is important both because it demonstrates central nervous system injury from low-dose thimerosal, and also because it shows that this damage seems to be genetically influenced.[14]

Other Effects of Thimerosal on the Immune System

Havarinisab et al. looked into the potential immunological importance of ethylmercury exposure in a couple of studies. Since methylmercury compounds have long been known to be strongly immunosuppressive, they hypothesized a similar effect from EtHg. They injected thimerosal (49% EtHg) into mice and found a 65% reduction in both B-cells and T-cells in the spleen within the first weeks of treatment. This was a stronger immunosuppressive effect than was seen with similar doses of MeHg. After thirty days, thimerosal induced immunoproliferation (excess immune cells) and the formation of autoantibodies to fibrillarin proteins; this effect was more profound and occurred later than after MeHg exposure. They also found that inorganic mercury was a more potent stimulator of autoimmune activation than either EtHg or MeHg.[15] This could be important in light of the large deposition of inorganic mercury in the brain after thimerosal injections seen by Burbacher in the primate study, bearing in mind that the inorganic form lingers indefinitely on the wrong side of the blood-brain barrier.

In a second study, Havarinisab characterized the immunoprolifera-
tive effect of thimerosal as a shift to a TH2-type immune response.
A similar activation was seen with inorganic mercury; his results suggest that the rapid conversion of EtHg to inorganic mercury could be
responsible for this secondary autoimmune effect. MeHg does not have
a similar immuno-stimulatory response, nor is it converted to inorganic
mercury at anything near the same level as EtHg.[16]

A 2006 study from the MIND institute at UC Davis showed the
exquisite sensitivity of dendritic cells to toxic effects from nanomolar
concentrations of thimerosal. (Remember from chapter 6 that dendritic
cells are antigen-presenting cells active in the body's innate immune
system, where they regulate inflammatory cytokine production.) A ten-
micromolar exposure killed 90% of the dendritic cells in twenty hours.
A fifty-nanomolar exposure to thimerosal lasting a few minutes disrupted the calcium channel on the dendritic cell membrane, which is
the main signaling pathway used by the cell to perform its tasks. Thimerosal altered the dendritic cell cytokine secretion pattern by causing
an early excessive output of IL-6 (Th-1), which was followed by an
overall suppression of cytokine secretion.[17]

Thimerosal Inhibits Methylation

Waly et al. showed that thimerosal is a potent inhibitor of methionine synthase (MS), a critical enzyme in the methylation cycle (chapter
12). At concentrations as low as 1 nM/L, MS activity is completely disrupted in neuronal cells. This is at concentrations much lower than have
been demonstrated in the blood of infants after exposure to TCVs. He
also showed a similar but less potent disruptive effect from other metals,
including aluminum (present in vaccines) and lead.[18]

Thimerosal Depletes Intracellular Glutathione in Brain Cells

James et al. studied the effect of thimerosal exposure on the glutathione (GSH) status of two types of brain cells, astrocytes and neurons.[19]

Because the brain is unable to produce cysteine, the rate-limiting step of GSH production, it's dependent on the transport of cysteine from the liver. Also, the neurons are dependent on astrocytes for GSH production in the brain since they're unable to absorb the oxidized form of cysteine (called cystine) from the plasma.

In the first phase of the study, both kinds of cells were exposed to thimerosal in increasing doses. As the dose increased, so did the percentage of cell death.

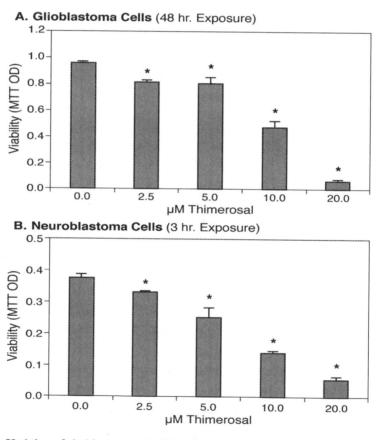

Fig. 2: Viability of glioblastoma cells (A) and neuroblastoma cells (B) with increasing concentrations of thimerosal in the media. Asterisks indicate significant differences from control cells without thimerosal treatment ($n - 3$, $p < 0.01$). Source: James, *Neurotoxicology*, 2005.

Although it took forty-eight hours of exposure for astrocytes to reach their toxic threshold, neuronal cells were affected within three hours, indicating a much higher sensitivity to thimerosal toxicity.

James pretreated the cells in the second phase of the study with several different GSH precursors (N-acetylcysteine, cystine, and methionine), and with GSH itself. Methionine was used as a control since it was not expected to affect cysteine concentrations in brain cells. Their results were as follows:

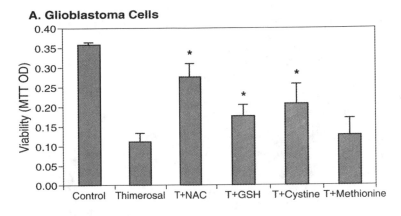

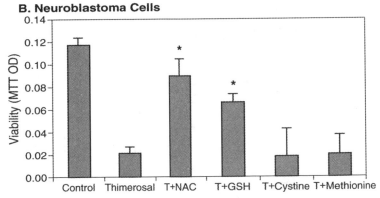

Fig. 3: Viability of glioblastoma cells (A) and neuroblastoma cells (B) without (control) and with exposure to 15 microM/L thimerosal alone for 48h or thimerosal treatment after a 45 min pretreatment with 100 microM/L of N-acetyl cysteine (NAC), glutathione ethyl ester (GSH) cysteine, or methionine. Asterisks indicate significant differences between cells treated with thimerosal alone and cells pretreated with indicated nutrients ($n - 3$, $p < 0.05$). Source: James, *Neurotoxicology*, 2005.

The James study showed that pretreatment with GSH-related substrates had a protective effect; in both types of cells, N-acetylcysteine (NAC) was the most protective. As expected, methionine showed no protective effect. Results showed that exposure to thimerosal for one hour caused less than a 50% decline of intracellular GSH in the astroglial cell line, but an eight times greater decrease in the neuroblastoma cells, once again demonstrating how exquisitely sensitive neurons are to thimerosal. The baseline level of GSH was also much lower in the neurons, which might account for their sensitivity. Pretreatment with NAC and GSH prevented thimerosal-induced GSH depletion.

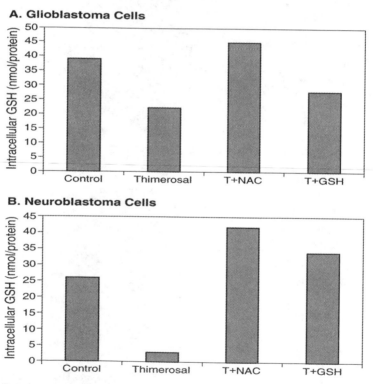

Fig. 4: Concentration of intracellular GSH in 10 to the sixth glioblastoma cells (A) and neuroblastoma cells (B) without (control) and with 15 mmol/L Thimerosal alone or Thimerosal after pretreatment with100 mmol/L of N- acetyl cysteine (NAC), GSH ethyl ester (GSH) in a representative experiment that was repeated with similar results. Source: James, *Neurotoxicology,* 2005.

A similar study was done by Ueha-Ishibashi et al. using thymus cells from rats. A concentration-dependent depletion of intracellular GSH from thimerosal exposures in micromolar amounts was reported. Pretreatment with L-cysteine was partially protective. They demonstrated that cells undergoing oxidative stress (induced with hydrogen peroxide) were three times more likely to die when exposed to thimerosal.[20]

Another study by the same authors showed that in rat brain neurons thimerosal induces an increase in intracellular calcium associated with GSH depletion, leading to increased oxidative stress and cell death. This toxic effect was compared with that of methylmercury, and found to be quite similar.[21]

Other Effects of Thimerosal

Other studies have reported toxic effects from thimerosal on a variety of body tissues. Alexandre et al. demonstrated a complete shut down of cell division and damage to the microtubular system in primary oocytes within minutes after exposure to micromolar concentrations of thimerosal (microtubules are protein structures found within cells, one of the components of the cytoskeleton; they are crucial for cell division).[22] Westphal et al. demonstrated that thimerosal was genotoxic (causing damage to DNA that can result in mutations) to human lymphocytes at concentrations as low as 0.6 mcg/ml. Concentration in the tissues at the injection site of TCVs will be much higher than this since vaccines have concentrations of 25 -50 mcg/ml. These authors also remarked on the wide variability of toxic effects among participants in their study.[23]

Autistic Children and Mercury Exposure

Several studies have examined the mercury burden in children with autism. Holmes et al. investigated mercury levels from baby hair samples in ninety-four children with autism compared to forty-five age- and gender-matched neurotypical controls.[24] All of the children had received the full schedule of TCVs. The researchers registered maternal mercury exposures from fish ingestion, dental amalgams, and Rho(D) immunoglobulin injections.

Although hair is a minor pathway of mercury excretion compared with stool and urine, the use of first-cut baby hair samples made it possible to measure mercury excretion relatively soon after a known mercury exposure from vaccines. Hair has been used in other mercury toxicity studies; it reflects exposure over a much longer period (several months) compared with blood levels (less than a month). The results of the study were initially surprising in that there was a highly significant difference between the hair levels of mercury in autistic children compared to the controls—but it was the normal children who had higher hair mercury (p value < .0000004). The children with the lowest hair mercury levels were the most severely autistic (based on the opinion of the clinician—not standardized). These low mercury levels occurred in spite of the fact that the mothers of the children with autism had higher mercury exposures (more amalgams, higher percentage of Rho(D) immunoglobulin injections).

This was the opposite of what the researchers expected to find, but it made sense when they considered that hair is solely a measure of excretion; its accuracy as a measure of exposure assumes that everyone excretes mercury at a similar rate. Previous mercury studies clearly demonstrate a wide variability of excretion capacity. If the autistic children were poor excretors, the mercury would remain bound in their tissues rather than exiting the body via the hair follicle. Further evidence of an atypical excretion pattern in the autistic children is demonstrated in figure 5.

The neurotypical children with higher maternal exposures had higher mercury hair levels (in fact, these children had levels of mercury above what is considered normal, perhaps reflecting a general increase in environmental exposures to the population). As is shown, the autistic children did not follow this same pattern; hair excretion remained low regardless of increasing maternal exposure.

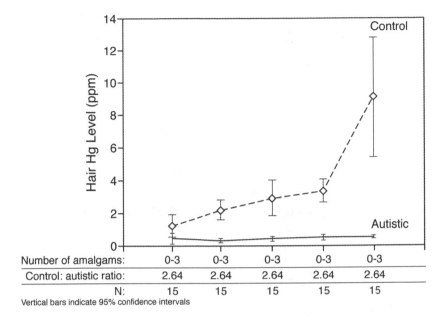

Vertical bars indicate 95% confidence intervals

Fig.5: A plot of the birth hair mercury levels of non-autistic (control) children versus autistics compared to the grouped numbers of dental amalgams of the birth mothers. N equals the number of subjects and the control-to-autistic ratio for each subset is presented. Source: Homes, *International Journal of Toxicology*, 2003.

Figure 6 shows the pattern of actual excretion vs. mercury exposure in both the study group and the control group. The line represents the predicted pattern of excretion based on exposure. The control children follow this predicted value almost exactly, and the autistic children do not.

The study suffers from some methodological flaws—there is a potential selection bias in that in both groups, parents who suspected mercury issues might have been more likely to participate, and the study population might not be representative of the entire autism population. In any case, the study strongly suggests that children with autism have an abnormal pattern of mercury excretion compared with neurotypical children; low hair mercury despite known exposure could reflect a decreased excretion capacity and an accompanying increased body burden of mercury.

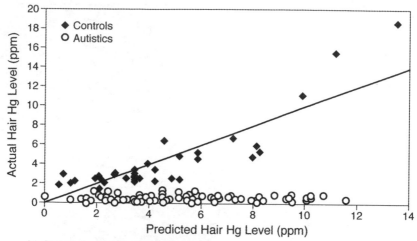

(1) Statistically significant (P<0.000000002)
(2) Statistically significant (P<0.00002)
(3) Statistically significant (P<0.02)

Fig. 6: Actual hair levels in autistic children and controls are compared to a predicted value. The predicted value is obtained using the regression equation for controls: birth hair mercury level = (5.60) + 0.04 (amalgam volume [(1)]) + 1.15 (fish consumption [(2)]) + 0.03 (vaccine [(3)]) R^2 = .79. Perfect prediction of actual hair levels by the regression model is represented by the dashed line. Filled diamonds represent individual non-autistic subjects and open circles represent autistic subjects. Source: Homes, *International Journal of Toxicology*, 2003.

Bradstreet et al. also examined whether children with autism had a higher burden of heavy metals compared with neurotypical children. They measured the excretion of mercury and other toxic metals following a three-day oral challenge of DMSA, a heavy metal chelator.[25] They evaluated 221 autistic children in their autism specialty clinic and compared them to eighteen children without developmental delays whose parents were concerned about unspecified possible heavy metal exposure.

All of the autistic children had received a full schedule of TCVs. Ten of the control children had been vaccinated and eight had not because of the parents' religious beliefs. None of the children in either group had dental amalgams. The group of children with autism had much higher urine excretion of mercury (p<0.0002). When age- and gender-matched, the autistic children still showed much higher mercury excretion ($p<0.002$). An interesting sub-analysis compared vaccinated controls to unvaccinated controls and found near-equivalent metal excretion. This suggests that neurotypical vaccinated children are able to adequately excrete the mercury from their systems in spite of presumably higher exposure from the vaccine, i.e., it was not retained, as it was in the autistic children.

This study has methodological weaknesses including its retrospective design and the inability to control for exposures of environmental mercury other than thimerosal and dental amalgams. The control group might not be representative of the normal population because they were being evaluated for possible heavy metal toxicity, but if anything this would have weakened the results of the study because the control group would have been skewed towards a higher heavy metal burden. Yet the results remain highly statistically significant, clearly suggesting that autistic children have a problem processing mercury.

Environmental Mercury Exposure and Autism

Two groups of researchers have looked for a geographical association between autism rates and sources of environmental mercury. Palmer et al. studied environmental pollution data from Texas in the EPA's Toxic Release Inventory (TRI),[26] as well as information regarding developmental disabilities per school district from the Texas Education Agency (TEA). Autism diagnoses were made either by special education psychologists or qualified outside personnel.

Palmer's team showed that for every thousand pounds of mercury released into the environment, there was a 61% increase in the rates of autism, and a statistically significant increase in special education rates (43%). This association was independent of the number of children served in the district, district wealth, ethnic make-up, and community type.

The increase in autism alone accounted for the increase in special education rates in association with rising levels of mercury—other learning disabilities did not increase. The authors point out that this doesn't establish a causal relationship, and that school-based diagnosis might not reflect the entire autistic population in the community. It is however an important observation that warrants further study, especially when considering legislation to control the emission of toxic substances.

The second study considering a possible association between autism and environmental pollutants was done by Windham et al. in California, as part of a broader environmental surveillance program initiated by the CDC (Centers for Disease Control and Prevention).[27] Several states are monitoring specific environmental impacts on case rates of autism. This particular study reflects data on children born in 1994 in six San Francisco area counties; all children with an autism diagnosis before their ninth birthday were included, and diagnostic criteria were verified. They included a total of 284 children with ASD and 657 age-matched controls.

Using EPA Hazardous Air Pollutants data, they examined twenty-five chemicals that theoretically could be relevant to autism. They found a 50% increase in autism in areas with the highest levels (top quartile) of environmental exposure to chlorinated solvents and heavy metals, particularly mercury, cadmium, nickel, trichloroethylene, and vinyl chloride. They concluded that living in areas with higher ambient levels of these hazardous chemicals during pregnancy or early childhood results in an increased risk of developing autism.

The Institute of Medicine (IOM) Report

In 2001, the IOM (a branch of the National Academy of Sciences) was commissioned by the CDC to review the available research on the possibility of a connection between developmental disorders and TCVs. The IOM concluded:

> Although the hypothesis that exposure to thimerosal-containing vaccines could be associated with neurodevelopmental disorders is not established and rests on indirect and incomplete information, primarily from analogies with methylmercury and levels of maximum mercury exposure from vaccines given in children, the hypothesis is biologically plausible. The committee also concludes that the evidence is inadequate to accept or reject a causal relationship between thimerosal exposures from childhood vaccines and the neurodevelopmental disorders of autism, ADHD, and speech or language delay.

They described the removal of thimerosal from pediatric vaccines as "prudent" and said that "full consideration should be given to removing thimerosal from any biological or pharmacological product to which infants, children, and pregnant women are exposed." They called for further policy review and biomedical research regarding the issue.[28]

Three years later, there was a surprising reversal of this opinion. The CDC and the NIH gave the IOM over $2,000,000, asking them to re-examine the vaccine issue because of the "significant number of studies" that had been published in the three years since their last recommendations (only one was done by the CDC). This time the IOM was asked to narrow the focus to the question of whether TCVs cause autism. The IOM reviewed the epidemiological studies (presented in Ch. 10), discarded the studies which showed a positive association because of "methodological flaws," but applauded the negative association studies as "well-designed," and concluded that the epidemiological evidence was sufficient to reject a causal relationship between thimerosal and autism.

They dismissed all of the biological research regarding thimerosal and its potential role in causing autism as "theoretical" and "unproven" because of the "early stage of scientific understanding about the cause of autism." The IOM suggested that there is no evidence that immune system abnormalities play a part in the neuropathogenesis of the disease, and that no studies have documented immune abnormalities or brain inflammation in autistic subjects (even though the majority of the nearly two hundred papers on immune dysfunction in autism cited in Ashwood's paper had already been published). The IOM concluded, "In the absence of experimental or human evidence that vaccination affects metabolic, developmental, immune, or other physiological or molecular mechanisms that are causally related to the development of autism, the committee concludes that the hypotheses generated to date are theoretical only."[29]

Based on my own review of the literature concerning the toxicity of thimerosal, the known biological abnormalities of autism, and the relative strengths and weaknesses of the epidemiological studies, I find the IOM conclusion both confusing and contradictory. Frankly, from a scientific perspective, it doesn't make sense. Their conclusions were based entirely on a few epidemiological studies that are critically flawed in my estimation and in the estimation of many other physicians and scientists. They even acknowledged that "determining causality with population-based methods such as epidemiological analysis requires either a well-defined at-risk population or a large effect on the general population." Autism has neither a well-defined at-risk population nor a large population effect. "Absent biomarkers, well-defined risk factors, or large effect sizes, the committee cannot rule out, based on epidemiological evidence, the possibility that vaccines contribute to autism." And yet in their conclusion, ruling out the connection was exactly what they did.

The hypothesis linking thimerosal and autism is that there is a small subset of the population who are at risk genetically. The panel commented that little is known about the cause of autism or the biological mechanisms of the disease, but then they seemed quite comfortable asserting that thimerosal is not related, in spite of the acknowledged "theoretical" plausibility. The committee further recommended that, "from a public health perspective," no further investment should be made on the theoretical risk of vaccines and autism but instead "more promising" areas of research should be explored—there were no suggestions as to what areas they considered more promising nor why the "theoretical" risk should not be explored further. Regardless of the part thimerosal might play in causing the epidemic of autism, it seems clear that mercury, ethylmercury in particular, affects many of the biological systems known to be abnormal in autism. Further study of these interactions is sure to add a critical piece to the autism puzzle.

The IOM's conclusions (however peremptory) and the publicity that followed effectively killed any substantial research funding related to mercury or detoxification abnormalities in autistic children. The committee went on to suggest a variety of ways that trust in vaccine safety could be reestablished in the lay community. They justified their recommendation by saying that "using an unsubstantiated hypothesis to question the safety of vaccination and the ethical behavior of those government agencies and scientists who advocate for vaccinations could lead to widespread rejection of vaccines and inevitable increases in incidences of serious infectious disease." But they are apparently unwilling to do the research necessary to effectively confirm or refute the hypothesis.

I propose that this lack of transparency, as well as the perplexing lack of scientific integrity in the studies and the conclusions by the IOM, other government agencies, and vaccine manufacturers, is the true reason for the loss of confidence by the public. I believe that the way to regain trust is, to acknowledge the possibility of error and to diligently study the negative effects on our children that might have occurred.

Scientists base their conclusions on data; the IOM seems to have done the opposite, basing their data on a pre-conceived conclusion. In early meetings of the IOM committee, Marie McCormick, the chairperson, was quoted as saying that the CDC "...wants us to declare,well, these things are pretty safe...." She went on to say, "...we are not ever going to come down that [autism] is a true side effect of [vaccine exposure]."

And Dr. Kathleen Stratton, a member of the IOM and the study director of the Immunization Safety Review Committee, commented, "We said this before you got here, and I think we said this yesterday, the point of no return, the line we will not cross in public policy is to pull the vaccine, change the schedule... We wouldn't say 'compensate,' we wouldn't say 'pull the vaccine,' we wouldn't say 'stop the program.'" All of these statements were made before the panel members had reviewed any of the research.

Not surprisingly, the CDC, the NIH, the FDA, and the AAP applauded the IOM conclusions; the endorsements were widely publicized by news conferences, reassuring the public that the issue had been put to rest and that the safety of TCVs had been conclusively proven. The fact that this report considered only autism was not mentioned, even though their previous review had shown positive association with some other neurodevelopmental disorders. Autism advocacy groups were angered and alarmed by the thin logic upon which the conclusion was based, and by the exposed conflicts of interest of the committee members.

Even members of Congress expressed concern, most notably David Weldon (Florida), who is also a physician. He said, "If it is eventually determined that an entire generation of kids was essentially poisoned, a class-action suit against the federal government could be on the order of hundreds of billions of dollars, and so there's very good reason for them to try to cover this up.And then when they appear as though they are covering it up, it makes you suspicious that it's all true."[30]

The repercussions of the IOM reversal of opinion are far-reaching. Thimerosal-free vaccines are no longer given preference over TCVs for influenza, in spite of the fact that six-month old babies and pregnant women are urged to get the shot. Because of the new influenza recommendations, thimerosal exposure is creeping back to pre-2001 levels, which will muddy any assessment of autism rates following the removal of thimerosal from the rest of the US pediatric schedule. Nor are thimerosal-free vaccines given preference for shipment to other countries—a potential diplomatic time bomb.

More evidence for thimerosal-related toxicity continues to emerge despite the political and financial difficulty in continuing research. I believe that the evidence as it stands is strong enough that regardless of whether a positive or negative association with autism is ultimately proven, no form of mercury whatsoever belongs in vaccines given to children.

chapter 13

AUTISM AND THE BRAIN

WHILE AUTISM HAS BEEN VIEWED AS A BRAIN DISEASE FOR MANY decades, surprisingly little is actually understood about the brains of autistic patients. Various studies have looked at the structural and physiological differences in the autistic brain, but the results are inconsistent. This probably reflects the differences among subgroups of children with autism, all labeled with a common behavioral symptom complex but possibly stemming from different etiologies.

Neuroanatomy (Brain Structure)

With computerized tomography (CT) and magnetic resonance imaging (MRI) scans, we're now better able to study the anatomy of autistic brains (researchers used to have to work from scarce autopsy specimens). Functional PET (positron emission tomography) scans and Functional MRIs provide information not only about the structure but also the function of different brain regions. As expected, these technological innovations have revealed many abnormalities in the brains of autistic children. Some features are consistent, but there's wide individual variation of pathology.

A frequent finding is that autistic children have larger-than-normal head circumferences, correlating with larger-than-normal brains.

During the first year of life there appears to be a period of rapid brain growth in autism, followed by a plateau, and then a period of slower-than-normal growth extending into adolescence.[1] The rate of brain growth is different in different regions of the brain, with the cerebellum and cerebral cortex most consistently involved. Growth of white matter has been found to be more extensive than gray matter.[2] In the cerebral cortex, there is also a front-to-back distribution of growth rate with the frontal cortex growing much more rapidly than the occipital lobe.[3]

Other studies found growth abnormalities that didn't fit these patterns: one study detected abnormal enlargement in the cerebral cortex but not in the cerebellum;[4] another study isolated cortical enlargement to the temporal, parietal, and occipital lobes, but not the frontal lobe;[5] others have found abnormalities in the limbic system, the brain stem, the basal ganglia, and the corpus collosum.[6] In some studies there was evidence of both enlargement and reduction of certain brain regions in different participants. For example, studies of the cerebellum show that while the majority of cases have a smaller than normal cerebellar vermis, a minority are larger than average (16%).[7] Up to 50% of autistic patients in other studies had normal cerebellar size.[8]

On the microscopic level, there appears to be a disruption of the normal cellular structure and organization in particular regions of the brain. A consistent abnormality is the loss of Purkinje cells and granular cells in the cerebellum.[9 10 11 12] The cerebellum is thought to be responsible for affect, motivation, social interaction, learning, and the processing of motor and sensory information.[13] It is also responsible for tasks that require rapid shifts in attention—difficulty shifting attention could contribute to autistic behaviors.[14]

The majority of studies find abnormalities in the limbic system of the autistic brain, including increased cell-packing density and smaller neuronal size, consistent with an arrest in normal maturational development.[15] The limbic system (the hippocampus, the amygdala, the cingulate gyrus, and the septal nuclei) takes part in the integration of memory and emotional behavior and accompanying changes in physiology, including heart rate, respiratory rate, and blood pressure.

More than half of the studies show cerebral cortex abnormalities,[16] thought to result from a defect in the migration of neurons during the first six months of fetal development. One study showed a reduction of cerebral blood flow to the frontal cortex in three- and four-year-old autistic children that was no longer present in the same children when they were six and seven.[17] Abnormalities in the frontal lobe and in its connection to the limbic system can result in difficulty with "theory of mind," the ability to intuit what other people are thinking.[18] The frontal lobe and the cerebral cortex are responsible for other higher-function social and language skills and information processing.[19]

It has been hypothesized that the accelerated period of brain growth and the cellular abnormalities in autistic children represent a dysregulation of the brain development processes, which normally have both progressive and regressive processes that can occur simultaneously. Progressive events (most of which occur prenatally) include the formation of new nerve cells (neurogenesis), axon guidance, and the formation of synapses and neurotransmitter receptors. It's believed that the vast majority of the neurons are formed by seven months gestational age.

Normal regressive events include apoptosis (normal programmed cell death), axon pruning, and synapse elimination. These mostly postnatal events are influenced by experience and "learning." Disruptions in the balance of these two patterns result in abnormal brain construction and disorganization.

Because there is a wide variability in the pathology seen in autistic brains, the exact developmental timing of the abnormalities is not clear. Some studies point to the early part of the first trimester of pregnancy, whereas others suggest it's more likely between the first and second year of life.[20][21] In reality, it's likely different for different children.

Abnormal Neurochemistry

Part of the difficulty of studying neurochemistry is that the chemicals that are active in the brain as neurotransmitters are also found in regions outside of the brain. For example, the GI tract has its own nervous system, complete with its own production of neurotransmitters that can act entirely independently of the central nervous system. Many of these neurotransmitters are structurally identical to those in the brain. Serotonin, a brain chemical that helps to regulate mood and sleep, is also the main neurotransmitter in the gut, so assessing levels of neurotransmitters from the blood or from the urine might tell very little about what's happening inside the brain.[22]

There is evidence of complex interactions between chemical signals in the brain and those of the immune system. Just as there are chemical messengers (cytokines and chemokines) used by the immune system to modulate and integrate immune response, there are chemical messengers in the brain called neurokines that signal neuronal pathways. Interestingly, there seems to be extensive cross-communication between the immune system and the nervous system using these same chemical messengers. For example, it has been shown that cytokines and chemokines from the immune system can affect cognitive and behavioral processing and can modulate the nervous system response to inflammation, infection, and injury.[23]

Also there is evidence that many of the pro-inflammatory cytokines (such as IL-1, IL-6, IL-12, IFN-γ, and TNF-α) play an important part in neurodevelopment.[24] Cytokines can affect mood, sleep, appetite and nutritional uptake, exploratory behavior, and social interaction,[25] and can also increase neurotransmitter metabolism in certain brain regions, and alter the synapses that can affect memory and learning. Some cytokines, like IL-6, have a profound impact on brain development by inducing changes in the neurons and glial cells, such as proliferation, survival, death, neurite outgrowth, and gene expression. Cytokines have been shown to not only cross but to impair the blood-brain barrier, thus allowing access to neurotoxins that otherwise would be shut out. Cytokines can access and affect the peripheral nervous system structures as well.[26]

Conversely, neurotransmitters and neuropeptides can affect the development of many organ systems in the body, especially the immune system (including the spleen, thymus, bone marrow, and lymph nodes).[27]

Several neurotrophins (nerve growth factors, including neuropeptide Y, substance P, calcitonin gene-related peptide (CGRP), vasoactive intestinal peptide (VIP), brain-derived neurotropic factor (BDNF), and NT4/5) have profound immunomodulatory actions.[28] These have all been implicated in the development of ASD.[29] Neuropeptides play a part in recruiting the innate immune system, including the migration of dendritic cells.[30] If you recall, these cells activate the appropriate immune response to an antigen, and they could have a role in the neuroinflammatory abnormalities found in autistic patients.[31] Any study of cytokines and neurokines in patients with autism must consider the workings of both the immune and the neurological system when trying to ascertain the reasons for neurochemical abnormalities.

Many neurotransmitter abnormalities have been detected in patients with autism, but the studies often conflict.[32][33] One of the most studied neurotransmitters in relation to autism is serotonin. Famous as the "feel good" neurotransmitter, it has a wide range of effects on normal physiological functions, including circadian rhythms, mood, sleep, anxiety, motor activity, pain recognition, and cognition. It's found not only in the neurons in the brain, but also in platelets and lymphocytes, and it's the primary neurotransmitter of the enteric (GI) nervous system; in fact, over 95% of the body's serotonin is made in the bowel.[34] It can exert either proliferative or suppressive effects on immune cells, depending on its concentration.

Serotonin metabolism in the brain is affected by cytokines such as IL-1 β, IFN-γ, and TNF-α.[35] It is known that some pro-inflammatory cytokines can affect the activity of a serotonin transport gene, but the studies looking for abnormalities of this gene in autistic subjects have been inconclusive.[36][37] Elevations of serotonin have been detected in the blood (specifically in the platelets, which are serotonin transporters) in about one-third of autistic patients.[38] Other studies have found high levels of serotonin metabolites in the urine.[39] However, levels of serotonin metabolites in the CSF in autistic patients were normal.[40] Some studies, but not all, have reported autoantibodies against serotonin receptors in autistic patients.[41][42] A couple of studies have shown a decreased capacity to synthesize brain serotonin in autistic children relative to controls, specifically in the frontal cortex, the thalamus, and the cerebellum.[43][44]

Treatment studies with medications that target serotonin pathways have also been inconclusive.[45] L-dopa and fenfluramine (both of which lower blood serotonin) did not show a consistent benefit. Some behavioral improvements were demonstrated in a study of autistic adults using fluvoxamine (Luvox), a selective serotonin reuptake inhibitor (SSRI).[46] To date there has been only one study, from Japan,[47] showing positive results in autistic children from treatment with an SSRI, yet they are the most widely prescribed medications for this disease.[48]

In October 2006 the FDA approved risperidone for treatment of children with autism. Risperidone is an atypical antipsychotic that can increase serotonin levels. Several double-blinded, placebo-controlled studies have now been completed that show modest improvements in some behaviors such as aggression, hyperactivity, and self-stimulatory behavior,[49] but there is also a high rate of adverse reactions, including drowsiness (52%), headache (38%), and weight gain (36%). Depression, attempted suicide, anxiety, dystonia (involuntary, sustained muscle contractions), emotional lability (mood swings), gynecomastia (excessive male breast development), and constipation have also been reported.[50] The longest safety studies on risperidone for children lasted only fifty-four weeks,[51][52][53] so long term reactions have not been characterized. Aggression and self-injury almost always improve in children once the underlying cause of this behavior is addressed, particularly if it's gut pain. Obviously it makes a lot more sense to address the source of the behavior before proceeding with psychoactive drugs that might be injurious.

Dopamine, another neurotransmitter of particular interest in autism, is thought to be involved in a wide spectrum of neurobehavioral functions, including cognition, motor function, brain-stimulation reward mechanisms, eating and drinking behaviors, sexual behaviors, neuroendocrine regulation, and selective attention. Interest in dopamine and autism arose from the observation that some dopamine-blocking agents (antipsychotics) seemed effective in the treatment of some aspects of the disorder, particularly stereotyped behaviors, aggression, and self-injury. One study looking at peripheral blood levels of dopamine metabolites did not show any difference compared with controls,[54] while another showed elevated levels of dopamine derivatives in the urine.[55] Several studies have looked for elevated dopamine metabolites in the CSF, but the majority of them didn't find evidence of abnormal values.[56]

Norepinephrine is a neurotransmitter derived from dopamine that plays a critical part in attention, filtering of irrelevant stimuli, stress response ("fight or flight"), anxiety, and memory. With the exception of elevated levels in the blood, studies looking for abnormal levels of this neurotransmitter in people with autism have been negative. Since norepinephrine is a short-lived neurotransmitter that increases with any stress response, it's likely that elevated levels in the blood are a result of patient stress brought on by getting blood drawn. Medications that target this neurotransmitter pathway haven't been consistently helpful with core autistic symptoms.[57]

Some early research on the neurotransmitter acetylcholine looked for abnormalities in the brains of autistic subjects. The cholinergic system plays a role in the development and function of cognitive abilities, particularly the ability to focus on the environment and achieve a coherent behavioral response. Acetylcholine is a primary neurotransmitter in the autonomic nervous system (ANS), the part of the neurological system that works without our conscious control. Many symptoms of autism can be understood when explained as the dysfunction or imbalance of the ANS. Autonomic functions include heart rate, blood pressure, bowel motility, bladder function, sweating, pupil dilatation, and others. The ANS comprises the sympathetic and the parasympathetic system. Each has unique neurotransmitters and neuromuscular receptors that originate in different parts of the spinal cord. The functions of these two opposing systems frequently balance each other out. For example, the sympathetic system is responsible for "fight or flight" reactions (elevated heart rate, dilated pupils, elevated blood pressure, erection of the hairs on our skin, etc.), enabling us to be on high alert in situations that might be dangerous. The parasympathetic system lowers heart rate, lowers blood pressure, and constricts pupils when we are safe.

The ANS orchestrates bowel and bladder function; the parasympathetic part induces bowel contraction and times the contraction of the bladder muscle and relaxation of the urethral sphincter to allow the bladder to empty. Sympathetic nerves do the opposite—they decrease bowel motility and prevent bladder contraction. In children with autism, the ANS is dysregulated—there seems to be an overall imbalance favoring the sympathetic system. Common signs and symptoms seen in autism that can be explained by autonomic dysfunction include elevated heart rate or blood pressure, feeding problems, dysphagia (difficulty swallowing), nausea, recurrent vomiting, abdominal bloating, constipation or diarrhea, dark/light intolerance, dry eyes, dilated pupils, sleep apnea, abnormal sweating patterns, dry skin, flushed skin after eating, unexplained high fevers, altered perception of pain, sensory defensiveness, self-mutilation, insomnia, bed-wetting, difficulty urinating, difficulty potty-training, poor socialization skills, anxiety, phobias, tics, and emotional lability.[58]

It is still not clear if the problem is an overproduction of catecholamines (epinephrine, norepinephrine), an underproduction of acetylcholine, or a problem with the receptors on the post-synaptic membrane. The receptors could be in short supply or could be injured or blocked, from antibodies, toxins, or infections. A few studies have shown abnormalities in some of the acetylcholine receptors in autistic brains, and there have been some positive effects reported from studies using medications that increase acetylcholine in the synapses between neurons.[59][60]

Oxytocin and vasopressin are neuropeptides that influence social behavior and are shown to be abnormal in autism.[61][62][63] Oxytocin is also shown to modulate autoimmune response.[64] Not enough research on the role of these substances in autism has been completed to offer conclusions.

Glutamate is a neuroexcitatory transmitter in the brain. It's metabolized into gamma-aminobutyric acid (GABA), which acts as an inhibitor and maintains a normal glutamate balance. If glutamate is excessive, it causes excitotoxic damage or death to neuronal cells. There is evidence that impaired intracellular energy metabolism increases neuronal vulnerability to glutamate, and might be responsible for many chronic neurodegenerative conditions.[65] High levels of glutamate have been associated with seizures, which are common in autistic patients.

Several studies have detected an abnormal glutamate-to-GABA balance in the brains of autistic patients. For example, in one study done on postmortem brain specimens from autistic patients, there was a 48-61% decrease in an enzyme critical in converting glutamate to GABA.[66] But the few studies done to evaluate the use of GABAergic medications (those that increase available GABA) report results that are modest at best.[67]

Several studies have documented autoimmune antibodies against brain proteins (chapter 7), although the clinical significance of these antibodies remains in question. Specific autoimmune damage to brain structures has yet to be proven. One review indicates that receptors (on circulating T-cells) targeting brain proteins might be benign until triggered by bacteria or a virus, at which point they become activated, resulting in neuroinflammation and subsequent damage.[68]

Opioid peptides and opioid receptors are modulators of neuronal development, influencing migration, proliferation, and differentiation within the CNS (central nervous system). One study showed that opioid peptides can inhibit the development of neurons and glial cells in the brain.[69] Opioid peptides are produced by the gut, lung, placenta, testis, lymphoid tissue, and immune cells, as well as from food. Studies show that opioids behave like cytokines and can act on immune cells, including the glial cells in the brain.[70] It's also been shown that these opioids can influence the immune response directly, enhancing the production of cytotoxic T-cells, NK cells, and antibody synthesis, and acting as chemoattractants for monocytes and neutrophils.

The precise mechanism is unclear, but it's postulated that opioids act as cytokines by attaching to receptors on peripheral blood and glial cells. Several studies have shown excessive levels of diet-derived opioids in autism, and it's thought that these have detrimental effects on brain development and behavior. It is probable that these food-derived opioids bind to the opioid receptors in the brain, causing chronic nerve cell stimulation. These peptides are derived from gluten- and casein-containing foods in particular—this might be why so many children with autism improve on gluten-free, casein-free diets.[71][72][73][74] Naltrexone, a potent opiate antagonist commonly prescribed for the treatment of alcohol and drug addiction, induced some improvement in self-injurious behavior in 80% of the patients treated, although the benefits were generally short-lived.[75]

Seizures

Studies have reported frequencies of epilepsy (defined as greater than one seizure not induced by fever) in autistic children ranging between 11 and 39%.[76] Older children and those with greater cognitive impairment are more likely to have seizures.[77] Some studies have also linked a higher risk of epilepsy in autistic children with the regressive form, an older age of symptom onset, and a family history of epilepsy.[78] Autistic children with epilepsy are more likely to have partial motor seizures than grand mal (generalized) seizures. This can make diagnosis difficult, because periods of social unresponsiveness and stereotyped repetitive behaviors could be either a primary manifestation of autism or a partial motor seizure. Accurate diagnosis requires EEG monitoring. Tuchman et al. demonstrated that there was abnormal epileptiform (epileptic-like) activity on sleep EEGs in 68% of autistic children with known epilepsy and in 15% of the autistic children without epilepsy.[79] Kawasaki et al. did serial sleep EEGs in 158 children with autism over several years and found that 60% of these children had abnormal activity on one or more tests. The EEG abnormalities were most commonly focal, and located in the temporal or frontal lobes.[80]

Tuchman points out that there's no evidence showing that epilepsy is the cause of regression in autism, nor that treatment of the seizures results in any improvement in the cognitive or behavioral symptoms of autistic patients.[81] There have been no controlled studies showing a positive benefit from antiepileptic medications in autistic patients. Anecdotal and open label studies report mixed results. Those that have shown a positive response found an equally positive response in the placebo group. Treatment of autistic children with abnormal EEG spikes but without clinical seizures has not been proven to be beneficial.[82]

Sleep Disturbances

Parents commonly report that their autistic children have abnormal sleep patterns, including difficulty falling asleep, early arousal times, and frequent night awakenings. Children with autism have increased muscle activity during sleep rather than normal muscle atonia (paralysis of voluntary muscle movement). These sleep disturbances aren't surprising in light of the abnormalities documented in the serotonin system, which is normally responsible for controlling REM (rapid eye movement) sleep and arousal cycles.

Melatonin is a hormone produced in the pineal gland; it controls normal circadian body rhythms, and is derived from serotonin by methylation. Abnormalities in the daily rise and fall of the melatonin secretion, as well as generally low levels of the hormone, have been documented in autistic children and young adults. A number of studies have documented improved sleep patterns with supplemental melatonin.[83 84]

Children with autism also have a higher degree of obstructive sleep apnea caused by enlarged tonsils and adenoids, interrupting sleep due to frequent hypoxic episodes in the night. Seizures have also been correlated with sleep disturbances, both as a cause and a result.[85] With the recent appreciation of the influence of GI abnormalities in autism, sleep disturbances have also been correlated to GI disease (such as reflux) that might be easily missed because of communication deficits in these children. Any child with frequent nighttime wakening deserves a full GI workup.

My experience has been that many children also have problems sleeping as a result of food allergies and sensitivities. When these foods (such as cow's milk) are removed, the children sleep better.

Treatment of sleep disturbances in autism isn't simple. It requires accurate diagnosis of the underlying cause as well as behavioral, nutritional, or pharmaceutical support, and sometimes surgical management (e.g., removing tonsils and adenoids).

chapter 14

THE AUTISM WEB— MAKING SENSE OF THE DISEASE

AUTISM HAS BEEN AROUND FOR OVER SIXTY YEARS, YET MOST OF what's known about its widespread effects on the body has been learned in the last decade. Our understanding of the illness has increased dramatically now that the focus of research has at last turned toward the metabolic and physiologic abnormalities in autistic children rather than the behavioral abnormalities.

There is much yet to learn. We still don't know the underlying cause, or if there might be some unifying mechanism. Whatever the cause or causes, it should be clear to anyone reading this book that what we think of as *autism* is simply one of many symptoms of what is in fact a disease complex; the diagram on page 180 demonstrates the intricate interactions among the affected body systems. This complexity makes it difficult to isolate a single cause or even a single pathway that sets off the cascades of events leading to the disease state. There are several reasonable event devolutions, all of which are likely to start with genetic susceptibility.

The first possibility is that the disease is primarily neurological, with secondary effects on other organ systems. In this hypothesis there is a disruption of normal neuronal development resulting in disordered cellular structure in several brain areas. These might differ depending on the timing of the original neurological insult (probably prenatal). If the brain's capacity to reorganize and weed out cells during postnatal development is compromised, the result is abnormal brain growth coinciding with autistic regression. The abnormal brain development creates dysregulation of neurotransmitters, neurotrophins, and neurokines—neurochemical aberrations that will have adverse effects on the developing immune system.

The neurological disruption in the brain affects the GI tract (resulting in motility issues and inflammation) because neurotransmitters in the brain are the same as those in the gut. The gut houses most of the immune system, and the neurochemical confusion triggers abnormal cytokine production that results in autoimmune reactions and chronic organ damage. Gut inflammation leads to "leaky gut" syndrome, allowing toxins to enter the body through the bloodstream. The overburdened detoxification system results in oxidative stress and tissue damage. Abnormal cytokines and oxidative injury create a porous blood-brain barrier, allowing toxins into the brain that set off a vicious cycle of brain inflammation; ongoing neuronal damage ensues.

A second possible sequence begins in the gastrointestinal tract. Subtle GI abnormalities can begin shortly after birth; the baby has difficulty processing food proteins, leading to colic, reflux, constipation, or loose stools, and the gut sustains further injury with the introduction of solid foods and cow's milk, creating an inflammatory condition that's initially localized and superficial. When the inflammation leads to micro-damage to the mucosal surface, normal digestion is compromised, resulting in a leaky gut. Harmful substances trespassing the body now stimulate a widespread immune response. Some of these substances, like dietary opioids, directly affect the brain and the immune system by acting as false neurotransmitters and cytokines. Other substances trigger immune responses, resulting in further inflammation that causes yet more damage to the GI tract.

The baby's immature immune system misinterprets the chronic inflammation, starting a pattern of ongoing systemic immune dysregulation that has secondary effects on the brain and that begins to allow persistence of enteric viruses, including those introduced through vaccination. The resulting matrix of systemic inflammation and immune abnormalities leads to such illnesses as sinusitis and ear infections that are treated with antibiotics, which in turn allows resistant gut bacteria and yeast to overgrow. These organisms produce neurotoxins that directly affect the brain and produce further negative effects on the GI tract. As in the first hypothesis, abnormal functioning of gut and brain barriers allows toxins access, overwhelming the detoxification system so that further damage is sustained and compounded.

A third possible course of events stems from early and repeated damage from toxic substances in our environment. Because of a genetically weak detoxification system, babies who develop autism are more susceptible to toxins, even at low doses. The developing fetus is exposed to mercury through maternal amalgams, fish consumption, or thimerosal-containing injections (flu shots and Rho(D) immunoglobulin). As you may recall, thimerosal is a mercury-based preservative that was common in childhood vaccines until concerns emerged regarding its safety (chapters 11 and 12). Other placental toxins have a synergistic effect, causing neurological damage and immune dysregulation to the growing baby while it's still in the womb. On the day of birth, the newborn is given hepatitis B vaccine (with mercury, aluminum, and other additives), and exposed to anesthetics, inducing agents, pain medications, or antibiotics given to the mother during delivery. The baby's capacity to detoxify is minimal at best, so the toxins begin to accumulate in its small body. Over the course of the next six months, many immunizations with doses of thimerosal that far exceed safety limits for adults are given. And the baby is even exposed to toxins existing in formula or breast milk.

Thimerosal disrupts dendritic cells (chapter 6) in the baby's immune system and interrupts methylation, leading to abnormal neurotransmitter function and decreased ability to form glutathione. To make matters worse, babies are given acetaminophen for pain and fever the day before and for several days after the immunizations, further depleting glutathione (chapter 10) and leaving brain and gut cells even more liable to toxic injury.

As these struggling babies confront other common exposures, autoimmune reactions are triggered and inflammation increases. Because the dendritic cells' function has been disrupted by thimerosal, they don't kill foreign invaders such as viruses and bacteria efficiently, leading to chronic ear infections and frequent upper respiratory tract infections. Repeated courses of antibiotics further injure the gut through the destruction of beneficial bacteria. Abnormal bacteria and yeast erode the gut lining and a leaky gut ensues.

Now the tiny body is flooded with new food antigens and harmful chemicals that previously weren't absorbed. The detoxification and immune systems are at the tipping point when the baby develops a viral illness or is given a live-virus vaccine. In fact, babies are exposed to three, sometimes four live viruses at once; MMR (measles, mumps, rubella) and the chicken pox vaccine all contain viruses known to have immunosuppressive and neurological effects. This event can be more than a small body can handle—the brain is now injured and the child regresses into autism.

All three scenarios are easily defended by the medical literature, but the third, implicating environmental toxins as the underlying cause of autism, is the most logical in light of the epidemic rise in the numbers of autistic children. As with most things, toxic capacity is likely distributed in a typical bell curve. As our environment becomes more toxic, more people reach their personal toxic tipping point, resulting in more and more chronic immunological disease. In spite of the "miracles" of modern medicine, chronic diseases like asthma, diabetes, multiple sclerosis, lupus, and rheumatoid arthritis are on the rise—modern diseases outpacing modern medicine. All of these involve excess inflammation or autoimmune reactions or both. Chronic neurological or neurodegenerative diseases such as Alzheimer's disease, Parkinson's, ADHD, and autism are also on the rise, and I'd include depression, anxiety, obsessive compulsive disorder, dyslexia and other learning disabilities in that category as well.

Both as a medical community and as a society, it's imperative to invest in our understanding of how the immune system responds to our increasingly toxic environment. I believe that understanding autism will give us the key to unlock the mysteries of many other modern diseases.

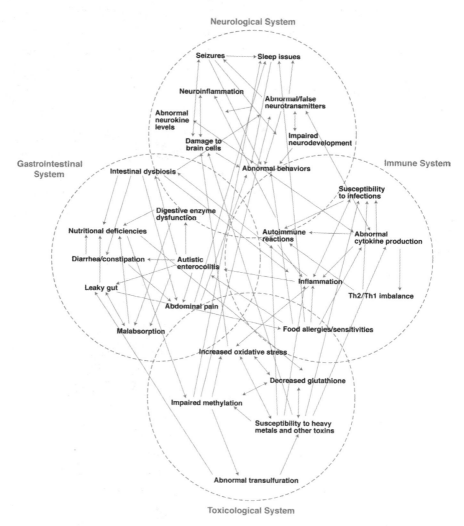

chapter 15

TREATING AUTISM

HISTORICALLY AUTISM HAS BEEN CONSIDERED AN UNTREATABLE disease. Traditional management consisted of prescribing a variety of psychoactive medications designed to control behaviors. While occasionally effective at decreasing some of the more difficult issues like aggression and self-injury, these medications don't address the core symptoms of autism, and side effects can be prohibitive. Treatment of autism, therefore, was an ongoing process of managing behavior and balancing medication side effects. Little or no attention was paid to the underlying cause of the illness, the reason for the abnormal behaviors, or symptoms related to other affected organ systems. Not surprisingly, most people with autism didn't get any better, and most spent their lives in institutions. Until very recently, this was the unquestioned expectation.

With the advent of behavior management strategies like ABA (applied behavioral analysis), children given intensive therapy began showing improvement in many core autistic behaviors, and we began to see that with early intervention children with autism could improve to lead productive lives, outside of institutions. This shift in expectation led to the push for early intervention programs, but while many children with autism make progress, for most children behavior management is not enough.

Newly armed with the understanding that autism is in fact a metabolic disease affecting multiple organ systems (not just the brain), many physicians are treating autism effectively by addressing these underlying physiological factors. As the body begins to heal, so does the brain. Through the combination of medical treatment and intensive behavioral interventions, children with autism are achieving a higher degree of functioning than was ever thought possible. In fact, although a true cure still eludes us, many have dropped their diagnosis and are indistinguishable from their peers. Most of these recovered children have medical issues that require ongoing management, but they're leading essentially normal lives. This recovered group is still the minority; nonetheless, when appropriately treated most children improve measurably, and any gain makes an impact on the quality of life for the children and for their families.

As our understanding of this disease improves, the treatments become more effective—and more children will recover. The remainder of the book will focus on the principles of treating autism, given the scientific information we have so far. This book isn't meant to be a treatment protocol; I intentionally leave out dosages of medications and nutrients because I strongly believe the first requirement of effective treatment is the help of a physician who is trained in treating autism. Each child has a unique biochemical makeup. What works for one child could make another worse. The Autism Research Institute has compiled a survey of now over 20,000 parents regarding the efficacy of various interventions from the parents' perspective, ranging from nutritional supplements to psychoactive medications. I have included the results as an appendix. It is reported as a ratio of the number of children that improved versus the number that got worse after each given intervention. The results may be quite surprising to some. Weeding through these treatment options to find the right combination for a given child can be challenging. This requires a detailed history and physical exam, appropriate lab tests, and carefully monitored clinical treatment trials. In addition, the treatment of autism is changing rapidly and some of the treatments that we use today will be replaced by more effective methods. However, some universal principles and strategies in autism treatment are likely to endure.

The Multi-Tiered Treatment Approach

Treatment has three components: replace what the child is missing, remove what is causing harm, and break the inflammatory cycle. All of the interventions that I use in treating autism fall into one or more of these categories. The order of these treatments depends on the patient's history. In the early stages, I usually follow a fairly consistent pattern, with a first tier of nutritional support and diet changes; this sets the foundation for higher-tiered interventions. Many vitamins and minerals act as coenzymes in critical enzymatic pathways in body metabolism. Without corrected nutrition, it's unlikely that we'll ever correct abnormalities in the affected organ systems.

Diet changes often result in rapid improvements in both neurological and GI function, leading to better absorption of nutrients, decreased GI inflammation, and decreased immune system activation; subsequent improvement in sleep, bowel function, mood, and immunity follow. Changing the diet is probably the most difficult thing that parents are asked to do, but the improvements are often immediate, and when they are, give the parents enough hope and encouragement to continue with the changes.

The next step is usually to focus on the gut. GI inflammation causes pain; as pain decreases, behavior improves, sleep improves, and the children can gain more from their educational programs because they're no longer distracted. There's also strong evidence that GI inflammation triggers systemic inflammatory response, including inflammation in the brain. So, treating the gut treats the brain. A damaged gut is also a source of toxin exposure, so healing the gut will decrease the overall toxic and allergic burdens in the body. Higher-level treatments that address the detoxification, the immunological, and the neurological systems are then tailored to the child, based on symptoms.

Before starting any treatment program, there are some principles to consider. Since these differ for parents and physicians, I list them separately.

To Parents:

Find a good doctor who specializes in treating the medical needs of autistic children. For some, this will be easier said than done. Since we've only recently come to understand that autism is a treatable medical condition, few doctors have experience or the specialized knowledge that comes from focusing on this disease. Because of its multi-organ system involvement and complicated pathophysiology, autism doesn't fit neatly into the box of any other currently recognized medical specialty. Although many doctors claim to know how to treat autism, few are doing so full-time. When looking for a doctor, be sure it's someone who continues to attend autism-specific medical conferences and remains up-to-date. Research about the medical aspects of autism is published regularly, so physicians can't rely on what we knew even six months ago. Reading published research alone is insufficient, since the publishing lag can be years long; the networking of information is how most doctors learn which autism treatments are effective. Look for someone who networks with other autism specialists around the world.

Don't rely on your doctor to know everything. Almost every significant advance in autism treatment has been the result of parents either pushing their doctors into action, or taking it upon themselves to figure things out. You are your child's best advocate. Learn about the disease. Study. Take what you learn to your doctor. Much of what is required of you to treat your child will require a lot of effort. Without understanding why a particular treatment is necessary, you might be tempted to give up too soon. Arming yourself with research and with the understanding of the biological rationale behind the treatment strategy for your child is likely to help you gain the support of your primary care physician. It will also help you to educate family members, school personnel, and neighbors about supporting you in your child's treatment.

Don't start everything at once. You have learned here how very complex the physiological abnormalities in autism are. The treatment of these abnormalities is complex as well. Your child will eventually be taking multiple nutritional supplements and is likely to be placed on a variety of medications depending on the particular part of their biochemistry that's being targeted. Often, the response of your child to an intervention tells us more than lab reports. Keeping a journal is the best way to record your child's response so that you can report to your doctor. Not every child responds the same way to a given treatment. A child might have a negative response to an intervention that helps the majority. These negative behaviors are unpredictable, but are usually temporary. If too many things are started at once, we can't tell which treatment caused which response, positive or negative. Generally, several days or weeks between new interventions will reveal any immediate positive or negative effects. A good doctor can help you work efficiently through the options shown to be useful in other autistic children.

Remember that the treatment of autism is like a marathon, not a sprint. It usually takes several years to reverse the physiological dysfunction. Although there are many anecdotes about patients responding dramatically and immediately to a single treatment, this is not the norm. In fact, most of the "overnight" responders have had concurrent therapies that were subtly beneficial, laying the groundwork for amazing improvement. Most autistic children have cycles of progress followed by plateaus and sometimes even short regressions as treatment is tailored to suit their needs, but you should see an encouraging trend overall. Autism is a chronic disease, and the management is likewise ongoing. Do not give up if immediate results don't meet your expectations. Younger children generally respond more rapidly, but older children and adults also improve. There is no age cut-off when you should discontinue therapy. *Never* give up hope, at any age. The more scientists and physicians learn about autism, the more effective the treatments will become.

To Physicians:

Keep an open mind. Much of this information is new, and much is foreign to our previous understanding about the disease. We're taught in medical school to be skeptical and to evaluate things with a critical eye—this skepticism should stimulate our minds to look deeper, not prevent us from doing so.

Do your own research. Do not rely on what others tell you, including me. This is why I've presented the current research and references in this book. I hope you'll review the literature for yourself and formulate your own opinion—but review the entire studies, not just the abstracts, and pay attention to the study methods. Look for hidden sources of bias that could affect study results. Put new information about autism in the context of the information that's already available to be sure that it makes sense physiologically. Question dogma. We all know many examples when long-standing dogma in medicine has been disproved with evidence-based medicine.

Treat the entire body. Whatever your thoughts on the various hypotheses on the etiology of the disease, it is no longer possible to argue that autism only affects the brain, so a treatment approach that exclusively targets the neurological symptoms is illogical. This is akin to treating AIDS by surgically removing skin lesions. The patient might look better, but the underlying illness is untreated.

Get training. Understanding the autism disease complex requires a lot of effort. Learning the nuances of treatment for individual children is even more difficult, and takes experience. I strongly recommend attending some medical conferences such as the Defeat Autism Now (DAN!) Conference held biannually. DAN! Conferences usually include a practitioner-training seminar. The latest medical research and treatments are also explored and discussed at many other conferences held in the US and in other countries. If possible, it's useful to spend time with an experienced autism physician. If you are in a country where help is not immediately available, you might be able to access educational services remotely. Thoughtful House Center for Children in Austin, Texas *(www.thoughtfulhouse.org)* is committed to educating other physicians so that people with autism worldwide can get the help that they need.

Listen to the parents. They are with your patient night and day, and they are the ones who are implementing the therapies that you prescribe. Be willing to educate them and to be educated by them. They will teach you a great deal about autism that you can't learn from attending a seminar or from reading a book. Effective treatment requires a partnership between you and the parents.

A Note about Laboratory Testing

Many laboratories offer a variety of tests that are touted as useful in autism treatment. Many such tests aren't currently reimbursed by insurance companies, and parents can easily spend thousands of dollars on information that might or might not be helpful in guiding therapy. If you're not sure whether test results will yield information that could help determine treatment decisions for the child, it's better to use precious financial resources elsewhere. Often, an empiric trial is still the only way to know if a particular intervention is appropriate for an individual child. (Some of the laboratory data that is presented in research settings is not currently available through commercial labs.)

chapter 16

CORRECTING NUTRITIONAL DEFICIENCIES

BEFORE I BEGAN TREATING AUTISTIC CHILDREN, LIKE MANY OF MY medical colleagues I thought that supplements were an unnecessary waste of time and money; we're taught that if you eat a normal, varied diet, your body will get everything it needs. The truth of this rests on several assumptions: first, that you're in fact eating a variety of nutritious foods. Second, that you have normal digestion and can break food down to a form that's easily absorbed. Third, that there's a healthy mucosal surface in the bowel that will absorb nutrients and screen out things that are harmful. And last, that the chemistry of the body is functioning in such a way that you're able to utilize nutrients.

Running counter to this bias against supplements are many examples of illnesses in which nutrients are central to the treatment prescribed by mainstream physicians. For instance, in emergency medicine, vitamin B1 (thiamine) is part of the "coma cocktail" that's given to anyone brought to the hospital "unresponsive without known cause." In the

Emergency Department it's not uncommon to treat late-stage alcoholics, who are notoriously thiamine-depleted because they often go for days without eating and because they tend to have damaged livers, where B vitamins are stored. Alcohol also destroys the absorptive surface of the gut, preventing uptake of whatever nutrients they do eat. Vitamin B1 has a powerful effect on the nervous system; a severe deficiency can actually induce a coma, which can be reversed with an injection of thiamine.

Doctors are recognizing that many conditions require supplemental nutrition, including cancer, HIV, malabsorption syndromes, short-bowel syndrome, anorexia, old age, and pregnancy. These conditions have in common a decreased oral nutrient intake, an abnormal GI tract, a change in metabolism, or a combination of the above. Autism shares these characteristics as well.

Children with autism will very often eat only a narrow range of foods.[1] It's not unusual for me to see children who refuse to eat anything except french fries, chicken nuggets, and cheesy crackers. These children don't take in enough nutrients to maintain normal cell function. Children with autism also have abnormal enzyme function, and consequent inadequate digestion.[2][3] Abnormal bowel motility, inflammation of the mucosal lining, and leaky gut syndrome all interfere with absorption of the limited nutrients that they do eat (chapter 9).

Autistic children have abnormalities in cellular biochemistry that would prevent utilization, even if they ate normally. For example, pyridoxal kinase is an enzyme known to function abnormally in autism that converts vitamin B6 (pyridoxine) into P5P (pyridoxal-5-phosphate), the metabolically active form of the vitamin. Weakness in this enzyme causes functional B6 deficiency, even if there's adequate intake and normal or even high blood levels of B6. This weakness can be overcome through oral intake of very high amounts of B6[4][5]—it could be why many autistic children respond favorably to high-dose B6 supplementation.[6][7](More on the efficacy of B6 later in this chapter.)

Whether autism-associated deficiencies are a cause or a result of abnormal metabolism is not clear, but in either case, the foundation of an appropriate treatment strategy is to re-supply the nutrients the child's body needs to perform more normally. Vitamins and minerals as coenzymes are essential to drive biochemical reactions forward in cellular metabolism. Without adequate coenzyme levels, these processes stall, or function less efficiently. Effective treatment requires nutritional correction in order to maximize cell function and to speed the healing process.

In the sections that follow, I describe the nutrients that are used in the treatment of autism, and the rationale for their use. This is not a comprehensive list of all the nutrients the human body needs, rather it is a list of those nutrients that so far have been found to be particularly applicable in the treatment of autism.

Vitamins

Vitamin A

Vitamin A fights infection by activating the immune system's natural killer cells. It helps activate T-cells and B-cells in the adaptive immune system, thereby supporting immune memory. Vitamin A protects against viruses, including measles virus. Its metabolites are involved in the normal function of retinoid receptors in the eye. It's critical not only for vision, but for sensory perception, language processing, and attention skills. It's also necessary for cell growth and differentiation, especially in the epithelial tissues of the gut and the brain.[8][9]

It's best to take vitamin A in its natural cis- form, most abundantly found in cold-water fish like salmon and cod, and in milk fat. Most nutritional supplements, including baby formulas, use vitamin A palmitate, the synthetic version. Absorption of the palmitate form is impaired if there are mucosal or pH problems in the gut, common in autistic children. Also, vitamin A palmitate can deactivate the control switch of many metabolic pathways involved in vision and cell growth, and can disrupt metabolism and hormonal regulation of lipids, proteins, and glycogen.

Dr. Mary Megson hypothesized that some autism symptoms are related to disruption of G-proteins, which control many metabolic processes in the cells and are dependent on vitamin A. This G-protein blockade can be reversed through a combination of cod liver oil and urocholine (a cholinergic agonist). Megson noted significant, often immediate improvement in visual perception, attention, and language after these supplements were given.[10]

Vitamin B1 (thiamine)

Thiamine plays a part in such metabolic processes as carbohydrate metabolism, antioxidation, and biosynthesis of neurotransmitters and nucleic acids (DNA). TD (thiamine deficiency) results in a diffuse decrease in cerebral glucose utilization, meaning that the brain is starved for fuel. The frontal lobe, the mammillary bodies, and the basal ganglia are particularly vulnerable to TD.

TD causes Wernicke's encephalopathy, a neurological disorder in adults (usually alcoholics), which is characterized by confusion, ataxia, and oculomotor disturbances. In children, TD is usually the result of chronic malnutrition from cancer, GI disease, or anorexia nervosa; it manifests as vomiting, nystagmus (rapid eye movements), purposeless movement of the extremities, and sometimes convulsions. Damage to neurons is likely a result of impaired oxidative metabolism in susceptible regions of the brain. Reactive oxygen species such as nitric oxide can then accumulate in the brain tissues and eventually lead to nerve cell death. Active inflammatory response in the brain by microglial cells is a further manifestation of thiamine deficiency—this contributes to damage, both to the cells and to the blood-brain barrier.[11][12]

Interestingly, lead poisoning is known to induce TD, and supplementation of thiamine is a useful adjunct to chelating agents in the removal of lead and other metals from the body.[13] In a pilot study by Lonsdale et al. on the use of thiamine tetrahydrofurfuryl disulfide (TTFD) in autistic children, 30% of the patients had intracellular thiamine deficiency. Eight of the ten children improved on the autism rating scale while receiving TTFD.[14]

Vitamin B2 (riboflavin)

Riboflavin, or its metabolite FAD (flavin adenine dinucleotide), is a cofactor for the folic acid cycle enzyme MTHFR (methylene tetrahydrofolate reductase), described in chapter 10. MTHFR also regulates the folate metabolism pathway, influencing the generation of nucleic acids, the building blocks of DNA. Minor mutations in the MTHFR enzyme are common in the normal population, and even more frequent in autism. These mutations can decrease the activity of the MTHFR enzyme, and so could be partly responsible for the methylation abnormalities in autism.[15] A deficiency of riboflavin will also contribute to MTHFR dysfunction.[16]

Vitamin B3 (niacin)

Niacin and its coenzyme forms (NAD, NADP) act as hydrogen carriers in hundreds of different enzymatic reactions involving the synthesis and degradation of carbohydrates, fatty acids, and amino acids. It acts as a peripheral vasodilator and is thought to have some positive effects on cerebral blood flow. Niacin deficiency can result in neurological disturbances that include dementia, hallucinations, and psychosis.[17] A NAD deficiency can result in the abnormally low cellular energy production and elevated lactate seen in some children with autism.[18]

Vitamin B6 (pyridoxine)

B6 and its metabolite P5P (pyridoxal 5-phosphate) are vital nutrients in the body. P5P is a known cofactor in 113 enzymes, including those responsible for the formation of serotonin, dopamine, norepinephrine, and other neurotransmitters.[19] It's involved in the conversion of glutamic acid, an excitatory neurotransmitter, to GABA, an inhibitory one.[20] As mentioned in chapter 13, it's been shown that children with autism have an elevated glutamate-to-GABA ratio that can result in excitotoxic damage to brain cells. B6 deficiency might be one explanation for this abnormality. P5P plays yet another key role in the detoxification pathway, in the synthesis of cysteine.[21] A functional B6 deficiency can therefore cause disruption in many biochemical pathways relevant to treating autism.

Decades ago, Bernard Rimland reported improvement in autistic children following high doses of vitamin B6,[22] an observation that was followed by many controlled studies documenting the symptomatic improvement as well as the safety of this treatment.[23 24 25 26 27 28 29] Areas of improvement included better social engagement, decreased tactile sensitivity, improved language, more appropriate facial expressions, decreased stereotyped behaviors and obsessions, and improved eating habits. The abnormally elevated urine excretion of homovanillic acid (HVA, a derivative of dopamine) was decreased in the children given B6. This suggests that B6 supplementation had a direct effect on neurotransmitter metabolism in these patients. A very small percentage of the patients had increased excitability and nausea in a few of the studies. Other side effects, such as increased irritability, sound sensitivity, and enuresis (bed wetting), were noted in earlier studies but disappeared entirely with the addition of magnesium supplements.[30]

A meta-analysis by Kleijnen et al. reviewed large, double-blinded, randomized, placebo-controlled studies on the use of high-dose vitamins in the treatment of a variety of neurological conditions, including autism. They showed consistently positive effects with the combination of high dose Vitamin B6 and magnesium in autistic children—the benefit in other neurological conditions was less conclusive.[31]

High serum levels of B6 have been documented in autistic children (not receiving supplements) compared to neurotypical children.[32 33] But in the same study group, P5P, the major metabolite of B6, was much lower in children with autism compared to controls. This is highly suggestive of dysfunction in the enzyme pyridoxal kinase (responsible for converting B6 to P5P), most likely related to a genetic polymorphism. Since this polymorphism decreases binding affinity of the enzyme to B6, the weakness can be overcome by increasing the amount of vitamin B6 available to be bound.

Vitamin B12

Two enzyme processes in the body are known to be dependent on B12 (cobalamin). Methylcobalamin catalyzes the conversion of homocysteine to methionine in the methylation cycle (chapter 10). The other enzyme reaction uses adenosyl-cobalamin to convert methylmalonic acid into succinyl-CoA, which is further metabolized to produce cellular energy, or used in the synthesis of porphyrins.[34]

It's estimated that 40% of the general population has insufficient dietary intake of vitamin B12 and folate. Vitamin B12 deficiency in adults is a well-known cause of neurological or psychiatric symptoms, including slow cerebration (thinking), confusion, memory changes, delirium with or without hallucinations and delusions, depression, acute psychotic states, mania, and even reversible schizophrenia-like conditions. B12 deficiency can cause peripheral neuropathy (numbness or pain in extremities) and pernicious anemia. It can also cause early developmental regression in infants. Treatment with B12 improves areas of language and cognition, although it rarely reverses chronic dementia in adults. Interestingly, the treatment of dietary B12 deficiency in infants can produce unusual but temporary muscle twitching at the same time as improved cognition and awareness.[35][36]

Diagnosing B12 deficiency can be difficult. Relying on low serum B12 levels alone will miss about 50% of cases. A more sensitive indicator is elevation of methylmalonic acid and homocysteine, both of which will back up in cases of B12 deficiency. But in autism, because of blocks in other parts of the methylation cycle, it's uncommon to see an elevated homocysteine level, in spite of good clinical and metabolic response to methylB12 supplementation.[37] Often, a clinical treatment trial of methylB12 (by injection because of poor absorption in the gut[38][39]) is the best test to detect occult B12 deficiency.

Vitamin C (ascorbic acid)

Vitamin C is one of the most potent non-enzyme antioxidants (more on antioxidants in chapter 18). It enhances selenium utilization in the cells[40] and preserves the antioxidant function of vitamin E.[41] It plays a part in metal metabolism; lead toxicity alters vitamin C metabolism, and supplementing vitamin C increases lead excretion with heavy metal chelators.[42]

Scurvy results from severe vitamin C deficiency. Symptoms of incipient scurvy are weakness, irritability, weight loss, and vague muscle pain, followed by a skin rash and swelling of the lower extremities. Untreated, advanced scurvy produces severe pain in the bones, shortness of breath, easy bruising, gum disease, loosening of the teeth, jaundice, and generalized edema (swelling). Death can result from high output heart failure secondary to anemia, bleeding into the chest cavity, or organ failure.[43]

Full-blown scurvy is rare where there is good access to fruits and vegetables high in vitamin C; nonetheless this deficiency remains a common and often unrecognized problem. Several studies have documented decreased levels in otherwise healthy American populations at rates between 2% and 30%.[44] Deficiency rates are much higher in smokers (33-50%) or the acutely ill (35%).[45][46][47][48][49] The depletion in ill patients most likely reflects the nutrient's role as an antioxidant.

Vitamin C can be rapidly depleted by physiological stress or by increased detoxification requirement, and children with autism have both conditions. Adams et al. showed that autistic children had much lower blood levels of vitamin C compared to national controls. Supplementation of moderate-dose vitamin C only partially resolved the relative deficiency.[50] Another study done in the early 1990s showed that autistic children responded to high doses of vitamin C with favorable overall behavioral scores and reduced sensory motor disturbances (self-stimulatory behavior). The researchers postulated that the benefits resulted from direct inhibition of dopamine pathways in the brain by vitamin C (mechanism shown in other studies), rather than from correction of nutritional deficiency, as none of the children in their study was clinically deficient in vitamin C.[51]

Vitamin D

Vitamin D, a fat-soluble vitamin, is a regulator of calcium status. We get it through oral intake or by the action of sunlight on the skin. The average daily intake is 500 IU/day (minimal requirement has been set at 100 IU/day, although adequacy of this number has been questioned[52]). Severe deficiency can lead to rickets, a bone disease caused by low calcium levels.

Vitamin D is converted into its active form in the kidney by parathyroid hormone, which is secreted in response to low calcium levels in the plasma. Vitamin D then increases calcium levels by stimulating transcellular absorption of calcium in the small intestine, increasing calcium resorption from the bone, and decreasing calcium excretion from the kidney. Since the majority of calcium is absorbed between the cells, the role of Vitamin D in calcium levels is still relatively minor except in cases of poor dietary calcium intake. Vitamin D helps to regulate calcium transport into the cells and is partially responsible for maintaining the high extracellular concentration gradient of calcium that is critical for normal cell function.[53 54 55 56]

To my knowledge, vitamin D deficiency hasn't been documented in autism specifically. But because their food choices are so often limited, or because of prescribed dietary restrictions and, in some cases, decreased sunlight exposure, autistic children might be at risk, and so adequate vitamin D intake should be ensured. An excellent source is cod liver oil. It's also been shown that toxic metals such as lead, cadmium, aluminum, and strontium can interfere with normal vitamin D metabolism,[57] a fact that could be important in autism in light of the heavy metal detoxification abnormalities.

Vitamin E

Vitamin E (alpha-tocopherol) is the main membrane-bound antioxidant. It is fat soluble, and concentrated in vegetable oils and wheat germ. It scavenges free radicals that cause damage to cell membranes (lipid peroxidation), but is less effective against oxidative stress in the cytosol (the fluid within cells). Damage to cell membrane lipids can have a profound effect on cell function. Many of the chemical reactions inside the cell are coupled with membrane-bound proteins that act as signaling molecules. This is particularly important in the neurological system, since function of any neurotransmitter is tightly regulated by its release and subsequent uptake by cell membranes at the neuromuscular synapse. Vitamin E supplementation is effective in alleviating some of the cell membrane damage, with improvement of symptoms in diseases such as schizophrenia and Tourette's disorder. It's estimated that it takes as long as six months for vitamin E treatment to increase levels in the brain and to restore levels of membrane lipids, so long-term therapy is essential.[58][59][60]

Folic Acid

Folic acid is required both for regulating neurogenesis (birth of neurons) and its opposite, apoptosis (programmed cell death). Deficiency of folic acid has been associated with slowly progressive neurological dysfunction in adults (stroke, Alzheimer's, and Parkinson's) and children. This deficiency causes degeneration of cells that produce dopamine, and results in motor dysfunction (as with Alzheimer's). Depression is more common in patients with folic acid deficiency. Supplementation of folinic acid (a metabolite of folic acid) has been shown to improve clinical symptoms in some of these patients.[61][62][63]

Folic acid is active in one-carbon (methyl group) transfers, and is linked with the methylation cycle described in chapter 10. The folic acid cycle is also a source for single carbon transfer used in the formation of the purines and pyrimidines that make up the structure of DNA.[64] Folic acid deficiency in pregnant women is linked to neural tube defects in their fetuses.[65]

Folic acid cycle abnormalities are common in patients with autism. James et al. have shown that supplementation of folinic acid in combination with betaine (trimethylglycine) partially reversed methylation defects in children with autism.[66] A more recent study by James et al.

shows that some children with autism have genetic polymorphisms in their folic acid cycle that put them at higher risk of methylation and detoxification problems.

Vitamin K

Vitamin K (fat soluble) is a cofactor for proteins that both support (factor VII, factor IX, factor X, prothrombin) and regulate (protein C, protein S) blood coagulation.[67] Deficiency causes abnormalities in blood clotting and increases risk of hemorrhage. Vitamin K is also important for the carboxylation of osteocalcin, a protein within the bone matrix that helps to bind calcium and to retain it. Deficiency can contribute to calcium loss and lead to osteoporosis.[68]

Vitamin K also functions in conjunction with vitamin E in protecting cell membranes from oxidative stress damage.[69] Its antioxidant effect has been shown to prevent cell death specifically associated with glutamate toxicity and intracellular glutathione (GSH) depletion in neurons.[70]

Vitamin K has also been shown to decrease inflammation by suppressing IL-6 production.[71] It also suppresses inflammation induced by E. coli bacteria-derived LPS (lipopolysaccharide).[72]

Green vegetables (especially spinach) and fermented foods are sources of vitamin K; it is also generated by microorganisms in the gut. People with inflammatory bowel disease, fat malabsorption syndromes, or intestinal dysbiosis from frequent antibiotic use will be at risk of deficiency.[73]

Since children with autism meet all of the above criteria, they're in a high-risk group for vitamin K deficiency. Although I'm not aware of any studies specific to vitamin K and autism, supplementation of this nutrient is no doubt beneficial as an antioxidant and as an anti-inflammatory, and also in preventing long-standing calcium loss from the bones.

Minerals

Zinc

Zinc is a component of more than eighty different enzymes; it's needed for the development and maintenance of the brain, adrenal glands, GI tract, and immune system. Both serotonin and melatonin synthesis rely on zinc-activated enzymes. DNA synthesis and repair is zinc-dependent, as is GABA formation. Zinc is an essential cofactor for antioxidation pathways and proteins needed for growth and homeostasis.[74][75][76][77]

Zinc metabolism is coupled with copper metabolism; zinc deficiency is often associated with elevated copper levels. Although copper has several functions involving antioxidation and neurotransmitter metabolism, elevated levels of copper can be harmful. Excess free copper is a pro-oxidant, catalyzing reactions producing high levels of free radicals, and inhibiting antioxidant enzymes.[78] High copper impairs further uptake of zinc, reducing the activity of zinc-dependent enzymes.

The protein that controls zinc-to-copper ratios is called metallothionein, also necessary for the immune system, neuronal development, and detoxification of heavy metals. Walsh et al. at the Pfeiffer Institute in Illinois studied blood chemistry profiles of 503 patients with autism spectrum disorder, and found that 85% had significantly elevated copper/zinc ratios compared to healthy controls. Of the forty-nine patients who had normal copper-to-zinc ratios, forty-five were using zinc supplements at the time of the blood sample, so it's likely that these children also had abnormal baseline levels. The authors hypothesized that children with autism have a metallothionein defect that's contributing to the findings of elevated copper/zinc, immune system abnormalities, behavioral issues, and problems with heavy metal detoxification.[79]

Diagnosing zinc deficiency isn't easy, because normal homeostasis keeps the serum level within a tight range in spite of intracellular zinc depletion. I usually measure zinc with an intracellular (erythrocyte) mineral test, and it's almost always low in my autistic patients. Physical signs of zinc deficiency include: eczema, acne, psoriasis, poor wound healing, oral or leg ulcers, white lines in fingernails, growth retardation, delayed sexual maturation, poor taste acuity, hair loss, and chronic immunodeficiency or frequent infections (especially with Candida albicans). Treatment is with oral zinc supplements.[80 81]

Magnesium

Magnesium is a critical intracellular ion acting as a coenzyme in over three hundred enzyme reactions; it particularly influences energy transfer in the cells. It's important for the formation and regulation of many proteins, nucleic acids (DNA), and neurotransmitters (dopamine, norepinephrine, serotonin, etc.).[82 83] It acts as a cell membrane stabilizer, as a regulator of the ion channels in the membrane, and it inhibits the glutamate NMDA (N-methyl-D-aspartate) receptor on brain cells—the receptor that allows influx of calcium into the cell, which in excess can lead to excitotoxic damage and apoptosis.

Magnesium deficiency decreases blood flow to areas of the brain, potentially resulting in damage from ischemia (oxygen deprivation). Symptoms of mild magnesium deficiency are irritability, sound sensitivity, hyperexcitability, anxiety, and mood changes. With greater deficiency, patients can develop twitching, tremors, irregular pulse, insomnia, muscle weakness, jerkiness, and leg cramps. It's common to see one or more of these symptoms in autistic patients.[84]

Magnesium deficiency has been frequently documented in children with autism and ADHD (up to 77% of ADHD children in one study), and supplementation has been shown to improve neurological symptoms.[85 86] A study by Mousain-Bosc et al. found low intracellular (erythrocyte) magnesium (Ery-Mg) in the majority of children with ADHD and PDD,[87 88] in spite of normal serum magnesium levels in many. This is strongly suggestive of an abnormality of magnesium transport into the cell, or preservation of serum levels in spite of overall body depletion. They also showed that the Ery-Mg levels of the parents of the children with ADHD and of the children with PDD were low compared to controls. In each of the studies, magnesium levels rose with treatment and behaviors improved. Upon discontinuation of the magnesium, Ery-Mg levels dropped, and abnormal behaviors returned.

These studies point out that diagnosing magnesium deficiency can be difficult; relying on the typical serum ranges could grossly underestimate the level of deficiency. Liebscher suggested that a serum value of 0.9 mmol/l (millimoles/liter) (rather than the more typical 0.7 or 0.8 mmol/l) is more appropriate for ruling out this deficiency in the normal population.[89]

Calcium

Calcium is the most abundant mineral in the body, and bone is the main source for metabolic processes. Plasma levels of calcium are regulated by controlling bone absorption/resorption through the actions of parathyroid hormone, calcitonin (a polypeptide hormone from the thyroid gland that lowers the level of calcium in the blood plasma), and vitamin D. Calcium is primarily an extracellular mineral, and cell entry is tightly controlled. Neither plasma calcium nor intracellular calcium levels are accurate measures of total body calcium supply. It's primarily absorbed in the lower half of the small intestine by paracellular absorption (passing in between the mucosal cells). In situations of low oral calcium intake, it can be absorbed through the cells (transcellular) with the assistance of vitamin D.[90]

The concentration of ionized calcium in the extracellular fluid is maintained at a very high value compared to the intracellular concentration (over 10^{-4}). This concentration is achieved via an active cell transport mechanism that is maintained with vitamin D. The concentration differential from inside to outside the cell membrane allows rapid entry of calcium into the cells when the calcium channels are opened. The influx of calcium signals cell functions that include secretion, neuromuscular impulse, contractions, or clotting, depending on the type of cell. High or persisting levels of intracellular calcium can cause damage or death to the cell.[91]

Because autistic children frequently have a narrow, self-limited diet, they're unlikely to get adequate calcium. Coupled with associated deficiencies in vitamin D and vitamin K, this puts them at risk of calcium deficiency, so supplementation is required. A casein-free diet would also increase the risk if calcium were not supplemented.

Selenium

Selenium helps to spare vitamin E, and is critical for pancreatic enzyme function. It's known to be protective against oxidative stress, particularly in heart disease (prevents abnormal lipid breakdown and plaque formation) and drug metabolism.[92][93] Selenium is important for immune function—deficiency affects the occurrence, virulence, or progression of some viral infections, including Coxsackie viruses and influenza.[94] It is thought to protect against cancer, and we know it's an antioxidant based on its position in the binding site of GSH peroxidase. Studies have shown benefits from selenium for patients under severe oxidative stress, as in sepsis, trauma, burns, and pancreatitis.[95]

Although most patients with this deficiency are asymptomatic, it's been associated with pediatric cardiomyopathy, and an unusual cartilage growth defect in regions of China where selenium is lacking in the soil. Deficiency is associated with muscle pain, abnormal liver function enzymes, and fingernail bed abnormalities in infants. It appears that the need is much higher in infants and children compared to adults, because of their rapid growth and metabolism.

Children with a low-protein diet or abnormalities in protein metabolism can become selenium-deficient. Many children with autism consume little protein and have trouble with protein digestion and catabolism (break-down), and so are at risk.

There are other reasons why children with autism can be selenium-deficient. Its bioavailability is impaired if there's an associated methionine deficiency, or deficiencies in B2, B6, or vitamin E. Heavy metals like arsenic, mercury, and cadmium also contribute to the deficiency.

Selenium status needs to be monitored, because of the potential of toxicity at high levels. Plasma selenium is rapidly responsive to changes in intake, while selenium erythrocyte levels are more indicative of chronic exposure. Symptoms of selenium toxicity include garlic odor of the breath, skin rashes, hair loss, fingernail abnormalities, dyspepsia, diarrhea and anorexia, all of which typically manifest after years of chronically high exposure. A level of 8-11 mcg/kg/day has been suggested as the upper level of chronic selenium exposure, but this is recognized as conservatively low.[96] Other sources have suggested the upper limit of supplementation to be between 400-450 mcg/day (for adults).[97]

Molybdenum

Molybdenum is a cofactor for the enzyme sulphite oxidase, which takes part in creating sulfate from cysteine. Children with autism commonly have low plasma sulfate and excessive sulfate urinary loss (chapter 18). Supplementing molybdenum can decrease urinary wasting of sulfate-containing proteins in about a third of children with autism.[98]

Omega Fatty Acids

Long-chain fatty acids such as EPA (eicosapentaenoic acid) and DHA (docosahexaenoic acid) play a part in neurological health.[99] EPA and DHA, omega-3s, are linked with many aspects of neuronal function, including neurotransmitter function (particularly dopamine), membrane fluidity, ion channel and enzyme regulation, and gene expression. DHA is the predominant omega-3 fatty acid in the brain, linked to development of both visual and auditory processing systems. EPA modulates the activity of the immune system through modification of the production of cytokines; it's known to shift the balance of the immune system response from pro-inflammatory to anti-inflammatory. In contrast, arachidonic acid (AA), an omega-6 fatty acid, is a pro-inflammatory agent. Omega-3s decrease damage from oxidative stress, possibly by speeding up the repair of the injured phospholipid membranes.

Besides neurological symptoms, other clinical indicators of omega-3 deficiency include excessive thirst, frequent urination, dry skin or hair, and atopic rashes (like eczema). Sleep disturbances and visual abnormalities can also be related to omega-3 deficiencies.

EPA and DHA can be produced in the body by their precursor, alpha-linolenic acid (ALA), but this mechanism is not very efficient in humans, particularly males, so dietary sources are the most important. EPA and DHA are derived from animal sources, while ALA is found primarily in green vegetables and some nuts and seeds. Over the last century our Western diet has become more reliant on grains (high in omega-6 fatty acids) and grain-fed animal proteins than on fish and wild game, resulting in a relative lack of omega-3s. The use of vegetable oils high in omega-6 fatty acids has also contributed to the imbalance.

Studies show a link between deficiencies in these fatty acids and several neuropsychiatric diseases, such as attention deficit hyperactivity disorder (ADHD), Alzheimer's, schizophrenia, and depression. Supplementation of Omega-3s has yielded mixed results, but in general has shown a positive effect on many of the behavior aspects of the disorders.[100]

A few reports in the literature document low levels of omega-3 fatty acids in subjects with autism.[101][102] Others have reported fatty acid levels similar to controls.[103] A 2006 randomized, double-blind, placebo-controlled trial on the use of omega-3 fatty acid supplementation in autistic children showed measurable improvement in hyperactivity and stereotypy with no adverse reactions, at a dose of 1.5 grams per day (EPA 0.84 g/d, DHA 0.7 g/d).[104]

Omega-3 supplementation is considered safe, with side effects generally absent at doses below three grams per day. At higher doses, side effects include digestive symptoms such as nausea, belching, or loose stools. It is generally agreed that omega-6 levels are more than adequate in a typical Western diet, but that omega-3s are insufficient and should be supplemented.[105][106] An emerging issue concerning dietary intake of omega-3 fatty acids is that fish, the major source of the nutrient, is now contaminated with potentially high levels of mercury, so purified nutritional supplements are likely the safest method to address these deficiencies.

Essential Amino Acids

Increased energy requirements and metabolism mean that dietary intake of essential amino acids must be proportionately higher in infants and young children than in adults. Protein intake is essential to normal health because of rapid rates of protein turnover, and loss of protein in the urine. In conditions of metabolic stress, intake requirements for essential amino acids are even higher. A source for protein catabolism for energy production, amino acids are also building blocks for neurotransmitters, bile salts, enzymes, and hormones.[107]

A study by Aldred et al. compared blood levels of amino acids from autistic children and their families with a group of controls. Amino acid concentrations were greater than control values for glutamic acid, phenylalanine, asparagine, tyrosine, alanine, and lysine (p<0.05). Glutamine levels were low. Interestingly, amino acid levels of the parents were also different from controls, and similar to those of their autistic children. This is highly suggestive of a genetically inherited abnormality in amino acid processing. Elevated levels of phenylalanine and tyrosine can lead to higher concentrations of catecholamines such as dopamine, epinephrine, and norepinephrine, with subsequent effects on behavior. The authors also suggested that the abnormal balance between glutamic acid and glutamine might imply an abnormal downregulation of the glutamate receptor in cells (including neurons), which could lead to an increase in brain glutamate levels; excess glutamate in the brain causes excitotoxic damage to the cells. Low glutamine can also have negative effects on gut function because it's important for maintaining a healthy gut mucosa.[108]

Another study retrospectively reviewed plasma amino acid levels measured as part of the initial diagnostic workup in autistic children. Some of these children (n=10) were on a parent-imposed (not medically supervised) restricted diet (usually gluten-free, casein-free). Others were not on a restricted diet (n=26). They were compared to age-matched controls with developmental delays but not autism (n=24). Results showed that about 60% of autistic children had at least one deficiency in essential amino acids, regardless of diet, compared to only 4% of the control children, suggesting protein malnutrition. In both autistic groups, certain amino acid deficiencies (valine, leucine, phenylalanine, and lysine) reached statistical significance.

There were a few individual amino acid levels that were different between autistic children on restricted diets compared with those on unrestricted diets (e.g. tryptophan) and between the diet-restricted children and the controls (e.g. isoleucine), but patterns were inconsistent. There was also a trend toward lower amino acid levels (not statistically significant) in the autistic children on diets, compared to autistic children not on diets. This led the authors to conclude that most autistic children have a baseline state of protein malnutrition that could be made worse by medically unsupervised restricted diets.[109]

Taurine

Taurine is considered a semi-essential amino acid since it can be manufactured in the body through the metabolism of cysteine, but this pathway is often not sufficient to maintain adequate taurine stores, so taurine must be supplemented in the diet.Taurine helps form bile salts, which improve fat absorption by the gut and stimulate bile flow.[110] Bile acid aids in digestion and detoxification.Taurine is also a potent antioxidant, an osmotic buffer, a pro-homeostatic neurotransmitter, and an immunoprotectant.[111][112][113] It's also been shown to have some anti epileptic properties and is thought to counteract excitatory neurotransmitter excesses, particularly glutamate.[114] Taurine is frequently low in autistic patients, possibly due to abnormalities in taurine synthesis from cysteine, or inadequate dietary sources.[115][116]

Glutamine

Glutamine is an amino acid energy source for enterocytes in the small intestine and lymphocytes in the immune system. It helps form nicotinamide for energy transfers and glucosamine for connective tissues. It's an ammonium donor for the formation of purine and pyridamine nucleotides for DNA and RNA synthesis. It's one of the three components of the GSH molecule, critical for antioxidation and detoxification and is also thought to help prevent enterocolitis.[117][118][119] Supplementation could help in children with low levels or gastrointestinal symptoms.

Arginine

Interest in arginine supplementation stems from its role in NO (nitric oxide) metabolism in the body. Arginine is the substrate for NOsynthase, which controls NO generation. NO is thought to play a part in smooth muscle relaxation and blood flow, and might be a factor in conditions such as gastroesophageal reflux, pyloric stenosis (narrowing of the lower part of the stomach, causing forceful vomiting), and IBD.[120] NO levels have been shown to be abnormal in children with autism; high levels are toxic.[121] Arginine is also used to build creatine, which is the main transporter of energy molecules within the cell.[122]

Other Nutrients

Creatine

Creatine is an amino acid involved in energy transfer in the muscle and in the brain. It's synthesized from arginine and glycine and methylated by SAMe. In children with abnormal methylation or decreased supply of precursors in the diet, creatine can become depleted. Low cellular creatine in the brain will adversely affect cellular communication—the brain's primary energy-consuming task.[123] Whitely et al. showed that children with autism have low excretion of urine creatinine, which is the waste product of normal creatine metabolism.[124] Low creatine has been documented in regions of the brain in autism. It's not clear whether this is a regional supply issue, or related to some other mechanism.[125]

Creatine is also critical for normal muscle development, and supplements have been used at very high doses by body-builders. Since some children with autism have associated hypotonia and low muscle mass, creatine supplementation is reasonable.

Carnitine

Carnitine is a cofactor in the utilization of fat reserves under conditions of fasting and stress. It aids in the transport of long-chain fatty acids to the mitochondria in the cell, where they undergo oxidation for energy production. Children with autism frequently appear to have a mild to moderate carnitine deficiency without the clinical picture of other known primary carnitine deficiency syndromes. Autistic children also frequently have elevated ammonia, low pyruvate with normal or elevated lactate, and elevated alanine. Taken together, this is suggestive of a mild mitochondrial disorder.[126] Carnitine supplementation is considered a safe method of improving this deficiency.[127]

Coenzyme Q10

Coenzyme Q10 (CoQ10) is one of the substances most commonly used to improve mitochondrial and energy metabolism dysfunctions. Evidence of mitochondrial disorders, including elevated lactate and pyruvate, has been shown in autism; supplementation with CoQ10 can lower these markers and result in clinical improvement.[128][129]

Providing a Good Diet

Many diets are being tried on children with autism other than the gluten- and casein-free diet, including the specific carbohydrate diet (SCD), the body ecology diet (BED), the low oxalate diet (LOD), the yeast-free diet, and the Feingold diet. Making a decision about whether any of these diets is appropriate can be difficult, and is best done in consultation with a clinical nutritionist experienced in working with children on the autism spectrum. Knowing what foods to give a child is as important as knowing what to restrict. Because autistic children are already nutritionally compromised, we have to ensure that whatever they eat meets their metabolic needs.

Food is also a source of exposure to chemicals, preservatives, and toxins that are either contaminants in the food or are introduced during the manufacturing process. Since children with autism have impaired detoxification capacity, it is best to choose food that's less processed and clean of chemicals and toxins. Organic foods from trustworthy sources should be free of these toxins and carry a much higher nutrient content per gram.Whenever possible, organic food is preferred. Tap water is a major source of heavy metals, so using a good filtering system or buying filtered water is a good idea too.

Correcting nutrient deficiencies is a necessary foundation for other interventions in autism. To overcome absorption and utilization issues, high dose supplementation is often required, but should be undertaken with clear understanding of potential side effects and risk of toxicity for each nutrient, and with the guidance of a physician or nutritionist.

chapter 17

TREATING THE GUT

SEVENTY TO EIGHTY PERCENT OF CHILDREN WITH AUTISM HAVE gastrointestinal symptoms, including abdominal pain, diarrhea, constipation, abdominal bloating, or abdominal posturing (applying pressure to the abdomen for pain relief). When their GI system is treated, the children have less pain, feel much better, and consequently have improved behaviors. There is also evidence of a strong gut-brain link in autism, in which case treating the GI disease would have a direct effect on the brain.

Treating Dysbiosis

Dysbiosis is an imbalance of the normal microflora in the GI tract and is often found in children with autism (chapter 9). It is fair to assume that this is caused by a combination of frequent oral antibiotics (especially as infants when normal microflora patterns are established), changes caused by local inflammation, and an abnormal immune system that allows harmful organisms to persist. The dysbiosis starts a vicious cycle of increased inflammation and damage to the GI mucosa, further discouraging growth of beneficial bacteria.

The injury to the bowel wall contributes to absorption issues and nutritional deficiencies. Lack of good bacteria can contribute to specific nutritional abnormalities such as vitamin K deficiency. Many of the harmful organisms that are frequent inhabitants in the bowels of autistic children (e.g. clostridium and candida) are also known to produce endotoxins that can have harmful effects locally (inflammation and damage to the mucosal surface) and systemically (throughout the body), including the brain. Re-balancing the gut flora by killing harmful organisms and then supplementing beneficial bacteria with probiotics can produce significant clinical improvement.

Probiotics

Lactic-acid bacteria, including *Lactobacilli, Bifidobacteria,* and *Enterococci,* are the most commonly used probiotic agents. *Lactobacilli* are known to produce molecules that fight pathogenic bacteria (bacteriocidins), lower the pH of the stool, and form oxidants that discourage harmful bacteria from colonizing.[12]

Saccharomyces boulardii is a harmless, antibiotic-resistant yeast that encourages growth of beneficial bacteria at the same time that it discourages growth of pathogenic (disease-causing) bacteria and yeast.[3] [4 5 6] It's also been shown that *S. boulardii* can increase the activity of digestive enzymes along the mucosal lining and enhance secretion of secretory IgA in the intestinal fluid, providing immune protection.[7] It also produces a soluble anti-inflammatory factor that inhibits the pro-inflammatory cytokine, IL-8.[8]

Studies show probiotics can shorten the duration of acute diarrhea in children,[9] eradicate *Clostridium difficile* infections that have withstood multiple courses of antibiotics,[10] prevent nosocomial (contracted in a hospital) diarrhea, and shorten the shedding of rotavirus in hospitalized children.[11] They've also been shown to improve antigen-specific and total serum IgA antibody levels in children infected by rotavirus.[12] Probiotics are useful in decreasing food-derived inflammatory markers and symptoms (including eczema) in people with lactose intolerance and milk allergies.[13 14 15 16] They can also induce and maintain remissions of IBD.[17]

Some laboratories will test stool levels of beneficial bacteria and help guide selection of the appropriate probiotic. I use probiotics to re-colonize the GI tract of any child who's been on an oral antibiotic, or who has documented dysbiosis.

Antifungals

To date there are no published, controlled studies on the use of antifungals in the treatment of autism, yet because they often bring about behavioral improvement, many physicians who specialize in treating children on the spectrum put antifungals high on the list of effective treatments. The question is unresolved as to whether the medications (fluconazole, itraconazole, ketoconazole) work by killing yeast, decreasing the levels of yeast-produced neurotoxins, or by directly affecting a metabolic pathway. Labs that test yeast-derived organic acids in the urine of autistic children often report high numbers, and it's not uncommon to see mild-to-moderate levels of yeast growth in stool culture.

These children typically respond to antifungal medications with symptomatic improvement and a decline in laboratory values, but this is often preceded by a transient worsening of behaviors thought to be caused by a "die-off" reaction. (As the yeast are being killed and their cells rupture, their neurotoxins are absorbed into the bloodstream and reach the brain.) This negative reaction usually lasts for less than a week, and is followed by significant behavioral improvement.

Anti-yeast medications that work through different mechanisms (such as nystatin) and yeast-inhibiting natural products such as caprylic acid, oil of oregano, and grapefruit seed extract can all be effective, so it seems likely that the improvement is a result of the inhibition of yeast growth. It's also possible that even if the levels of yeast in the GI tracts of autistic children are not necessarily higher than controls, autistic children are more sensitive to the neurotoxins produced by yeast because of their detoxification and metabolism issues. Based on the many positive anecdotal reports of behavioral improvement with antifungal therapy in autism, it's an area that is in great need of good clinical trials.

Antibiotics

It has been documented in the literature that children with autism often have elevated levels of potentially harmful and toxin-producing bacteria in the GI tract. The most common of these is from the Clostridium family. This bacterium is difficult to grow in the lab, so diagnosis often requires evidence of toxin in the stool or the urine. Since these are anaerobic organisms (existing in the absence of oxygen), treating them requires the use of an antibiotic that specifically targets anaerobes such as metronidazole (Flagyl).

Getting a stool culture and sensitivity report (estimates the effectiveness of particular antibiotics/antifungals against a given organism) can also guide therapy for other pathogenic organisms that might be present. In clinical practice, we often see measurable behavior and GI symptom improvement with a short course of targeted antibiotics and antifungals, which we follow with a rebalancing effort using probiotics and natural inhibitors such as herbs and *Saccharomyces boulardii.*

Changing the Diet

Some diets that are in common use in the autism community attempt to heal the gut through manipulation of foods that are thought to contribute to intestinal dysbiosis. The most popular of these originated as a treatment for inflammatory bowel disease and is called the Specific Carbohydrate Diet (SCD, designed by Elaine Gottschall, a researcher in biochemistry and cell biology).[18]

Gottschall's theory was that yeast and abnormal bacteria cause or contribute to GI inflammation and absorption problems through the overproduction of mucus, preventing contact of nutrients with the cell's absorptive surface. By starving the yeast and bacteria of complex carbohydrates (their preferred food source), the dysbiosis will be corrected and the gut will heal. SCD is limited to protein, fats, and simple carbohydrates.

Others have suggested a low sugar or a yeast-free diet. The yeast-free diet eliminates sugars, fruit (which is frequently contaminated with surface yeast), or foods like bread that incorporate yeast in the manufacturing process. The theory is that eliminating ingestion of yeast (or decreasing sugars that feed yeast) will lower their content in the bowels.

To my knowledge no controlled studies have been published evaluating these diets for treatment of autism, but there are many positive anecdotal reports.

Digestive Enzymes

Children with autism have low activity of disaccharidase enzymes (necessary to break down carbohydrates) in the digestive tract;[19] [20] abnormal function of pancreatic digestive enzyme secretion has also been documented.[21] Other research has shown that DPP-IV (diaminopeptidase IV, the enzyme that breaks down casein and gluten peptides) is frequently deficient in children with autism.[22] Low levels of amino acids have also been reported, suggesting protein maldigestion.[23]

In light of these abnormalities, it seems reasonable that treatment with digestive enzymes would be beneficial for autistic patients. I'm aware of only one unpublished pilot study that looks specifically at the use of digestive enzymes in autism.[24] In a survey of parents and teachers, significant improvements were reported in 87% of the children who remained enrolled in the study. Areas of improvement included neurological symptoms such as mood, attention, eye contact, socialization, and GI symptoms. However, over a third of the original study population dropped out before completion for reasons including "experienced adverse symptoms and/or no change in symptoms were noted," and these patients were not included in the final analysis. The study was not placebo-controlled, so based on this particular study it's difficult to make any inferences on the benefit of digestive enzymes in autism. This is another area in sore need of good clinical trials. I have many patients in my practice whose parents report improvement in both GI and neurological symptoms from using digestive enzymes. I do not feel that digestive enzymes are a substitute for appropriate dietary changes, however.

Fixing a Leaky Gut

Many factors, often occurring simultaneously, contribute to a leaky gut. Correction of the problem is also multifactorial, with the common goal to improve the function of the tight junctions between the cells. First, remove food proteins that are known to damage tight junctions—a gluten-free diet might be beneficial. Next, supplementation with omega-3 fatty acids is known to strengthen the junctions, and supplementation with the amino acid glutamine has also been shown to help. Abnormal intestinal bacteria can damage the mucosal cell layer and the tight junctions; so treating dysbiosis is critical in reversing leaky gut syndrome. Decreasing inflammation in the bowel helps to reduce damage as well.[25] Calcium and sulfate are part of the structure of the proteins in the tight junctions, and correcting deficiencies in these nutrients will improve leaky gut symptoms.[26]

Treating Constipation

Afzal and others report a high frequency of both constipation and loose stools in children with autism, suggesting a bowel motility disorder.[27] Most often the consistency of the stool is soft or mushy in spite of the fact that there are several days or even a week between stools. (A normal bowel would absorb most of the water out of the stool if it sat in the colon that long, and they would come out as hard pellets). This reflects an underlying bowel disease.

Children with autism rarely complain of pain because of difficulty with communication, and often because of unusually high pain tolerance. Abdominal discomfort usually manifests as unexplained irritability, unusual postures that apply pressure to the abdomen, self-injurious behavior, or difficulty sleeping. I believe that abnormal neurotransmitter function in the bowel also impairs normal smooth muscle function in children with autism, contributing to GI motility problems (impaired movement through the bowel, resulting in diarrhea or constipation), and creating issues with bladder emptying as well. This could explain why autistic children have a difficult time potty training.

In my practice, I encourage a daily bowel movement, often accomplished by diet changes (especially the removal of dairy), digestive enzymes, dysbiosis treatment, and nutrient support such as oral magnesium, fiber, and vitamin C. In many cases, intermittent bowel "clean-outs" are necessary, with magnesium citrate, mineral oil, senna, polyethylene glycol, bisacodyl suppositories, or sodium phosphate enemas. *The Journal of Pediatrics, Gastroenterology, and Nutrition* has published a clinical practice guideline in treating children with constipation, and although autistic children have some unique challenges based on their underlying GI and neurological disease, many of the principles are the same.[28]

Keep in mind that in children with autism, constipation might manifest as a sudden change to liquid stools. Because of fecal impaction in the colon, only loose stools can get around the blockage and be excreted. When in doubt, an abdominal X-ray can show the impaction and guide treatment.

Treating Reflux

An upper endoscopy frequently documents gastritis and esophagitis in autistic children.[29] Biopsies show a high rate of lymphocytic and eosinophilic infiltration of the mucosa, suggesting an autoimmune or allergic origin.[30][31] Symptoms of reflux in autistic children can include abdominal pain, refusal to eat, unexplained irritability, vomiting, coughing or wheezing, pounding on the chest, or frequent night-time waking. Erosions of the teeth and frequent ear infections can also be symptoms of reflux disease.[32] Treatment includes diagnosing and removing food allergens, addressing inflammatory responses, and decreasing injury to the esophageal mucosa with acid-reducers.

Treating Autistic Enterocolitis

Autistic enterocolitis has strong corollaries with classic pediatric IBDs (inflammatory bowel disease) such as Crohn's disease and ulcerative colitis; like autism, pediatric IBD prevalence is on the rise, apparently also from a combination of genetic and environmental factors. Pediatric IBD is associated with nutritional abnormalities, growth delays, and psychiatric symptoms (e.g. depression and anxiety); there is a male predominance in young children diagnosed with IBD. A correlation exists between Crohn's disease and abnormal microflora of the gut (antibiotics are often used as adjunctive therapy in pediatric IBD), and food antigens might also play a part in its development.[33]

The most essential part of treating autistic enterocolitis is making the correct diagnosis, and at this point the only accurate way to do that is through endoscopy and biopsy. Endoscopy can help to locate the disease and characterize its severity. This will modify treatment decisions. To date, there are no clinical treatment trials on the specific treatment of autistic enterocolitis, although these are forthcoming. Management of autistic enterocolitis is based on experience with Crohn's disease and ulcerative colitis in children. The medications described below are standard pediatric IBD treatment.

Medications for IBD

5-aminosalicyclic acids. 5-ASAs (sulfasalazine, mesalamine, balsalazide) are the standard first-line medications used to treat IBD. They are salicylate-based medications that are thought to have a mostly topical effect on the bowel lining (they're related to aspirin, which is acetylsalicylic acid). They're generally well tolerated and safe. One issue when using sulfasalazine for treating autistic enterocolitis is that it's known to induce depletion of folic acid.[34] Since autistic children are already folate-deficient, supplementation is critical to maintain folate status.

Corticosteroids. Corticosteroids (prednisone, prednisolone) are considered the standard for inducing clinical remission in children with moderate or severe IBD. They're inappropriate and ineffective as maintenance therapy, and long-term use is associated with many complications, including abnormal bone density, delayed growth, hypertension, cataracts, thin skin, abnormal fat deposition, and psychological effects.

Immunomodulators. Immunomodulators (6-mercaptopurine, methotrexate, azathioprine) are the primary agents used for maintenance treatment of moderate to severe IBD. They've been shown to decrease the rates of relapse and the need for corticosteroids in children with Crohn's disease. These medications are not without side effects though, including pancreatitis, bone marrow suppression, allergy, infection, and hepatitis. Methotrexate can also induce depletion of folic acid. During therapy, drug metabolites as well as organ function must be closely monitored via blood levels.

Infliximab. Infliximab (Remicade) is a TNF-α blocker that's been used for refractory (resistant to treatment) cases of Crohn's disease in children. It's associated with a high degree of clinical response but a high relapse rate, and re-treatment failures are common. Infliximab has also been associated with a higher risk of infections, including upper respiratory infections, urinary tract infections, and shingles. Reactions to the medication infusions (it's given intravenously) are seen at rates ranging from 16-38% of children. [35]

Other Therapies

Enteral nutrition. Restricting oral intake to elemental (predigested proteins) or polymeric formulas (proteins as intact polypeptides) is gaining popularity as a first-line treatment for inducing remission in children with flare-ups of IBD. It's administered via nasogastric tube or directly through a surgically inserted gastric tube. It is associated with a high degree of success in controlling the bowel symptoms, but is generally not considered for long-term treatment because of compliance and maintenance issues.[36][37][38]

Omega-3 fatty acids. Several studies show that omega-3 fatty acid supplements can successfully maintain clinical remissions in IBD. Omega-3s competitively inhibit the production of arachidonic acid, which is thought to be the primary source of inflammation.[39][40][41]

Oral IG. Schneider et al. did a pilot study using an oral preparation of human immunoglobulin on children with autism and GI disease, postulating that the anti-inflammatory properties would improve GI symptoms. (It's been effectively used in other acute and chronic GI conditions to alleviate symptoms, including rotavirus-induced diarrhea, necrotizing enterocolitis, and chronic non-specific diarrhea.) They showed a significant improvement in GI symptoms in 50% of children in their small study. There was also a positive trend in behavior improvement. The improvements did not persist after the medication was discontinued.[42] A larger clinical trial on the use of oral IG in children with autism has recently been completed, but is not available for review at the time of this writing.

chapter 18

DETOXIFICATION

TREATING THE DETOXIFICATION SYSTEM IN AUTISM INVOLVES several factors: antioxidants to prevent injury from oxidative stress, methylation cycle and transsulfuration pathway support, and removal of toxic substances.

Preventing Oxidative Stress

Oxidative metabolism is a critical and unavoidable part of biochemistry. During normal mitochondrial energy transfer, molecules called reactive oxygen species (ROS) are produced which can cause damage to both the surface and the interior of cells. The damage from ROS is called oxidative stress. Normally, the body is well equipped with antioxidants to prevent this damage. The primary antioxidant enzymes are superoxide dismutase (SOD), catalase, and GSH (glutathione) peroxidase (GPx). GSH reductase and glucose-6-phosphate dehydrogenase are secondary antioxidant enzymes. To optimize their function, these all require cofactors, including selenium, iron, copper, zinc, and manganese. Other antioxidant molecules include GSH, vitamin C, vitamin E, vitamin K, transferrin, ceruloplasmin, and carotenoids.[1]

The brain's high energy requirement and limited inherent antioxidation capacity make it particularly sensitive to oxidative stress. Since it's mainly composed of lipids (including the neuronal cell membranes and synaptic junctions), and lipids are especially vulnerable to oxidative stress, the brain is a high-risk organ. Damage to the brain's lipid membranes could be one reason why people with neurological disorders respond well to omega-3 supplementation; the major fatty acid component of the brain's cell membranes is DHA, so it can help to repair injured membranes.[2] Neurons can't manufacture GSH (it must be imported from the liver) and are therefore particularly sensitive to damage from toxins.[3]

We know that children with autism have high levels of oxidative stress; a study by Chauhan et al. showed that these children had higher levels of lipid peroxidation (an indicator of damage to lipid membranes) compared to their non-affected siblings.[4] Other studies confirm abnormally elevated oxidative stress markers in autistic patients.[5][6][7][8][9] A recent study by James et al. has shown that autistic children have significant differences in ratios of the active (reduced) form of GSH and the inactive (oxidized) form, GSSG, a measure highly indicative of oxidative stress.[10] Several studies have shown abnormal levels of other antioxidants in autism, including GPx,[11][12][13][14] GSH,[15] catalase,[16] SOD,[17][18] ceruloplasmin,[19] and transferrin.[20]

The function of the methylation cycle depends on the degree of oxidative stress in the cell. Many of the enzymes in the methylation cycle are down-regulated in response to oxidative stress, so if it's high it could be one cause of methylation issues in autistic children.[21]

Treatment of oxidative stress in autism primarily involves the use of supplemental antioxidants. Many of these, including vitamin E, vitamin C, and vitamin K, were discussed in chapter 17. It's equally essential to supply the antioxidant coenzymes such as zinc and selenium. Omega-3 supplementation can help to repair damage, and correcting methylation cycle dysfunctions will help to produce more intracellular GSH.[22]

Supporting the Detoxification Pathway

Children with autism have impaired detoxification systems. They are genetically at risk for this because of polymorphisms (common small genetic mutations) in their methylation and detoxification pathways.[23][24][25] Methylation cycle dysfunction can impact metabolic systems negatively, including the transsulfuration pathway, which is one of the main detoxification mechanisms. The building blocks of transsulfuration come from the methylation cycle, derived from homocysteine. Under conditions of oxidative stress or toxic exposure, homocysteine metabolism is shifted away from methylation and toward detoxification, at which point it's converted to cysteine in two steps, each dependent on vitamin B6 (P5P). Cysteine can then cross the cell membrane and form GSH. Or it can become taurine, sulfate, or metallothionein, depending on the need. Deficiencies in each of these molecules have been documented in children with autism.[26][27][28] Treatment consists of correcting methylation issues and supplementing transsulfuration components.

Correcting Methylation

Dr. Jill James has shown that supplementing methylation cofactors for autistic children can normalize their methylation cycle parameters, increase intracellular reduced GSH levels, and correct oxidative stress markers.[29] James used a combination of oral betaine (TMG), oral folinic acid, and methylB12 (methylcobalamin) injections in the study. Both doctors and parents who have used methylB12 injections for autistic children consistently report significant clinical improvements.[30] More formal studies on the effectiveness of methylB12 in autism are currently underway.

Cysteine

Cysteine is a sulfur-bearing amino acid that plays a critical part in many enzyme systems in the body. It also has a central role in detoxification and is one of the three components of the GSH molecule. It is the rate-limiting step in the formation of GSH. Cysteine readily crosses the blood-brain barrier and brain cell membranes. Since the brain doesn't produce GSH, it's through this active transport of cysteine and its subsequent assembly inside the cells that the stores in the neurons are maintained and the detoxification capacity supported.

Cysteine acts directly on the brain as an excitatory neurotransmitter and indirectly as an inhibitor of brain activity by inducing an analgesic affect through the opioid receptors.[31] The best way to supply cysteine in children with autism appears to be through the form of N-acetylcysteine, or as GSH. Giving cysteine itself often results in negative behaviors, possibly because of its activity as an excitatory neurotransmitter.

N-acetylcysteine (NAC)

NAC is a readily bioavailable amino acid derivative of cysteine that's used in medicine for a variety of indications. One of the most common is as an antidote for acetaminophen toxicity (chapter 11). Acetaminophen is detoxified in the liver via the transsulfuration pathway. In an overdose, the body's supply of GSH is rapidly depleted and the toxic metabolite of acetaminophen can accumulate and damage the liver. Oral or IV NAC replenishes the GSH stores and allows the remaining acetaminophen to be metabolized to a non-toxic form and excreted. Alberti et al. showed autistic children to have an impaired ability to detoxify substances such as acetaminophen via the transsulfuration pathway.[32]

NAC has been shown in other studies to protect cells against toxin-induced cell death.[33][34] One study showed that the combination of NAC and DMSA (a chelating agent) can restore the biochemical profiles altered by lead toxicity more rapidly than with DMSA alone.[35] NAC has also been shown to effectively chelate mercury, cadmium, boron, and arsenic.[36] Abnormal transsulfuration could be at least part of the reason that autistic children have lower detoxification capacity and seem to be at particular risk of heavy metal injury.

Besides detoxification, NAC might be applicable as an anti-inflammatory agent, in that it's been shown to suppress several proinflamma-tory cytokine pathways.[37] In addition, NAC is now understood to be protective against glutamate toxicity in the brain, and to prevent gluta-mate release at the synaptic junctions of neurons. Glutamate receptor function is evidently abnormal in the brains of autistic patients (chapter 13), predisposing them to neurotoxicity related to this excitatory imbal-ance, so NAC might be addressing this issue as well. Studies done on the use of NAC in obsessive-compulsive disorders have shown benefit from its supplementation.[38]

Glutathione

Glutathione (GSH) is the most important molecule for the detoxifi-cation and elimination of environmental toxins.[39] It's the major extracel-lular and intracellular antioxidant, manufactured primarily in the liver and exported from there to other body tissues. It's composed of three amino acids (cysteine, glutamate, and glycine), but to pass through the cell membrane it usually needs to be disassembled into its constituent parts and then reassembled from intracellular components—although there is some evidence that there are specific transporters of intact GSH on cell membranes in some tissues.[40] Children with autism have low intracellular and plasma levels of GSH and benefit from supplementa-tion,[41] but the question remains as to what the best method of supplying GSH to the cells and tissues might be. We don't know for sure if it's better to supply its precursors through improved methylation function and NAC supplementation, or even if the GSH molecule given exog-enously can improve levels in the cells, particularly the brain.

Although the importance of GSH in disease processes is well char-acterized in the medical literature, surprisingly few studies have been done examining direct GSH supplementation, and none of these have involved autistic children. It's been used in nebulized (inhaled) form for diseases such as cystic fibrosis, [42][43] idiopathic pulmonary fibrosis,[44] HIV,[45] and asthma.[46] These studies showed improvement in GSH levels in the lung tissues and bronchial fluid, resulting in clinical improvement to the patients, but there was no apparent absorption into the bloodstream. One study on the inhaled form documented a decrease in oxidative-stress-induced injury to lung tissues and increased intracellular GSH concentrations in lung epithelial cells. This suggests that there is either an active transport of the GSH molecule across the cell membrane, or intracellular levels are increased from a greater supply of cysteine to the cell.[47]

GSH via nasal spray has been used in the treatment of chronic otitis media or effusion (excess pleural fluid) in children with positive results, with application required every three to four hours to maintain mucosal concentrations.[48] Studies on rodents show that oral GSH raised both plasma and tissue concentrations. On the same rodents, supplying oral forms of amino acid precursors of GSH (cysteine, glutamine, and glycine) had no effect on GSH tissue concentrations.[49][50][51] IV GSH has been beneficial in diseases such as chronic hepatitis C infection,[52] peripheral vascular disease,[53] and during liver transplantation,[54] and it has been shown in one pilot study to improve symptoms of patients with Parkinson's disease to a similar or greater extent than dopaminergic medications.[55]

Many doctors in the US are using various forms of GSH (IV, oral, and transdermal) on autistic patients, reporting positive improvements in neurological function. It's often reported that the best improvements are from IV GSH; it can result in hyperactivity or irritability when given orally.

Supplying Sulfate

Sulfation is the process of attaching a sulfate group (-SO4) to an existing molecule, changing its solubility and its metabolism. This is done by enzymes called sulphotransferases. When a sulfate molecule is attached to a substance, it creates a water-soluble sulfate salt that is readily excreted; sulfation is therefore an important detoxification process. Sulfate in the gut is part of the body's first line of defense, neutralizing various substances before they can be absorbed. For example, by modifying the structure of phenolic compounds derived from food, sulfate can prevent them from acting as false neurotransmitters.

Sulfate bonds form the tight junctions between mucosal cells in the GI tract, denying bloodstream entry to unwanted molecules. Sulfate takes part in the function of digestive enzymes, particularly gastrin and cholecystokinin (CCK). CCK stimulates secretin release, and their combination signals a release of other digestive enzymes from the pancreas.[56] (Abnormal secretin stimulation is documented in children with autism.[57]) Sulfation is part of the metabolism of many endogenous (produced in the body) substances including steroids (DHEA, progesterone), bile salts, and catecholamine neurotransmitters like dopamine and epinephrine.

The metabolism of cysteine is the largest source of sulfate with an estimated 20% or less coming from dietary sources. Increasing oral supplementation of sulfate (as with magnesium sulfate) generally results in diarrhea or GI distress. Sulfate metabolism is molybdenum-dependent, so a deficiency in this mineral could contribute to low sulfate levels.[58]

Children with autism have abnormally low plasma sulfate levels.[59] Abnormalities in the methylation cycle and transsulfuration pathway are the most likely cause, but it might be partially due to excessive wasting from the kidneys, where sulfate retention is dependent on adequate levels of sulfated molecules in the renal tubules. A deficiency can induce further sulfate wasting in the urine, starting a vicious cycle of depletion. Waring et al. found that in addition to high sulfate levels in the urine of autistic children (in spite of low plasma levels), there were high amounts of total urinary protein. This suggests a possible kidney injury leading to an inability to retain protein.[60]

Waring et al. have also shown decreased phenylsulphotransferase (PST) activity in children with autism.[61] PST is how food-derived phenolic amines are metabolized (chapter 10), and foods that are high in phenolic compounds (bananas, chocolate, cheese, apples, grapes, and tomatoes) can create abnormal behaviors in autistic children. This is of particular clinical interest because PST is the same substance whereby neurotransmitter amines (such as dopamine and epinephrine) are metabolized and excess levels are removed from the brain.[62][63]

In summary, abnormal sulfation has the strong potential of causing or contributing to many abnormalities commonly seen in autism, including leaky gut syndrome, detoxification abnormalities, and neurotransmitter dysfunction.

Because of the poor tolerance of sulfate given orally, most physicians treating this issue in autism supply sulfate transdermally, either through a cream (usually magnesium sulfate or zinc sulfate) or baths (Epsom salts).

Alpha Lipoic Acid

Lipoic acid is an essential cofactor for metabolism and a potent antioxidant. It has two sulfate bonds in its structure and looks very much like DMSA (see below). It's been used as a chelating agent in autism and other diseases, but when given orally it induces yeast overgrowth with subsequent negative behaviors in autistic children and should be used with caution. Transdermal preparations might bypass this negative effect.[64]

Removing Toxins
Lowering the Total Toxic Burden

As our worldwide environment becomes more toxic, it's increasingly difficult to eliminate exposures completely, but some simple things can be done: avoid thimerosal (mercury)-containing vaccines; don't eat fish (especially long-lived species that are high on the food chain); avoid or remove mercury-containing dental amalgams; have your house checked for lead, mold, and other toxins; drink filtered water; avoid antimony-containing fire retardants; eat organic food; avoid contact with arsenic-treated wood; avoid exposure to organopesticides, and use chemical-free cleaning products. The identification and treatment of the many environmental toxins are beyond the scope of this book.[65]

Chelation

We're exposed to heavy metals with known toxic profiles in the environment, including lead, mercury, antimony, arsenic, cadmium, aluminum, tin, chromium, nickel, and platinum. Heavy metals disrupt biochemical pathways such as the methylation cycle. They're also pro-oxidants (increase oxidative stress), trigger autoimmune reactions, and can otherwise alter the immune system. They can cause direct injury to sensitive cells in the brain and in the GI tract and disrupt neurotransmitter function. Studies show autistic children have particular difficulty metabolizing heavy metals.

The level of metal exposure considered "safe" is still unknown and is clearly different for different metals and different individuals at different ages. In the case of lead, neurotoxic injury has been proven at levels once considered safe.[66][67] Lead toxicity was once considered a medical issue only at blood levels above 60 ug/dl. Lanphear et al. did a meta-analysis of studies that compared blood levels of lead and lowering of IQ scores in pediatric patients. They found the effect on IQ was evident even in children with levels less than 10 ug/dl. In fact, the relative change in IQ scores was much higher in children with levels between 1 ug/dl and 7.5 ug/dl when compared to the change at higher lead exposures. In other words, the greater damage seems to happen early in lead exposure, and there is no truly safe level of lead. It's worth noting that this critical information was gathered well after the decrease of lead concentrations in the environment had begun, thanks to environmental protection mandates.[68]

How long will it take for us to pay attention to mercury and its effects on developing brains in low-level chronic exposures? Mercury is known to be more neurotoxic than lead, and its presence in the environment is on the rise. I'm afraid that we are inadvertently using our children as our "canary in the coal mine." Because of their developing brains and immune systems, they are the most susceptible to the effects of heavy metal and other toxins. The current CDC announcement of neurodevelopmental disorders in one of six American children should suggest to us that we are not doing a very good job of protecting them.

Because of the particular danger of heavy metal toxicity to autistic children, many physicians are exploring detoxification methods, resulting in anecdotal reports of neurological improvements from all over the US and elsewhere. The most common is the use of chelators with strong binding sites (usually composed of sulfate bonds) for heavy metals; a non-toxic complex of the chelator and the metal is formed. Chelation extracts heavy metals from the tissues, making them water-soluble so they can be excreted in the urine or stool. It has been in use for decades to treat both acute and chronic heavy metal poisoning cases. Lately it has become a popular integrative medicine modality to treat illnesses ranging from autism to coronary artery disease. At the time of this writing, thousands of autistic children have been chelated by various means, and anecdotal reports are favorable. To date, no controlled trials of chelation in autistic children have been published. One study on the use of DMSA in treating children with autism is currently underway, and another is to begin soon. It will be interesting to see if the results of these studies match the encouraging reports given by parents and by the physicians who use this treatment as part of the regimen for ASD (see ARI's parent ratings, appendix).

Many kinds of chelators have been used in medicine, each with different binding properties and side effect profiles. I'll discuss the three most commonly used in autism treatment. For further information about other chelators and other heavy metals, I refer you to an excellent review article by Blanusa and colleagues.[69]

DMSA (dimercaptosuccinic acid) is a less toxic derivative of dimercaprol (BAL), the original chelator used for lead toxicity. It's water-soluble and bioavailable if given orally (gastrointestinal absorption is variable but usually around 20%). It's effective against mercury and lead in particular, but also against arsenic, copper, antimony, and nickel. It has low toxicity and side effects are mild and transient; it was FDA approved in 1991 for the treatment of lead toxicity in children. The most common adverse effects are GI complaints such as abdominal cramps, diarrhea, nausea, and vomiting. Other side effects include a transient and reversible increase in liver function markers, various dermatologic symptoms (such as a rash, itching, hives, and sores), neurological symptoms (drowsiness, dizziness, neuropathies, headaches, tingling), and musculoskeletal symptoms (rib pain, back pain, leg pain). Blood abnormalities such as lowered neutrophils, anemia, increased platelets, or increased eosinophils are rarely reported. Studies have shown that DMSA doubles the excretion of zinc but has no effect on calcium, magnesium, and iron excretion, so adequate zinc supplementation must be given with any protocol using DMSA. There is no evidence that it can enter the cells at physiological pH.[70 71 72 73 74] There is research evidence that DMSA can remove lead and organic mercury from the brains of rodent animal models.[75 76 77]

DMPS (2,3-dimercaptopropane-1-sulphonic acid) is the most effective chelator for mercury; it's also effective against arsenic, copper, lead, and bismuth.[78] Pediatric dosing hasn't been established, nor is it FDA approved, but is approved for arsenic poisoning in China, and mercury and lead poisoning in Germany. It's generally well tolerated; the most frequent side effects include headache, fatigue, nausea, taste impairment, pruritis (itching), and rash. It can be given orally, IV, or as a suppository.

EDTA (Ethylenediaminetetraacetic acid) is primarily used as a lead chelator, and is also an effective chelator of aluminum and nickel;[79 80 81] it does not chelate mercury. EDTA has low gastrointestinal absorption and is commonly given IV. It binds with calcium and can induce a rapid decrease in serum calcium, so it's generally given as a calcium-disodium complex. Disodium EDTA (without calcium) has caused deaths due to irreversible hypocalcemia resulting in cardiac arrest.[82] It can also cause nephrotoxicity (kidney damage), which is usually reversible with cessation of the drug. Other adverse effects include headache, fatigue, fever, muscle aches, increased urination, liver injury, electrocardiogram changes, and GI symptoms. EDTA effectively removes lead from bones

(bones comprise 70% of lead stores in the body), resulting in a rise of soft-tissue concentrations that suggest the lead is redistributed from the bones to other organs and tissues. It is therefore recommended that EDTA be immediately followed by another chelator such as DMSA to "clean up" the unbound lead. EDTA is strongly associated with zinc depletion, so adequate zinc supplementation must be ensured.

Although currently chelation is widely used in the treatment of autistic children, many questions remain. The most important is, does it help? Although it has clearly been shown that tissue levels of heavy metals are decreased with the use of chelators, does this result in neurological improvements? Studies on chelation therapy in asymptomatic neurotypical children with moderate levels of lead in their blood have not documented changes in long-term neurological outcomes.[83 84 85 86] Despite this lack of documentation, the standard of care in cases of symptomatic lead toxicity is chelation therapy. Since it can be argued that autistic children are demonstrating neurological and immunological symptoms as a result of low-level, intermittent heavy metal exposures, carefully administered chelation therapy seems indicated.

A study done on lead-exposed rats showed that the use of DMSA chelation positively correlated with significant improvements in learning, attention, and arousal regulation, and a decrease of both blood and brain levels of lead in the animals that were exposed to low, moderate, and high levels of lead early in development. They also found that rats who were not lead-exposed but underwent chelation at this early developmental stage sustained lasting adverse effects on behavior. The authors suggest that in light of these results, chelation of autistic children (who they claim do not have elevated tissue lead levels) is dangerous. I agree that chelation should be done only when appropriate in children (autistic or not) that have documentable elevation of heavy metals. But in contrast with their conclusion, I believe that this provides even more evidence that removing heavy metals through chelation from children with neurodevelopmental disorders is not only appropriate, but indicated. The question of DMSA causing lasting harm if there are no metals present is an important one but cannot be determined using their study design since it appears that they did not provide these animals with minerals, antioxidants, or detoxification support supplements such as glutathione. It is very likely that the negative behaviors induced by DMSA in these animals were related to depletion in one or more of these areas and could have been prevented or reversed under better controlled circumstances.[87]

Other questions concern the most appropriate agent and route of administration. When physicians first started chelating autistic children, oral DMSA was the most commonly used form. Some of these children didn't tolerate oral DMSA due to GI symptoms and dysbiosis issues, so alternatives have been explored. Transdermal preparations of DMSA and DMPS reduce GI side effects, but it's unclear how well the active ingredient is absorbed. There are many anecdotal reports of behavior improvements with transdermal preparations, but no laboratory evidence of increased excretion of heavy metals in the urine after a single challenge dose.[88] Suppository forms of DMPS and DMSA (but not EDTA) are effective in removing large amounts of metals on a challenge. Intravenous DMPS and EDTA produce a large excretion of heavy metals but require IV access, which can be troublesome for some children with autism. No clinical trials have determined one best method in terms of neurological improvements.

Diagnosing heavy metal toxicity can be a challenge, with no universal standards for determining when an individual should be chelated, or for how long. Measures of unprovoked blood and urine reflect only acute, ongoing exposure, and do not assess tissue levels or total body burden. As the Holmes study[89] points out, low levels of mercury in the hair of autistic children might, in fact, reflect an abnormal excretion capacity, i.e., retention, rather than a low body burden. A provocation challenge with a chelating agent can provide clues about immediately accessible metals in the tissues, but there are no standards established for determining what level is abnormal or harmful in the general population. Because of compartmentalization of metals in the body, single provocation challenge tests can be misleading in determining total body burden. Serial challenge tests are a better indicator of metal excretion, and inferences can then be made regarding body burden.

A recent study by Nataf et al. has documented that children with autism have abnormal urinary levels of porphyrin metabolites, which are highly suggestive of heavy metal toxicity. (Metals can disrupt normal porphyrin metabolism resulting in elevation of certain subtypes in a pattern that is fairly toxin specific.) They proposed that urinary porphyrin markers could reflect body burden of specific toxins such as mercury, lead and organophosphates based on the pattern of the metabolites.[90]

My experience and that of many other physicians treating autistic children is that children with autism improve with chelation therapy, and that it's generally safe and well tolerated if done under appropriate medical supervision with mineral supplementation and monitoring of potential side effects. Chelation is promising, but needs to be further explored with quality research.

chapter 19

TREATING THE IMMUNE SYSTEM

CHILDREN WITH AUTISM HAVE DYSREGULATED, IMBALANCED immune systems that are prone to inflammation and autoimmune reactions, and inefficient at dealing with infections. These immune abnormalities are probably multifactorial, a combination of genetic susceptibilities and environmental exposures.

I divide therapies into three sections when addressing immune issues: supporting the immune system, removing immunological triggers, and breaking the inflammatory cycle. I believe this combined approach is required if we're going to truly correct the immune dysfunction.

Immune System Support

Reversing Nutritional Deficiencies

Many of the nutrients in chapter 16 are active in the immune system, especially vitamin A, vitamin C, zinc, and omega-3 fatty acids. Adequate levels of these nutrients are imperative if the immune system is to ever work correctly.

Colostrum

Colostrum is the thin fluid that comes from the breast three or four days before real milk production; it contains important immune factors that enable the newborn baby to handle the onslaught of exposures that confront it soon after birth. It contains immunoglobulins, antibodies, and other antiviral factors, and it also has glycoproteins that prevent attachment of unwanted bacteria to the baby's intestinal wall. It includes cytokines such as IL-10 that inhibit inflammation, and growth factors like TGF-β that promote cell growth and maturation of lymph and immune organs.[1]

Since colostrum is so important for newborn immune systems, it has been tried as a supplement to enhance immune function in diseases like multiple sclerosis and Alzheimer's disease, with some positive effects reported.[2][3][4] Most commercial colostrum supplements are from cows, but since many of the immune factors are similar to those in humans, it's thought to be useful. Note that when choosing a colostrum supplier for autism treatment, it's important to ensure that casein was removed.

Transfer Factor

Transfer factor is a small molecule produced by leukocytes (white blood cells) that is capable of transferring information about specific antigens to other cells in the immune system. It's been used in a number of diseases, ranging from viral infections to autoimmune reactions.[5][6][7][8] Fudenberg et al. did a study on giving autistic children transfer factor derived from the leukocytes of their parents. They reported that the majority showed significant improvements in behavior, decreased food sensitivities, decreased levels of rubella antibodies (excessively high to start with), and decreased candida (yeast) colonization.[9] Another study by Stubbs, et al. demonstrated clinical improvement in a child with autism caused by congenital cytomegalovirus infection.[10]

I've used commercially available transfer factor supplements that aren't human-derived with some of my patients, and it seems to help decrease the frequency of infections, but I haven't found any published studies on their use in autism.

IVIG

Human-derived IVIG (intravenous immunoglobulin) therapy improves immune function by giving the patient more antibodies to fight infection (passive immunity). It's also used to decrease autoimmune responses. Currently approved by the FDA for the treatment of congenital and acquired immune deficiencies, idiopathic thrombocytic purpura, and chronic leukocytic leukemia, it's been used for a variety of other autoimmune and neurological illnesses, including Guillain-Barre syndrome, multiple sclerosis, Kawasaki disease, chronic inflammatory demyelinating polyneuropathy, dermatomyositis, and multifocal motor neuropathy. It is thought to work by modulation of T and B cell function, by signaling immune cell receptors, and by activating the complement system. It's believed to decrease autoimmune reactions by providing regulatory antibodies.[11][12][13][14]

IVIG therapy is usually well tolerated. Side effects occur in less than 5% of study subjects (non-autistic), and include headaches, chills, nausea, fatigue, muscle aches, joint aches, back pain, and hypertension in individuals at risk. Because it's a human blood-derived product, there is a risk of transmitting blood-borne diseases such as HIV and hepatitis C, but this is extremely unlikely because of strict donor-screening methods and blood filtering techniques.[15] High cost, inconvenience (IV must be infused over several hours), and invasiveness limit its application for patients with autism.

Dr. Sudhir Gupta and colleagues at UC Irvine published an uncontrolled pilot study on the use of IVIG in ten children with autism who had either an immunoglobulin deficiency, evidence of autoimmunity, or suggestion of an infection-triggered regression. The children were given IV treatments of 400 mg/kg every four weeks for a minimum of six months. They showed variable improvements in areas of speech, social behavior, and eye contact, results that were based only on clinical impression and not validated by standard behavioral measurements. One child almost completely recovered speech during the trial period. In some of the patients, improvements reversed with discontinuation of the therapy. Although the children in this study had abnormal immune profiles in the initial blood evaluation, it was not reported if those profiles changed after treatment.[16]

Two other small studies had mixed results. A pilot study on five children by Delguidice-Asch et al. did not see any measurable difference in patients receiving IVIG over a six-month period.[17] A study by Plioplys on ten autistic children reported five with no improvement, four with mild improvement (not deemed sufficient to warrant further treatment) and one child with significant improvement who reverted back to baseline after IVIG was discontinued. There were no distinguishing laboratory or historical features in the child who responded favorably.[18]

A 2006 study by Boris et al. was done on twenty-seven autistic children given IVIG monthly over a six-month trial period. They reported a significant improvement (37%) in total aberrant behaviors (hyperactivity, inappropriate speech, lethargy, stereotypy) soon after receiving the first dose of IVIG. There was a gradual further decrease in the scores over the remaining five months of the trial, but the majority of the children regressed again two to four months after discontinuing the treatments.[19] These studies suggest that there's a subgroup of autistic children that respond to IVIG therapy, but the gains generally do not persist after the therapy is discontinued. Larger studies need to be done to determine if there is any long-term value in this treatment for children with autism.

Removing Immune Triggers

Removing Pathogenic Organisms

The presence of pathogens triggers an inflammatory reaction, followed by a mobilization of immune system resources, all joined in the effort to get rid of the offending organism. When the immune system function is abnormal, the immune response can be excessive and can persist long after the original trigger is gone. It's thought that autoimmune diseases including multiple sclerosis, Kawasaki disease, and Guillain-Barre syndrome are triggered by an infection.

Another example of a neurological disease triggered by an infectious agent is Pediatric Autoimmune Neuropsychiatric Disorder Associated with Streptococcus infection, or PANDAS syndrome. PANDAS is an autoimmune reaction to Group A streptococcus (the cause of strep throat), and is associated with a sudden increase in obsessive-compulsive behaviors, attention problems, and motor tics in children.[20][21][22] The treatment can be problematic because symptoms are caused by the abnormal immune response, and might persist even after the bacteria are gone. The treatment of the disease involves removing any remaining bacteria with antibiotics and treating the autoimmune response with IVIG or therapeutic plasma exchange. Although PANDAS is not specific to autism, sudden onset or worsening of OCD behaviors and tics is not uncommon in autistic children. I've seen many autistic children who fit this profile who have tested high for strep antibodies and have responded to treatment for PANDAS.

Autistic children have many organisms in their bowels—yeast, bacteria, and parasites—that can trigger inflammatory reactions. Treating these organisms is important if we're going to lower the inflammatory burden in the gut and prevent neurological effects from the toxins that they produce.

There is also evidence that some children with autism have persistence of immune- and neuroactive viruses, including measles, rubella, herpes, varicella (chicken pox), and cytomegalovirus, which were unsuccessfully dealt with on initial exposure and might have persisted to a chronic state. The presence of measles virus has been confirmed in the bowels and in the CSF of autistic children.[23][24]

Anecdotally, many autistic children have responded to anti-herpes virus medications such as valacyclovir hydrochloride (Valtrex); Epstein-Barr virus, varicella, and cytomegalovirus are also members of the herpes family. Although elevated IgG antibodies to viruses are common in autistic children, it's rare to see elevated IgM antibodies, indicating an acute infection. There is no evidence showing that valacyclovir is capable of treating a latent or non-replicating virus,[25] so in children who respond it's unclear whether it is because of suppression of active viruses or because the drug works directly on biochemical pathways in another way. It's most likely that valacyclovir is acting on the adenosine metabolism pathway, known to be abnormal in some children with autism.[26]

Unfortunately we still don't have an effective antiviral therapy specific to measles. Treatment involves supporting immune function to increase anti-viral activity, such as the use of vitamin A to decrease secondary inflammation.

Treating IgE-Mediated Allergies

Many of us produce excess levels of IgE antibodies in response to environmental allergens in foods, medicines, and environmental inhalants. These antibodies trigger immune cascade events that are designed to remove the noxious particle, but that sometimes go too far. The result is an immediate hypersensitive response, with the IgE antibodies signaling histamine release from the mast cells that are concentrated in mucosal tissues. Histamine causes what most of us recognize as allergy symptoms, including sneezing, runny nose, itching, hives, watery eyes, and nasal congestion. In a severe IgE-mediated allergy, there can be sudden life-threatening swelling of mucosal tissues in the airway, bronchoconstriction (narrowing of the air passages in the lung), a drop in blood pressure, and shock from lack of blood flow to vital organs (anaphylaxis). Triggers can be anything from food to bee stings to medications. This is a rare event, but the incidence is on the rise for reasons not yet explained by mainstream medicine.

Autistic children can have IgE-mediated allergies as part of their immune dysregulation syndrome. The first step in treatment is to remove the triggers from the environment, if possible. This might require air filters, or removing certain clothes, bedding, carpets, pets, or foods, and sometimes changing location.[27 28 29]

After reducing environmental triggers, I treat with medications that help to stabilize mast cells and decrease the production or the effects of histamine on the tissues. Examples of these medications include montelukast (Singulair), cetirizine (Zyrtec), fexofenadine (Allegra), and cromolyn sodium (Nasalcrom). Intranasal steroid sprays such as fluticasone (Flonase) can shrink swollen mucosal tissue. Controlling allergy symptoms often results in improvement in the behavior of children with autism, presumably because they feel better, but also possibly because of a more generalized anti-inflammatory effect on the gut and the brain.

Allergy Desensitization Therapies

Many allergists use a technique called allergen-specific immunotherapy to decrease symptoms in allergy-prone individuals. The idea is to increase immune tolerance to a particular allergen by exposing the patient to slowly increasing doses of the reactive substance. By making the substance less foreign to the immune system at smaller doses than what would trigger an inflammatory response, it's hoped that the immune system will learn to tolerate the antigen's presence. Once an individualized allergen profile is created, very low doses are introduced via allergy shots, nasal sprays, or sublingual drops. It can be very effective in alleviating allergy symptoms, but the initial testing must be done with medical supervision since there's a risk of triggering a rare life-threatening anaphylactic event. [30][31][32][33][34]

Remove Food Sensitivities

IgE-mediated allergies are not the most common abnormal immune activation in autistic children—it's much more common to see elevated levels of antigen-specific IgG antibodies. There is ongoing debate among mainstream allergist/immunologists about the relative importance of this type of immune response. It is not associated with histamine release or immediate life-threatening events, so it's often dismissed or ignored. However, evidence is emerging that IgG-mediated reactions are a common cause of disease symptoms ranging from eczema to headaches to behavior changes.

When biopsies are taken during endoscopy of autistic children, we consistently see eosinophilic infiltration in the mucosal tissues of the esophagus and duodenum. Eosinophils are increased in tissues in response to allergies; in the upper GI tract, this is most likely related to food, but obvious hypersensitivity reactions from food are uncommon in autistic children. It could be that the reactions are mild, or ignored because of communication issues, or that it's mediated through non-IgE antibodies.

Elevated IgG antibodies against various food proteins are very common in autism, and removing the foods results in clinical improvements that often are evident within days; deterioration follows shortly after reintroduction. A variety of laboratories offer IgG food sensitivity tests that utilize different measuring techniques. Although not validated, I use these tests as an indirect measurement of how reactive the patient's immune system is. I also use them as a guide to begin food elimination trials, which are how we look for clinical effects from the removal or reintroduction of a given food. In the end, I think elimination trials are the most accurate measure of a true sensitivity reaction.

Breaking the Inflammatory Cycle

In a normal immune response, inflammation results from recruitment of immune cells intending to quickly localize, isolate, and destroy the invader, and then resolve just as quickly; in a dysregulated immune system, inflammation can itself trigger more inflammation. Unregulated inflammation can cause a lot of damage to local tissues and bring about many of the adverse symptoms that we see during a disease process, such as swelling, pain, redness, warmth, and discoloration of the tissues.

Turning off the inflammatory cascade is the job of certain cytokines in the immune system, and in many diseases, including autism, these messengers don't appear to be working well. In fact, more and more diseases are recognized as related to abnormal inflammation: rheumatoid arthritis, diabetes, coronary artery disease, lupus, IBD, and others. Often the original inciting trigger is no longer even present, and it's only the abnormal immune response that is causing the ongoing symptoms. When removing triggers doesn't relieve the symptoms, it's time to focus on interventions that will break this vicious inflammatory cycle.

Anti-Inflammatory Medications

Many medications are designed to decrease tissue inflammation. Some, like ibuprofen, are considered relatively benign, while others can be quite dangerous. The choice of medication involves factors such as the location and severity of the inflammation. For IBD treatment, the effects of first line anti-inflammatories such as sulfasalazine and mesalamine (Pentasa) are mostly localized to the mucosal tissues in the gut. If these medications don't work we choose ones with systemic effects, like oral steroids. Unfortunately, since anti-inflammatories are immune suppressors they can lead to risk of infection and other serious side effects. Even over-the-counter drugs such as ibuprofen can cause GI bleeding and kidney problems with prolonged use or in predisposed individuals.

Anti-inflammatories with widespread actions might be necessary in treating autism, since excess inflammation seems to involve more than one organ system. An ideal anti-inflammatory drug to use in treating autism would break the inflammatory cycle without suppressing appropriate immune system activation. It would have effects both on the GI tract and the brain. It would be well tolerated, easy to administer, inexpensive, and without significant side effects. Such a drug might not exist, but there are several candidates under investigation.

PPAR Agonists

Peroxisome proliferator-activated receptors (PPAR) are hormone receptors on cell nuclei thought to be responsible for cell differentiation and gene transcription. A class of drugs called TZDs (thiazolidinediones) are PPAR-agonists, and include pioglitazone (Actos) and rosiglitazone (Avandia). These drugs are primarily used in patients with type-II diabetes mellitus because they make cells more sensitive to insulin. They also have anti-inflammatory effects (inhibit T-cell proliferation, block cytokine production, and induce apoptosis) on multiple cell types, and have been used in diseases such as atherosclerosis and IBD.[35][36]

PPAR-agonists block an intracellular signaling molecule called NFKB (nuclear factor kappa B), an important regulator of the inflammatory response.[37][38] NFKB is a particularly important regulator in brain astrocytes, which are known to be abnormally activated in autism.[39] It can be triggered in response to cytokines (such as TNF-α and IL-1), viral infections (e.g., HIV and measles), oxidative stress, and excitatory neurotransmitters. It's also a regulator of cell differentiation, proliferation, tumor growth, and cell death.[40] TZDs have been shown to reduce the activation of brain glial cells and stimulate them to increase the uptake of glucose, as well as to increase lactate production and improve mitochondrial functioning. These drugs are on trial in patients with multiple sclerosis[41][42][43] and Alzheimer's,[44][45] based on positive effects in animal trials. The beneficial immunological and neurological effects suggest that children with autism could also benefit from their use.

A pilot study by Boris et al. on the use of pioglitazone in twenty-five autistic patients has been submitted for publication at the time of this writing. Of the patients in the study, 76% responded with more than a 50% improvement in at least one of the five subgroup categories of the Aberrant Behavior Checklist. 56% responded with a better than 50% improvement in two subgroups and 40% responded at that level in three or more. There were no changes in blood analyses for insulin, glucose, or liver function, and no other significant side effects were reported.[46]

In October 2006, the same research group reported that they have now used pioglitazone in over seven hundred fifty autistic children, with improvement in behaviors and GI symptoms. In this group of children, side effects were as follows: hyperactivity (5%), periorbital edema (swelling around the eyes) (2.5%), and weight gain (9%). Mild change in CBC and/or liver function parameters was seen in 1%, and there were no incidents of hypoglycemia or hyperinsulinemia.[47] The safety and efficacy of pioglitazone has also been demonstrated in patients, including children, with other conditions.

Spironolactone

Spironolactone is a drug that's been in use for many years as a potassium-sparing diuretic and an aldosterone inhibitor. Because of its potent anti-inflammatory and immunomodulatory properties, it might be useful in autism. It also has inhibitory effects on the androgen (male hormone) pathways, which is interesting in light of findings suggesting that autistic children have elevated testosterone or DHEA (dehydroepiandrosterone) levels.[48 49 50]

Spironolactone is inexpensive and has a good safety profile in both children and adults. Studies show that it can markedly reduce TNF-α, MCP-1, and IFN-γ cytokines, all of which are elevated in autistic individuals. It's been used in juvenile rheumatoid arthritis, type 2 diabetes, hirsutism (excessive body hair growth), acne, and precocious puberty in both prepubertal boys and girls, with no significant side effects after long-term treatment. In a case report by Bradstreet et al., a 12-year old boy treated with spironolactone showed significant behavioral improvements, including reduction in irritability, lethargy, hyperactivity, and inappropriate speech. There was a twenty-one month gain in receptive language over a four-week period after starting the medication.[51]

Low-Dose Naltrexone (LDN)

Naltrexone, an opiate-blocking agent, has been extensively studied as a treatment for autism. These studies showed modest improvements in neurological functions, particularly in decreasing self-injurious behavior. The mechanism proposed by most authors was that the medication acts on the brain to prevent excess production or to block the effects of opiates that prevent normal neurotransmitter function.[52]

More recently, a new indication for the use of naltrexone in autism has been discovered. A paper by Agrawal et al. suggested that low-dose naltrexone (LDN) helped patients with multiple sclerosis by reducing levels of nitric oxide in the brain, preventing excitotoxic damage to the brain immune cells (oligodendrocytes).[53] It has been proposed elsewhere that the anti-inflammatory properties of the drug are the reason for improvement in autistic children.[54] Scifo et al. showed reduction in autistic behaviors in seven out of twelve autistic children in a study using LDN. They also saw normalization of the CD4/CD8 ratio (increase in CD4 helper cells and decrease in CD8 suppressor cells).[55]

Endogenous opiates are known to act on the immune system to stimulate cytokine production. It's theorized that in very low doses, naltrexone stimulates endogenous opiate production, which might be responsible for the immune effects that are seen. The true clinical utility of LDN on the immune system in autistic patients is still unknown because there are no large-scale, well-controlled studies. Many autistic children in the US are using a transdermal application (topical cream) of LDN and anecdotal reports are mostly positive, but it can induce some negative behaviors in other children. There is no evidence of any long-term or serious side effects.

chapter 20

TREATING THE BRAIN

THE PURPOSE OF THIS BOOK IS TO CLARIFY AUTISM AS A multi-system metabolic disease, not just a brain disorder. Interactions among the brain, the gut, and the immune system are intricate, and these systems are extremely sensitive to oxidative stress, damage from toxic substances, and uncontrolled inflammation. Traditional teaching—that autism is a result of brain injury that occurs in utero—presumes that any and all other symptoms are secondary. A thorough review of the published medical literature on autism reveals that this theory is antiquated and in need of revision. In light of rapidly increasing incidence and the rising percentage of children with the regressive form of the disorder, it seems ever more likely that it's the brain injury that is secondary. My own experience in treating children with this disease confirms this suspicion. Rather than focusing on "treating" the brain with various psychoactive medications (putting a Band-Aid on the problem), physicians who are approaching autism as a multi-system disease are having real success in reversing the disease process. Because of the complex interactions among the systems involved, treating the gut and the immune system is treating the brain. Detoxification is important for the neurological system. Providing basic nutrients is critical to brain function. *Stopping abnormal inflammation can help heal the brain.*

In this chapter, I focus on interventions that directly affect the brain and nervous system. And even here, we find evidence of the effects of these treatments reaching systems beyond the boundaries of the brain and nervous system.

Removing False Neurotransmitters and Neurotoxins

Diet-Derived Peptides

Molecules and proteins from food act on the brain. The opiate-like peptides found in foods that contain gluten and casein are particularly relevant to autism. A peptide is a particle of food protein that would normally be digested in the GI tract before being absorbed into the bloodstream. If digestive enzymes are abnormal and the gut lining is injured, peptides that normally would not be allowed can cross over into the bloodstream, i.e., leaky gut. Gluten and casein peptides can attach to opiate receptors in the brain and in the body. Opiates act as both neurotransmitters and immunomodulators. Exogenous opiates can interfere with our natural endogenous opiate (endorphin) function, changing the balance of neurotransmitters. Examples of other exogenous opiates are morphine, heroin, and other narcotics. Obviously these drugs have neurological effects and are addictive, but they also affect bowel function (slow motility) and weaken the immune system. Although food-derived opiates are not as strong as these drugs, the biochemical effects are similar, including how they make people feel.

An association between gluten and casein in the diet and autistic behavior in children was first recognized in the medical literature in 1980.[1] As with many new observations on autism, it was brought to scientific attention by parents of affected children. Since then, many studies have documented high levels of gluten- and casein-derived opioid peptides in children with autism, as well as clinical improvement in behavior after the removal of these foods. Each of these studies has some methodological flaws that preclude them from being considered definitive.[2] But in light of the positive clinical reports from doctors (including me) who are regularly prescribing this diet, as well as from parents, a clinical trial is warranted.

My experience has been that a trial of a strict GF/CF (gluten- and casein-free) diet for a minimum of several months is an important early intervention in the treatment of the disease. It's not uncommon to see immediate and obvious improvement in eye contact, attention, focus, behaviors, language, sleep, and bowel function. I also frequently see an immediate decrease in upper respiratory infections, sinusitis, ear infections, and eczema.

Because opiates are addictive, children with autism frequently self-limit their diet to foods that contain these proteins, or they binge on these particular foods and become very irritated and anxious if they don't have immediate access to them. Not unexpectedly, the improvements from eliminating them are often preceded by a short-lived behavioral regression, likely from symptoms of opiate withdrawal—and probably not dissimilar to how an addict feels coming off drugs.

Other foods can affect behavior in children. We discussed in chapter 18 how foods high in phenols can lead to negative behaviors in autism because of the decreased ability of the phenolsulfotransferase enzyme system that metabolizes the molecule. Phenol can then act as an excitatory false transmitter in the brain, so foods with a high content need to be guarded against. Avoiding food products that are high in chemicals and artificial colors is also important. These chemicals can be difficult to metabolize and could cause problems in children with weakened detoxification systems. Children with autism should eat an organic diet. In addition to having fewer chemicals, organic foods have higher nutrient value per gram compared to non-organic foods.

Treating Gut Dysbiosis

Dysbiosis has been discussed in detail in other chapters, but I want to stress that there is clear evidence that abnormal pathogens in the bowel can affect the brain. Many of these organisms produce neurotoxins as part of their normal metabolic waste, and these byproducts can affect neurotransmitter function. I frequently see immediate neurological improvements and decreased autistic behavior when the bowel flora is corrected.

Removing Toxic Substances

There is nothing controversial or new about the statement that substances such as lead, mercury, and organophosphates have negative impacts on brain function. Because of high lipid content (many toxins are fat soluble), poor internal antioxidation capacity, and dependence on other organs to provide nutrients and detoxification support, the brain is particularly sensitive to the damaging effects of environmental toxins. Every effort must be made to prevent exposure and to remove toxins from the body.

Modulating Neurotransmitters

The nervous system is the communication center of the body. It talks with the other organs through chemical messengers called neurotransmitters. The production, recycling, distribution, and then destruction and disposal of these neurotransmitters are all a required part of normal neurological functioning; in autism this process is disrupted, so that some neurotransmitters are found in high amounts and others are low. It seems that, very much like the disarray in the immune system, it's a problem of dysregulation rather than dysfunction. Correcting neurotransmitter issues can be very complex, and starts with addressing the problems that create the dysregulation in the first place.

Most of the psychoactive medications used in mainstream medicine change the balance of neurotransmitters in the brain, but without correcting underlying issues, they're unlikely to produce long-term improvements. I don't use them very often in my practice, but reserve them for instances when behaviors are dangerous or severely disruptive, and then only as a temporary measure. For those who are interested in learning more about these medications, I refer you to a review article by King et al.[3]

DMG (Dimethylglycine)

Present in food in small amounts, DMG is a molecule that acts as a methyl donor and has antioxidant properties.[4] It's closely related to the inhibitory neurotransmitter glycine, and is thought to be able to cross over the blood-brain barrier. Its potential action as a neurotransmitter is based on the fact that there is a binding site for glycine on the NMDA (N-methyl-D-aspartate) receptors on brain cells. The NMDA receptor is a type of glutamate receptor that controls entrance of calcium into the cells and has a role in the neuronal development of the embryonic nervous system, the formation of memory, and in mood maintenance.

It's hypothesized that DMG might play a regulatory role in the excitatory/inhibitory balance of neurotransmitters in the brain.[5] There have been a lot of anecdotal reports of DMG's benefit in treating autistic children.[6] Large-scale studies on the use of DMG with autism are lacking; Bolman et al. did a small trial of eight autistic patients on low doses of DMG and found no consistent beneficial effect. (It's worth noting their study was limited by small sample size, a wide range of ages and symptom severity, and low doses of DMG.)[7] Kern et al. did a larger trial of DMG in thirty-three autistic children and found that although there were positive benefits from DMG in some children, they were scattered effects, and didn't attain overall statistical significance when compared with placebo.[8]

My clinical experience with DMG is similar; some children definitely seem to respond with improvement in attention and language, while others seem to become distracted or hyperactive. However, since it seems to be safe and without significant long-term side effects, it's worth a clinical trial to see how an individual child will respond.

TMG (trimethylglycine), or betaine, acts as an alternate methyl donor to convert homocysteine to methionine in the methylation cycle.

This is a pathway secondary to the methionine synthase pathway catalyzed by methylcobalamin. After donating its methyl group, TMG becomes DMG, so betaine is one avenue of supply.

5-Hydroxytryptophan (5-HTP)

5-HTP is derived from tryptophan, an essential amino acid found in high amounts in turkey, among other foods. 5-HTP is further metabolized to serotonin, the neurotransmitter most commonly found to be abnormal in autism. 5-HTP can cross the blood-brain barrier and increase brain serotonin levels. Serotonin helps regulate sleep cycles, and is important for daytime attentiveness, mood, and bowel function. 5-HTP has been used as a therapeutic supplement in a variety of illnesses such as depression, fibromyalgia, insomnia, obesity, cerebellar ataxia, and chronic headaches.[9][10] 5-HTP is also a strong scavenger of free radicals that in at least one study had more potent antioxidant effect than vitamin C and melatonin.[11] I primarily use 5-HTP to assist children who have frequent nighttime awakenings, but have found that it can also help with attention during the day at lower doses.

Correcting Autonomic Dysfunction

Children with autism have many symptoms that can be explained as autonomic dysfunction (chapter 13), including elevated heart rate, higher than normal blood pressure, dilated pupils, anxiety, hyperactivity, constipation, and difficulty urinating. Autonomic dysfunction results from an imbalance between the two arms of the ANS, the sympathetic and the parasympathetic. In autism, there appears to be a shift toward excess sympathetic tone. It's not clear whether the problem is from too much sympathetic stimulation or not enough parasympathetic balance.

Medications targeting the ANS have been used in children with autism with some positive results. These include clonidine and guanfacine, which target the sympathetic system and are frequently used for attention deficit disorders, tics, and anxiety.[12] [13] Bethanachol is an acetylcholine (parasympathetic) analogue that's been shown to help some autistic children with bowel issues, and has improved cognition.[14] Supplying the acetylcholine precursors (choline or phosphatidylcholine) in the form of nutritional supplements is another option. As with all things related to autism, correcting ANS dysfunction will undoubtedly require a diversified approach.

Glutamate/GABA and Excitotoxicity

I briefly mentioned in chapter 16 that children with autism have elevated glutamate in the extracellular spaces in the brain. Glutamate, an amino acid that elicits an excitatory reaction in the neurons, creates cellular toxicity if too much accumulates. Neurons maintain a very high concentration gradient of calcium across their outer membrane with high extracellular calcium compared to low intracellular calcium. This is achieved by an active pumping mechanism that takes calcium out of the cell or sequesters it in particular intracellular compartments. On the cell membrane are gates that can open and allow calcium to enter the cell. Because of the high gradient across the cell membrane, calcium rushes in very rapidly when the gates open. This rapid intracellular increase in calcium (a positively charged ion) changes the electrical potential inside the cell and sets off a cascade of events resulting in a particular action by the cell, which in this case is neuronal firing, i.e., the active burst of the cell's potential. The calcium is then rapidly transported out of the cell and the whole process resets. Calcium, therefore, is the primary signal for neuronal cell function.

If the calcium signaling mechanism goes awry, several bad things can happen. One is that the cell is not able to reset and perform its function the next time. Another is that the cell continues to fire inappropriately. A third is that the cell is injured or killed because of the toxic effect of calcium remaining in the intracellular space. As mentioned in chapter 16, the NMDA receptor is one of the calcium channels in the cell membrane and is regulated by both glutamate and GABA. Glutamate opens the channel, and if unopposed, the channel remains open and too much intracellular calcium damages the cell. This is called excitotoxicity. GABA closes the channel and stops the cell from firing.

The glutamate-to-GABA ratio is very important, controlling the delicate balance of this calcium influx and allowing the neurons to fire only when it's appropriate. This ratio is controlled by an enzyme called GAD (glutamic acid decarboxylase), which converts glutamate directly into GABA. Anything that disrupts this enzyme could trigger an imbalance of the glutamate-to-GABA ratio and subsequently cause abnormal brain function. Vitamin B6 is an important coenzyme in the conversion of glutamate to GABA, and might be one reason why children with autism have excess glutamate. It has also been shown that thimerosal can disrupt glutamate transport systems, leading to excess extracellular glutamate.

Treatment involves supporting a normal glutamate-to-GABA ratio. For example, appropriate nutritional support of B6 and detoxification will help. Avoiding dietary sources of glutamate such as MSG (monosodium glutamate) is also important. Commercially available GABA supplements help some children, bringing about improved focus and less hyperactivity. An open-labeled study of a small group (n=18) of autistic children using Namenda (an NMDA receptor antagonist) showed modest improvement in the areas of social withdrawal and hyperactivity. Over a third of the patients reported negative side effects, including irritability, vomiting, rash, increased seizures, and excessive sedation. A much larger trial is required before any conclusions can be made regarding the efficacy and safety of this particular drug.[15]

Neurohormones

A hormone is defined as a substance, usually a peptide or steroid, produced by one tissue and conveyed by the bloodstream to another to effect physiological activity, such as growth or metabolism. Several hormones produced in the pineal gland affect the brain, and have been used in children with autism with beneficial effects.

Melatonin

Melatonin is a neurohormone derived from serotonin by methylation. One of its responsibilities it to induce sleep; supplementation is effective in treating sleep disorders in both normal and developmentally delayed subjects.[16][17] It's also a strong antioxidant, working as a free-radical scavenger and stimulating the production of other antioxidant enzymes such as glutathione peroxidase.[18][19] In addition, melatonin has beneficial effects on the immune system, the cardiovascular system, the GI system, and as a tumor-reducing agent.[20]

Sleep disturbances are commonly reported in children with autism, with a prevalence ranging from 40-80%. Not only is this very disruptive for the parents, sleep difficulties affect the child's daytime behavior. Melatonin metabolism abnormalities are one explanation for this problem, and studies on the use of melatonin to improve sleep patterns have been positive. There are no reported adverse effects or development of tolerance with supplemented melatonin, with the rare exception of daytime sleepiness, headache, or dizziness.[21]

Oxytocin

Another hormone, oxytocin, has generated interest because it's known to improve socialization and decrease fearful responses. Levels have been shown to be low in autistic children and to fail to increase during puberty, which they normally do in neurotypical children. A study published in 2006 showed mild gains in social appropriateness in autistic adults given oxytocin.[22] A case report by Bradstreet et al. showing benefit from the use of intranasal oxytocin in an autistic child has been submitted for publication at the time of this writing.

Secretin

Secretin, a gut hormone, induces secretion of pancreatic enzymes in response to pH changes in the small bowel during the digestive process. It's used in diagnostic GI procedures to assess pancreatic function. Interest in its possible use in autism arose when a mother whose child received intravenous secretin during a diagnostic procedure reported the child's sudden increase in language. This case report generated a lot of excitement in the autism community about the find of a potentially effective treatment.

Many studies followed,[23] using a number of methodologies (including double-blind, placebo-controlled trials), but most did not detect a difference between the study population and controls. In spite of these negative study results, many physicians treating autistic children report that a small subgroup of children has remarkable improvement with secretin infusions; the studies might not have been adequately designed to detect this subgroup. The studies did confirm that secretin is very safe and without significant adverse reactions.

Secretin receptors have been found in many brain regions including the cerebral cortex, the thalamus, the hypothalamus and the brainstem. The mechanism of action in autism could be from its direct neurotransmitter effect on the brain rather than through its action on the gut. One study suggests that it increases dopamine turnover in the brain, which is responsible for the improvement in symptoms.[24] Welch et al. propose that its main effect is through modulation of the stress response in the cerebellum.[25]

Since secretin receptors are found in many of the same brain regions that are affected in autism, and some children clearly seem to benefit, it still might be a reasonable treatment option.

Supply the Brain with Oxygen

Due to its high metabolic rate, the brain uses more oxygen per weight than any other organ; brain cells can't survive for more than a few minutes without it. We have learned from research on stroke cases that when a blood vessel in the brain is blocked, there is a nearly immediate loss of brain cells directly downstream. There is also an area adjacent to the dead cells that's injured, but not irreversibly. Stroke intervention targets these cells before they too are lost.

SPECT scan images done on the brains of autistic children have shown that some areas of the brain have decreased blood flow and presumably lower oxygen status.[26][27] Since MRIs don't show significant areas of cell death, the question is if there are brain cells existing in an inactive state due to decreased oxygen supply. Investigators wondered what would happen if the brains of children with autism were given more oxygen via hyperbaric oxygen therapy (HBOT).

Hyperbaric Oxygen Therapy

HBOT involves inhaling up to 100% oxygen at greater than 1 atmosphere absolute (ATA) in a pressurized chamber.[28] This procedure delivers increased oxygen to the tissues. HBOT has been used to treat a variety of conditions for decades. Its best-known uses are in treating carbon monoxide poisoning and in reversing decompression illness ("the bends") for deep sea divers. HBOT is also frequently used to increase oxygen to tissue in poor-healing wounds such as diabetic foot ulcers.[29][30] It's now commonly used to promote healing of surgical wounds or skin grafts, non-healing fractures, and serious skin infections. As physicians have gained understanding of the mechanisms and dynamics of oxygen in the tissues, the indications for HBOT have expanded to many other diseases, including IBD,[31] cancer (to ameliorate side effects from chemotherapy and radiation), acute myocardial infarction (adjunctive therapy),[32] fibromyalgia,[33] and complex regional pain syndrome.[34] It has also been used for neurological conditions such as cerebral palsy,[35][36] fetal alcohol syndrome,[37] brain injury,[38] multiple sclerosis,[39] and stroke.[40][41]

The rationale for HBOT for patients with neurological and developmental disorders is to relieve hypoxia, which often accompanies these conditions. The resulting oxygen increase leads to improvements in microcirculation and relief of cerebral edema. Other established effects that would apply to autism include lowering the presence of anaerobic bacteria in the gut, decreasing inflammation, and improving immune function (decreasing the proinflammatory cytokines, TNF-α and IL-1 β, and the transcription factor NFkappaB).[42][43] HBOT can also lower oxidative stress and increase intracellular glutathione.[44][45]

In 2006 a retrospective pilot study on six children with autism was published showing modest behavioral improvements, especially in the younger patients, according to parent assessment using various behavior scales. The children were given 40 one-hour sessions at 1.3 ATA (28-30% oxygen) over three months. No adverse reactions were reported.[46] The study was preliminary and not well controlled for other interventions, but it was suggestive that HBOT should be investigated further for autism treatment. Several larger, controlled HBOT studies are underway.

Treating Seizures

Seizures are not unusual in children with autism. They're caused by abnormal and repeated depolarization of neurons in the brain. Depolarization can be caused by trauma, low oxygen, low glucose, infection, toxicity, and metabolic imbalance, but most seizures are "idiopathic" (i.e., cause unknown). Seizures in autism are usually labeled idiopathic, but it should be evident from reading this book that the brain cells of an autistic child are exposed to many of the seizure-inducing abnormalities that I've just listed. Therefore, we can often gain control of seizures by treating infections, correcting metabolic abnormalities, relieving hypoxia, and removing toxins. Initially I continue seizure medications, weaning as tolerated, and monitoring EEGs.

A supplement that's sometimes used in autistic children with seizures is carnosine, a dipeptide amino acid that stimulates GABA function, with suspected anticonvulsant effects. A double-blind, placebo-controlled study in thirty-one autistic children using carnosine showed some significant improvements in language and social behavior.[47] I haven't found any studies specifically addressing seizure control in autism using carnosine. Carnosine should also be used with caution in children with abnormally elevated copper since it has the potential to introduce more copper into the body by binding to it in the gut.[48]

chapter 21

LESSONS FROM ISRAEL

MY FIRST VISIT WITH ISRAEL STARTED IN THE PARKING LOT IN front of my office, because he wouldn't get out of the van. During the entire first visit, about two hours, I saw his face for about two minutes. He held a pillow over his head the rest of the time and never spoke. Israel is a severely autistic adult whom I saw soon after starting my autism practice in Utah. Israel was the first adult I treated and was at the time the most profoundly autistic of any of my patients; he was institutionalized and heavily medicated. His father, Jim, said that the medications had taken away his son's personality, basically just sedated him—which was good for the institution, but not for Israel. When I met them, Jim had already begun exploring alternatives to medications and had started some nutritional interventions.

As I reviewed Israel's history, I was surprised by some of the things that Jim told me about him, about the things that Israel could do before. Prior to my involvement with autism, I would never have expected that this markedly autistic person could be capable of some of these things.

This is not a story about how much I helped Israel. In fact, I only consulted with them a few times after that. (The last time I heard from Jim, Israel was off of the medication and doing much better. He saw a reemergence of his personality, and Israel seemed to feel better.)

Instead, this is a story about what Israel taught me. His father told me that Israel loved to hike in the mountains, and knew how to ride a bike. After my first meeting with Israel, I was surprised that he had the motor skills or the balance to be able to do that. Jim said that Israel taught himself how to ride, but not in the conventional way. After watching other people, he picked up the bicycle and got on it. The first thing he did was to fall over on the ground. He picked himself up, got back on the bike and did it again. He fell over and over, and soon it became apparent to his father that he was actually trying to fall. After he had practiced falling, he got back on the bike, took off pedaling, and never fell again. He taught himself how to ski exactly the same way.

I find this story remarkable, and have thought about it many times. Israel is teaching us something about life. He wanted to ride a bike even though he was afraid of falling. So he practiced how to fall until his fear was gone. Then he never stopped pedaling. I think that all of us involved in any way with autism should remember this lesson. Many of us are so afraid of falling that we never get on the bike. Our autistic children are remarkable. They have courage. They want our help.

It is time that we take autism seriously, as a medical community and as a society. It is time that we invest in the kind of research and in medical treatment centers that are willing to look at autism in a new way. It is time to look beyond the brain and understand that autism is a complex but treatable medical disease. It is time to acknowledge the role of the environment in the rising rates of chronic diseases. We can no longer wait to completely understand all the complexities of autism before we act. Our affected children do not have that time. The oncoming, unborn generation does not have that time.

Israel taught me one more lesson. His father, a professional musician, was composing a symphony dedicated to his son. Jim asked Israel what he thought the symphony should be about. And, Israel, who is mostly non-verbal, said "love" and "peace on earth." Our autistic children, of all ages, deserve both. They deserve the chance to live healthy, happy, and functional lives. Our mission as physicians and our responsibility as parents—and as a society—is to see that they get that chance.

APPENDICES

APPENDIX A — PARENT RATINGS OF BEHAVIORAL EFFECTS OF BIOMEDICAL INTERVENTIONS

Autism Research Institute • 4182 Adams Avenue • San Diego, CA 92116

The parents of autistic children represent a vast and important reservoir of information on the benefits—and adverse effects—of the large variety of drugs and other interventions that have been tried with their children. Since 1967 the Autism Research Institute has been collecting parent ratings of the usefulness of the many interventions tried on their autistic children.

The following data have been collected from the more than 25,500 parents who have completed our questionnaires designed to collect such information. For the purposes of the present table, the parents responses on a six-point scale have been combined into three categories: "made worse" (ratings 1 and 2), "no effect" (ratings 3 and 4), and "made better" (ratings 5 and 6). The "Better:Worse" column gives the number of children who "Got Better" for each one who "Got Worse."

DRUGS	Got Worse^A	No Effect	Got Better	Better: Worse	No. of Cases^B
Adderall	42%	25%	33%	0.8:1	694
Amphetamine	47%	28%	25%	0.5:1	1246
Anafranil	32%	38%	30%	0.9:1	405
Antibiotics	32%	54%	14%	0.4:1	2039
Antifungals^C					
Diflucan	5%	42%	53%	10:1	505
Nystatin	5%	46%	49%	9.4:1	1229
Atarax	25%	53%	22%	0.9:1	502
Benadryl	24%	51%	25%	1.1:1	2924
Beta Blocker	17%	51%	32%	1.9:1	276
Buspar	26%	44%	30%	1.1:1	369
Chloral					
Hydrate	41%	39%	20%	0.5:1	443
Clonidine	21%	31%	47%	2.2:1	1441
Clozapine	37%	43%	20%	0.5:1	140
Cogentin	19%	55%	27%	1.4:1	176
Cylert	45%	35%	20%	0.4:1	618
Deanol	15%	57%	29%	2.0:1	206
Depakene^D					
Behavior	26%	43%	31%	1.2:1	1027
Seizures	12%	33%	55%	4.7:1	675

DRUGS	Got Worse^A	No Effect	Got Better	Better: Worse	No. of Cases^B
Desipramine	34%	33%	33%	1.0:1	82
Dilantin^D					
Behavior	28%	49%	23%	0.8:1	1097
Seizures	15%	36%	49%	3.3:1	422
Felbatol	20%	56%	24%	1.2:1	50
Fenfluramine	20%	52%	27%	1.3:1	473
Halcion	37%	42%	22%	0.6:1	65
Haldol	38%	28%	34%	0.9:1	1186
IVIG	10%	46%	44%	4.4:1	70
Klonapin^D					
Behavior	28%	39%	33%	1.1:1	224
Seizures	25%	60%	15%	0.6:1	60
Lithium	24%	45%	31%	1.3:1	441
Luvox	29%	37%	34%	1.2:1	203
Mellaril	28%	38%	33%	1.2:1	2088
Mysoline^D					
Behavior	41%	45%	14%	0.3:1	146
Seizures	19%	56%	25%	1.4:1	75
Naltrexone	20%	45%	35%	1.7:1	273
Paxil	30%	33%	37%	1.3:1	374
Phenergan	29%	46%	24%	0.8:1	291

DRUGS	Got Worse^A	No Effect	Got Better	Better: Worse	No. of Cases^B
Phenobarb^D					
Behavior	47%	37%	16%	0.3:1	1099
Seizures	18%	43%	39%	2.2:1	508
Prolixin	30%	41%	29%	1.0:1	97
Prozac	31%	32%	36%	1.2:1	1240
Risperdal	19%	27%	54%	2.9:1	912
Ritalin	44%	26%	29%	0.7:1	4029
Secretin					
Intravenous	7%	48%	45%	6.3:1	422
Transderm	10%	53%	37%	3.6:1	176
Stelazine	28%	45%	27%	0.9:1	431
Steroids	35%	33%	32%	0.9:1	111
Tegretol^D					
Behavior	25%	45%	30%	1.2:1	1492
Seizures	13%	33%	54%	4.2:1	814
Thorazine	36%	40%	24%	0.7:1	933
Tofranil	29%	38%	33%	1.1:1	766
Valium	35%	41%	24%	0.7:1	851
Zarontin^D					
Behavior	35%	45%	20%	0.6:1	148
Seizures	19%	55%	26%	1.4:1	104
Zoloft	32%	33%	34%	1.1:1	434

BIOMEDICAL/ NON-DRUG/ SUPPLEMENTS	Parent Ratings				
	Got Worse[A]	No Effect	Got Better	Better: Worse	No. of Cases[B]
Calcium[E]	2%	62%	35%	14:1	1871
Cod Liver Oil	4%	47%	49%	12:1	1389
Cod Liver Oil with Bethanecol	10%	50%	40%	4.2:1	105
Colostrum	6%	56%	38%	6.3:1	516
Detox. (Chelation)[C]	3%	24%	73%	25:1	627
Digestive Enzymes	3%	39%	57%	18:1	1223
DMG	8%	51%	42%	5.5:1	5601
Fatty Acids	2%	43%	55%	23:1	995
5 HTP	13%	51%	36%	2.8:1	254
Folic Acid	4%	54%	43%	11:1	1792
Food Allergy Treatment	3%	35%	62%	23:1	818
Hyperbaric Oxygen Therapy	6%	42%	52%	8.5:1	66
Magnesium	6%	65%	29%	4.6:1	301
Melatonin	8%	29%	63%	7.7:1	896
MT Promoter	13%	48%	38%	2.9:1	52
NAET	4%	52%	44%	11:1	77
P5P (Vitamin B6)	13%	37%	50%	4.0:1	418
Pepcid	11%	60%	29%	2.6:1	143
SAMe	17%	62%	21%	1.2:1	115
St. Johns Wort	17%	68%	16%	0.9:1	127
TMG	15%	43%	42%	2.9:1	683
Transfer Factor	10%	51%	39%	3.9:1	142

BIOMEDICAL/ NON-DRUG/ SUPPLEMENTS	Parent Ratings				
	Got Worse[A]	No Effect	Got Better	Better: Worse	No. of Cases[B]
Vitamin A	2%	59%	39%	19:1	990
Vitamin B3	4%	54%	41%	9.6:1	832
Vitamin B6/Magnesium	4%	48%	48%	11:1	6387
Vitamin B12	5%	34%	62%	14:1	688
Vitamin C	2%	56%	42%	17:1	2171
Zinc	2%	49%	49%	20:1	1736
SPECIAL DIETS					
Candida Diet	3%	43%	55%	19:1	867
Feingold Diet	2%	43%	55%	24:1	850
Gluten-/Casein-Free Diet	3%	32%	65%	20:1	2208
Removed Chocolate	2%	48%	50%	29:1	1944
Removed Eggs	2%	57%	41%	18:1	1290
Removed Milk Products/Dairy	2%	48%	51%	32:1	6113
Removed Sugar	2%	49%	49%	24:1	4014
Removed Wheat	2%	48%	50%	28:1	3565
Rotation Diet	2%	48%	50%	21:1	881
Specific Carbohydrate Diet	7%	28%	66%	10:1	195

A. "Worse" refers only to worse behavior. Drugs, but not nutrients, typically also cause physical problems if used long-term.

B. No. of cases is cumulative over several decades, so does not reflect current usage levels (e.g., Haldol is now seldom used).

C. Antifungal drugs and chelation are used selectively, where evidence indicates they are needed.

D. Seizure drugs: top line behavior effects, bottom line effects on seizures

E. Calcium effects are not due to dairy-free diet; statistics are similar for milk drinkers and non-milk drinkers.

ARI Publ. 34/Feb. 2007

APPENDIX B — DSM CRITERIA
DSM-III-R Criteria for Autism (1987)

Includes at least two items from item A, one from item B, and one from item C:

A. qualitative impairment in reciprocal social interaction (the examples within parentheses are arranged so that those first listed are more likely to apply to younger ormore disabled, and the later ones, to older or less disabled) as manifested by the following:

(1) marked lack of awareness of the existence or feelings of others (for example, treats a person as if that person were a piece of furniture; does not notice another person's distress; apparently has no concept of the need of others for privacy);

(2) no or abnormal seeking of comfort at times of distress (for example, does not come for comfort even when ill, hurt, or tired; seeks comfort in a stereotyped way, for example, says "cheese, cheese, cheese" whenever hurt);

(3) no or impaired imitation (for example, does not wave bye-bye; does not copy parent's domestic activities; mechanical imitation of others' actions out of context);

(4) no or abnormal social play (for example, does not actively participate in simple games; prefers solitary play activities; involves other children in play only as mechanical aids); and

(5) gross impairment in ability to make peer friendships (for example, no interest in making peer friendships; despite interest in making friends, demonstrates lack of understanding of conventions of social interaction, for example, reads phone book to uninterested peer);

B. qualitative impairment In verbal and nonverbal communication and in imaginative activity, (the numbered items are arranged so that those first listed as more likely to apply to younger or more disabled, and the later ones, to older or less disabled) as manifested by the following:

(1) no mode of communication, such as communicative babbling, facial expression, gesture, mime, or spoken language;

(2) markedly abnormal nonverbal communication, as in the use of eye-to-eye gaze, facial expression, body posture, or gestures to initiate or modulate social interaction (for example, does not anticipate being held, stiffens when held, does not look at the person or smile when making a social approach, does not greet parents or visitors, has a fixed stare in social situations);

(3) absence of imaginative activity, such as play-acting of adult roles, fantasy characters, or animals; lack of interest in stories about imaginary events;

(4) marked abnormalities in the production of speech, including volume, pitch, stress, rate, rhythm, and intonation (for example, monotonous tone, question-like melody,or high pitch);

(5) marked abnormalities in the form or content of speech, including stereotyped and repetitive use of speech (for example, immediate echolalia or mechanical repetition of a television commercial); use of "you" when "I" is meant (for example, using "You want cookie?" to mean "I want a cookie"); idiosyncratic use of words or phrases (for example, "Go on green riding" to mean "I want to go on the swing"); or frequent irrelevant remarks (for example, starts talking about train schedules during a conversation about sports); and

(6) marked impairment in the ability to initiate or sustain a conversation with others, despite adequate speech (for example, indulging in lengthy monologues on one subjectregardless of interjections from others);

C. markedly restricted repertoire of activities and interests, as manifested by the following:

(1) stereotyped body movements (for example, handflicking or twisting, spinning, head-banging, complex whole-body movements);

(2) persistent preoccupation with parts of objects (for example, sniffing or smelling objects, repetitive feeling of texture of materials, spinning wheels of toy cars) or attachment to unusual objects (for example, insists on carrying around a piece of string);

(3) marked distress over changes in trivial aspects of environment (for example, when a vase is moved from usual position);

(4) unreasonable insistence on following routines in precise detail (for example, insisting that exactly the same route always be followed when shopping);

(5) markedly restricted range of interests and a preoccupation with one narrow interest (for example, interested only in lining up objects, in amassing facts about meteorology, or in pretending to be a fantasy character);

D. onset during infancy or early childhood;

E. other symptoms that may occur with the syndrome:

(1) sensory disturbances as evidenced by atypical responses to stimuli (for example, touch, sound, light, movement, smell, taste). Responses may include overreaction, indifference, or withdrawal; and

(2) uneven acquisition of skills, and/or difficulty in integrating and generalizing acquired skills; and

F. the pupil's need for instruction and services mustbe supported by at least one documented systematic observation in the pupil's daily routine setting by an appropriate professional and verify the criteria categories in items A to D. In addition, corroboration of developmental or medical information with a developmental history and at least one other assessment procedure that is conducted on a different day must be included. Other documentation should include parent reports, functional skills assessments, adaptive behavior scales, intelligence tests, criterion-referenced instruments, language concepts, developmental checklists, or an autism checklist.

DSM-IV Criteria for Autism (1994)

A total of six (or more) items from (1), (2), and (3), with at least two from (1), and one each from (2) and (3):

A. (1) qualitative impairment in social interaction, as manifested by at least two of the following:

(a) marked impairment in the use of multiple nonverbal behaviors, such as eye-to-eye gaze, facial expression, body postures, and gestures to regulate social interaction

(b) failure to develop peer relationships appropriate to developmental level

(c) a lack of spontaneous seeking to share enjoyment, interests, or achievements with other people (e.g., by a lack of showing, bringing, or pointing out objects of interest)

(d) lack of social or emotional reciprocity

(2) qualitative impairments in communication, as manifested by at least one of the following:

(a) delay in, or total lack of, the development of spoken language (not accompanied by an attempt to compensate through alternative modes of communication such as gesture or mime)

(b) in individuals with adequate speech, marked impairment in the ability to initiate or sustain a conversation with others

(c) stereotyped and repetitive use of language or idiosyncratic language

(d) lack of varied, spontaneous make-believe play or social imitative play appropriate to developmental level

(3) restricted, repetitive, and stereotyped patterns of behavior, interests, and activities as manifested by at least one of the following:

(a) encompassing preoccupation with one or more stereotyped and restricted patterns of interest that is abnormal either in intensity or focus

(b) apparently inflexible adherence to specific, nonfunctional routines or rituals

(c) stereotyped and repetitive motor mannerisms (e.g., hand or finger flapping or twisting or complex whole-body movements)

(d) persistent precoccupation with parts of objects B. Delays or abnormal functioning in at least one of the following areas, with onset prior to age 3 years: (1) social interaction, (2) language as used in social communication, or (3) symbolic or imaginative play.

C. The disturbance is not better accounted for by Rett's disorder or childhood disintegrative disorder.

Reprinted with permission from the Diagnostic and Statistical Manual of Mental Disorders, Third and Fourth Edition, (© 2000). American Psychiatric Association.

NOTES

CHAPTER 2

1 Kanner, Leo. "Autistic Disturbances of Affective Contact," *Nervous Child* 2 (1943): 217-250. Reprinted in *Classic Readings in Autism,* ed. Anne M. Donnellan. New York: Teacher's College Press, 1985.

2 Ibid.

3 Ibid.

4 Ibid.

5 Ibid.

6 Ibid.

7 Prospects: the quarterly review of comparative education (Paris, UNESCO: International Bureau of Education), vol XXIII, no 1/2, 1993, P. 85-100.

8 Dolnick, Edward. *Madness on the Couch: Blaming the Victim in the Heyday of Psychoanalysis.* New York: Simon & Schuster, 1998, p.216.

9 Lovaas OI, Behavioral treatment and normal educational and intellectual functioning in young autistic children. *J Consult Clin Psychol.* 1987 Feb;55(1):3-9.

10 McEachin JJ, Smith T, Lovaas OI. "Long-term outcome for children with autism who received early intensive behavioral treatment." *Am J Ment Retard.* 1993 Jan; 97(4):359-72.

CHAPTER 3

1 Folstein S, Rutter M. Genetic influences and infantile autism. *Nature* 265, 726-728 (24) Feb 1977.

2 Bailey A, Le Couteur A, Gottesman I, Bolton P, Simonoff E, Yuzda E, Rutter M. Autism as a strongly genetic disorder: evidence from a British twin study. *Psychol Med.* 1995 Jan;25(1):63-77.

3   Ritvo ER, Freeman BJ, Mason-Brothers A, Mo A, Ritvo AM. Concordance for
     the syndrome of autism in 40 pairs of afflicted twins. *Am J Psychiatry*. 1985 Jan;
     142(1):74-7.

4   Le Couteur A, Bailey A, Goode S, Pickles A, Robertson S, Gottesman I, Rutter
     M. A broader phenotype of autism: the clinical spectrum in twins. *J Child Psychol
     Psychiatry*. 1996 Oct;37(7):785-801.

5   Steffenburg S, Gillberg C, Hellgren L, Andersson L, Gillberg IC, Jakobsson G,
     Bohman M. A twin study of autism in Denmark, Finland, Iceland, Norway and
     Sweden. *J Child Psychol Psychiatry*. 1989 May;30(3):405-16.

6   Folstein S, Rutter M. Genetic influences and infantile autism. *Nature* 265, 726-728
     (24) Feb 1977.

7   Jorde LB, Hasstedt SJ, Ritvo ER, Mason-Brothers A, Freeman BJ, Pingree C,
     McMahon WM, Petersen B, Jenson WR, Mo A. Complex segregation analysis of
     autism. *Am J Hum Genet*. 1991 Nov;49(5):932-8.

8   Bartak L, Rutter M, Cox A. A comparative study of infantile autism and specific
     development receptive language disorder. I. The children. *Br J Psychiatry*.
     1975 Feb;126:127-45.

9   Micali N, Chakrabarti S, Fombonne E. The broad autism phenotype: findings from
     an epidemiological survey. *Autism*. 2004 Mar;8(1):21-37.

10   Lotter V.; Epidemiology of autistic conditions in young children. I. Prevalence. *Soc.
     Psychiatry* 1966, 1; 124-137.

11   Spiker D, Lotspeich L, Kraemer HC, Hallmayer J, McMahon W, Petersen PB,
     Nicholas P, Pingree C, Wiese-Slater S, Chiotti C, et al. Genetics of autism:
     characteristics of affected and unaffected children from 37 multiplex families.
     Am J Med Genet. 1994 Mar 15;54(1):27-35.

12   Bailey A, Palferman S, Heavey L, Le Couteur A. Autism: the phenotype in
     relatives. *J Autism Dev Disord*. 1998 Oct;28(5):369-92.

13   Risch N, Spiker D, Lotspeich L, Nouri N, Hinds D, Hallmayer J, Kalaydjieva L,
     McCague P, Dimiceli S, Pitts T, Nguyen L, Yang J, Harper C, Thorpe D, Vermeer
     S, Young H, Hebert J, Lin A, Ferguson J, Chiotti C, Wiese-Slater S, Rogers T,
     Salmon B, Nicholas P, Petersen PB, Pingree C, McMahon W, Wong DL, Cavalli-
     Sforza LL, Kraemer HC, Myers RM. A genomic screen of autism: evidence for a
     multilocus etiology. *Am J Hum Genet*. 1999 Aug;65(2):493-507.

14   Konstantareas MM, Homatidis S. Chromosomal abnormalities in a series of
     children with autistic disorder. *J Autism Dev Disord*. 1999 Aug;29(4):275-85.

15   Szatmari P. Heterogeneity and the genetics of autism. *J Psychiatry Neurosci*.
     1999 Mar;24(2):159-65.

16   Nelson KB, Grether JK, Croen LA, Dambrosia JM, Dickens BF, Jelliffe LL,
     Hansen RL, Phillips TM. Neuropeptides and neurotrophins in neonatal blood of
     children with autism or mental retardation. *Ann Neurol*. 2001 May;49(5):597-606.

17   Korvatska E, Van de Water J, Anders TF, Gershwin ME. Genetic and
     immunologic considerations in autism. *Neurobiol Dis*. 2002 Mar;9(2):107-25.

18   Cook EH. Genetics of autism. *Ment Retard Dev Disabil Res Rev.* 1998 4:113-120.

19   Comi AM, Zimmerman AW, Frye VH, Law PA, Peeden JN. Familial clustering of autoimmune disorders and evaluation of medical risk factors in autism. *J Child Neurol.* 1999 Jun;14(6):388-94.

20   Sweeten TL, Bowyer SL, Posey DJ, Halberstadt GM, McDougle CJ. Increased prevalence of familial autoimmunity in probands with pervasive developmental disorders. *Pediatrics.* 2003 Nov;112(5):e420.

21   Molloy CA, Morrow AL, Meinzen-Derr J, Dawson G, Bernier R, Dunn M, Hyman SL, McMahon WM, Goudie-Nice J, Hepburn S, Minshew N, Rogers S, Sigman M, Spence MA, Tager-Flusberg H, Volkmar FR, Lord C. Familial autoimmune thyroid disease as a risk factor for regression in children with Autism Spectrum Disorder: a CPEA Study. *J Autism Dev Disord.* 2006 Apr;36(3):317-24.

22   Croen LA, Grether JK, Yoshida CK, Odouli R, Van de Water J. Maternal autoimmune diseases, asthma and allergies, and childhood autism spectrum disorders: a case-control study. *Arch Pediatr Adolesc Med.* 2005 Feb;159(2):151-7.

23   Campbell DB, Sutcliffe JS, Ebert PJ, Militerni R, Bravaccio C, Trillo S, Elia M, Schneider C, Melmed R, Sacco R, Persico AM, Levitt P. A genetic variant that disrupts MET transcription is associated with autism. *Proc Natl Acad Sci U S A.* 2006 Oct 19.

24   Folstein S, Rutter M. Genetic influences and infantile autism. *Nature.* 265, 726-728(24) Feb 1977.

25   Cook EH. Genetics of autism. *Ment Retard Dev Disabil Res Rev.* 1998 4:113-120.

26   Trottier G, Srivastava, Walker CD. Etiology of infantile autism: a review of recent advances and neurobiological research. *J Psychiatry neurosci.* 1999Mar;24(2):103-115.

27   Smalley SL. Genetic influences in childhood-onset psychiatric disorders: autism and attention-deficit/hyperactivity disorder. *Am J Hum Genet.* 1997 Jun;60(6):1276-82.

28   Cook EH. Genetics of autism. *Ment Retard Dev Disabil Res Rev.* 1998 4:113-120.

29   Cook EH Jr. Genetics of autism. *Child Adolesc Psychiatr Clin N Am.* 2001 Apr;10(2):333-50.

CHAPTER 4

1   Fombonne E. The epidemiology of child and adolescent psychiatric disorders: recent developments and issues. *Epidemiol Psichiatr Soc.* 1998 Sep-Dec;7(3)161-6.

2   Yeargin-Allsopp M, Rice C, Karapurker T, Doernberg N, Boyle C, Murphy C. Prevalence of autism in a US metropolitan area. *JAMA.* 2003 Jan 1;289(1)49-55.

3   Hoshino Y, Kumashiro H, Yashima Y, Tachibana R, Watanabe M. The epidemiological study of autism in Fukushima-ken. *Folia Psychiatr Neurol Jpn.* 1982;36(2):115-24.

4   Kanner L. Autistic disturbances of affective contact. *Acta Paedopsychiatr.* 1968;35(4): 100-36.

5   Rimland, Bernard. *Infantile Autism: The Syndrome and Its Implications for a Neural Theory of Behavior.* Prentice Hall: 1964.

6   Croen LA, Grether JK, Hoogstrate J, Selvin S. The changing prevalence of autism in California. *J Autism Dev Disord.* 2002 Jun;32(3):207-15.

7   Barbaresi WJ, Katusic SK, Colligan RC, Weaver AL, Jacobsen SJ. The incidence of autism in Olmsted County, Minnesota, 1976-1997: results from a population-based study. *Arch Pediatr Adolesc Med.* 2005 Jan;159(1):37-44.

8   Gillberg C, Wing L. Autism: not an extremely rare disorder. *Acta Psychiatr Scand.* 1999 Jun;99(6):399-406.

9   Burd L, Kerbeshian J, Klug MG, McCulloch K. A prevalence methodology for mental illness and developmental disorders in rural and frontier settings. *Int J Circumpolar Health.* 2000 Jan;59(1):74-86.

10 Steffenberg S, Gillberg C. Autism and autistic-like conditions in Swedish rural and urban areas: a population study. *Br J Psychiatry.* 1986 Jul;149:81-7.

11 Nylander L, Gillberg C. Screening for autism spectrum disorders in adult psychiatric outpatients: a preliminary report. *Acta Pxychiatr Scand.* 2001 Jun;103(6):428-34.

12 Wing L, Potter D. The epidemiology of autistic spectrum disorders: Is the prevalence rising? *Ment Retard Dev Disabil Res Rev.* 2002;8(3):151-61.

13 Croen L, Grether J, Hoogstrate J, Selvin S. The changing prevalence of autism in California. *J Autism Dev Disord.* 2002 Jun;32(3):207-15.

14 Jick H, Kaye JA. Epidemiology and possible causes of autism. *Pharmacotherapy.* 2003 Dec;23(12):1524-30.

15 Baron-Cohen S. The extreme male brain theory of autism. *Trends Cogn Sci.* 2002 Jun 1;6(6):248-254.

16 Baron-Cohen S. The hyper-systemizing, assortative mating theory of autism. *Prog Neuropsychopharmacol Biol Psychiatry.* 2006 Jul;30(5):865-72.

17 Silberman, Steve. "The Geek Syndrome." *Wired*, Issue 9.12, Dec 2001.

18 Byrd, Robert. MIND Institute. Report to the Legislature on the Principle Findings from The Epidemiology of Autism in California: A Comprehensive Pilot Study. UC Davis 17 Oct 2002. *www.dds.ca.gov/autism/pdf/study_final.pdf*

19 Croen L, Grether J, Hoogstrate J, Selvin S. The changing prevalence of autism in California. *J Autism Dev Disord.* 2002 Jun;32(3):207-15.

20 Blaxill MF, Baskin DS, Spitzer WO. Blaxill, Baskin, and Spitzer on Croen et al. (2002), the changing prevalence of autism in California. *J Autism Dev Disord.* 2003 Apr;33(2):223-6; discussion 227-9.

21 Croen LA, Grether JK. A Response to Blaxill, Baskin, and Spitzer on Croen et al. (2002), "The Changing Prevalence of Autism in California." *J Autism Dev Disord*, vol 33 April 2003, pp227-229(3).

22 Ritvo ER, Freeman BJ, Pingree C, Mason-Brothers A, Jorde L, Jenson WR, McMahon WM, Petersen PB, Mo A, Ritvo A. The UCLA-University of Utah epidemiologic survey of autism: prevalence. *Am J Psychiatry.* 1989 Feb;146(2)194-9.

23 Kirby RS, Brewster MA, Canino CU, Pavin M. Early childhood surveillance of developmental disorders by a birth defects surveillance system: methods, prevalence comparisons, and mortality patterns. *J Dev Behav Pediatr.* 1995 Oct;16(5):318-26.

24 Burd L, Fisher W, Kerbeshian J. A prevalence study of pervasive developmental disorders in North Dakota. *J Am Acad Child Adolesc Psychiatry.* 1987 Sep;26(5):700-3.

25 Bertrand J, Mars A, Boyle C, Bove F, Yeargin-Allsopp M, Decoufle P. Prevalence of Autism in a United States Population: The Brick Township, New Jersey, Investigation. *Pediatrics.* 2001;108;1155-1161.

26 Yeargin-Allsopp M, Rice C, Karapurker T, Doernberg N, Boyle C, Murphy C. Prevalence of autism in a US metropolitan area. *JAMA* 2003 Jan 1;289(1)49-55.

27 www.medicalhomeinfo.org/health/Autism%20downloads/AutismAlarm.pdf.

28 Gillberg C, Wing L. Autism: not an extremely rare disorder. *Acta Psychiatr Scand.* 1999 Jun;99(6):399-406.

29 Chakrabarti S, Fombonne E. Pervasive developmental disorders in preschool children: confirmation of high prevalence. *Am J Psychiatry.* 2005 Jun;162(6):1133-41.

30 Scott FJ, Baron-Cohen S, Bolton P, Brayne C. Brief report: prevalence of autism spectrum conditions in children aged 5-11 years in Cambridgeshire, UK. *Autism.* 2002 Sep;6(3)231-7.

31 Powell JE, Edwards A, Edwards M, Pandit BS, Sungum-Paliwal SR, Whitehouse W. Changes in the incidence of childhood autism and other autistic spectrum disorders in preschool children from two areas of the West Midlands, UK. *Dev Med Child Neurol.* 2000 Sep;42(9):624-8.

32 Charman T. The prevalence of autism spectrum disorders. Recent evidence and future challenges. *Eur Child Adolesc Psychiatry.* 2002 Dec;11(6):249-56.

33 Smeeth L, Cook C, Fombonne PE, Heavey L, Rodrigues LC, Smith PG, Hall AJ. Rate of first recorded diagnosis of autism and other pervasive developmental disorders in a United Kingdom general practice 1988 to 2001. *BMC Med.* 2004 Nov 9;2:39.

34 Fombonne E, Simmons H, Ford T, Meltzer H, Goodman R. Prevalence of pervasive developmental disorders in the British nationwide survey of child mental health. *Int Rev Psychiatry.* 2003 Feb-May;15(1-2):158-65.

35 Baird G, Simonoff E, Pickles A, Chandler S, Loucas T, Meldrum D, Charman T. Prevalence of disorders of the autism spectrum in a population cohort of children in South Thames: the Special Needs and Autism Project (SNAP). *Lancet.* 2006 Jul 15; 368(9531):210-5.

36 Magnusson P, Saemundsen E. Prevalence of autism in Iceland. *J Autism Dev Disord.* 2001 Apr;31(2):153-63.

37 Kadesjo B, Gillberg C, Hagberg B. Brief report: autism and Asperger syndrome in seven-year-old children: a total population study. *J Autism Dev Disord.* 1999 Aug;29(4):327-31.

38 Arvidsson T, Danielsson B, Forsberg P, et al. Autism in 3-6-year-old children in a suburb of Goteborg, Sweden. *Autism* 1997;1:163–73.

39 Gillberg C, Cederlund M, Lamberg K, Zeijlon L. Brief Report: "The Autism Epidemic". The registered prevalence of autism in a Swedish urban area. *J Autism Dev Disord.* 2006 Mar 28.

40   Kielinen M, Linna SL, Moilanen I. Autism in Northern Finland. *Eur Child Adolesc Psychiatry.* 2000 Sep;9(3):162-7.

41   Hviid A, Stellfeld M, Wohlfahrt J, Melbye M. Association between thimerosal-containing vaccine and autism. *JAMA.* 2003 Oct;290(13):1763-6.

42   Madsen KM, Hviid A, Vestergaard M, Schendel D, Wohlfart J, Thorsen P, Olsen J, Melbye M. A population-based study of measles, mumps, and rubella vaccination and autism. *N Engl J Med.* 2002 Nov 7;347(19):1477-82.

43   Madsen KM, Lauritsen MB, Pedersen CB, Thorsen P, Plesner AM, Andersen PH, Mortensen PB. Thimerosal and the occurrence of autism: negative ecological evidence from Danish population-based data. *Pediatrics.* 2003 Sep;112(3 Pt 1):604-6.

44   Lauritsen MB, Pedersen CB, Mortensen PB. The incidence and prevalence of pervasive developmental disorders: a Danish population-based study. *Psychol Med.* 2004 Oct;34(7):1339-46.

45   Fombonne E. Epidemiological surveys of autism and other pervasive developmental disorders; an update. *J Autism Dev Disord.* 2003 Aug;33(4)365-82.

46   Bryson SE, Clark BS, Smith IM. First report of a Canadian epidemiological study of autistic syndromes. *J Child Psychiatry.* 1988 Jul;29(4)433-45.

47   Fombonne E, Zakarian R, Bennett A, Meng L, McLean-Heywood D. Pervasive developmental disorders in Montreal, Quebec, Canada: prevalence and links with immunizations. *Pediatrics.* 2006 Jul;118(1):e139-50.

48   Icasiano F, Hewson P, Machet P, Cooper C, Marshall A. Childhood autism spectrum disorder in the Barwon region: a community based study. *J Pediatr Child Health.* 2004 Dec;40(12):696-701.

49   Sumi S, Taniai H, Miyachi T, Tanemura M. Sibling risk of pervasive developmental disorder estimated by means of an epidemiologic survey in Nagoya, Japan. *J Hum Genet.* 2006 Mar 25.

50   Honda H, Shimizu Y, Imai M, Nitto Y. Cumulative incidence of childhood autism: a total population study of better accuracy and precision. *Dev Med Child Neurol.* 2005 Jan;47(1):10-8.

51   Volkmar F, Bregman J, Cohen D, Cicchetti D. DSM-III and DSM-III-R Diagnoses of Autism. *Am J Psychiatry.* 1988 Nov 145:11;1404-1408.

52   Szatmari P. Thinking about Autism, Asperger Syndrome and PDDNOS. *PRISME,* 34:24-34, 2001.

53   Yazbak FE. Autism in the United States: a perspective. *JPANDS.* 2003 8:4:103-107.

54   Harrington JW, Rosen L, Garnecho A, Patrick PA. Parental perceptions and use of complementary and alternative medicine practices for children with autistic spectrum disorders in private practice. *J Dev Behav Pediatr.* 2006 Apr;27(2 Suppl): S156-61.

55   California Department of Developmental Services "Changes in the Population of Persons with Autism and Pervasive Developmental Disorders in California's Developmental Services System: 1987 through 1998." Report to the Legislature March 1, 1999:1-19.

56 Schattner A, Fletcher RH. Pearls and pitfalls in patient care: need to revive traditional clinical values. *Am J Med Sci.* 2004 Feb;327(2):79-85.

57 Fombonne E. Epidemiological surveys of autism and other pervasive developmental disorders; an update. *J Autism Dev Disord.* 2003 Aug;33(4)365-82..

58 Burd L, Fisher W, Kerbeshian J. A prevalence study of pervasive developmental disorders in North Dakota. *J Am Acad Child Adolesc Psychiatry.* 1987 Sep;26(5):700-3.

59 Burd L, Kerbeshian J, Klug MG, McCulloch K. A prevalence methodology for mental illness and developmental disorders in rural and frontier settings. *Int J Circumpolar Health.* 2000 Jan;59(1):74-86.

60 Nylander L, Gillberg C. Screening for autism spectrum disorders in adult psychiatric outpatients: a preliminary report. *Acta Psychiatr Scand.* 2001 Jun;103(6):428-34.

61 Gillberg C, Steffenburg S, Schaumann H. Is autism more common now than ten years ago? *Br J Psychiatry.* 1991 Mar;158:403-9.

62 Chang HL, Juang YY, Wang WT, Huang CI, Chen CY, Hwang YS. Screening for autism spectrum disorder in adult psychiatric outpatients in a clinic in Taiwan. *Gen Hosp Psychiatry.* 2003 Jul-Aug;25(4):284-8.

63 Blaxill MF. Any changes in prevalence of autism must be determined. *BMJ.* 2002 Feb 2;324(7332):296.

64 Blaxill MF, Baskin DS, Spitzer WO. Blaxill, Baskin, and Spitzer on Croen et al. (2002), the changing prevalence of autism in California. *J Autism Dev Disord.* 2003 Apr;33(2):223-6; discussion 227-9.

65 Ganz, Michael. "The Costs of Autism." *Understanding Autism: From Basic Neuroscience to Treatment.* Eds. Steven O. Moldin, John L R Rubenstein, CRC Press, 2006.

CHAPTER 5

1 Comi AM, Zimmerman AW, Frye VH, Law PA, Peeden JN. Familial clustering of autoimmune disorders and evaluation of medical risk factors in autism. *J Child Neurol.* 1999 Jun:14(6):388-94.

2 Sweeten TL, Bowyer SL, Posey DJ, Halberstadt GM, McDougal CJ. Increased prevalence of familial autoimmunity in probands with pervasive developmental disorders. *Pediatrics.* 2003 Nov:112(5)e420.

3 Perera FP, Rauh V, Tsai WY, Kinney P, Camann D, Barr D, Bernert T, Garfinkel R, Tu YH, Diaz D, Dietrich J, Whyatt RM. Effects of transplacental exposure to environmental pollutants on birth outcomes in a multiethnic population. *Environ Health Perspect.* 2003 Feb;111(2):201-5.

4 Reichrtova E, Ciznar P, Prachar V, Palkovicova L, Veningerova M. Cord serum immunoglobulin E related to the environmental contamination of human placentas with organochlorine compounds. *Environ Health Perspect.* 1999 Nov;107(11):895-9.

5 Longo LD. Environmental pollution and pregnancy: risks and uncertainties for the fetus and infant. *Am J Obstet Gynecol.* 1980 May 15;137(2):162-73.

6   Koos BJ, Longo LD. Mercury toxicity in the pregnant woman, fetus, and newborn infant. A review. *Am J Obstet Gynecol.* 1976 Oct 1;126(3):390-409.

7   Rice D, Barone S Jr. Critical periods of vulnerability for the developing nervous system: evidence from humans and animal models. *Environ Health Perspect.* 2000 Jun;108 Suppl 3:511-33.

CHAPTER 7

1   Ashwood P, Willis S, Van de Water J. The immune response in autism: a new frontier for autism research. *J Leuk Biol.* 2006 Jul:80;1-15.

2   Ashwood P, Anthony A, Torrente F, Wakefield AJ. Spontaneous mucosal lymphocyte cytokine profiles in children with autism and gastrointestinal symptoms: mucosal immune activation and reduced counter regulatory interleukin-10. *J Clin Immunol.* 2004 Nov;24(6):664-73.

3   Murch SH, Walker-Smith JA. Nutrition in inflammatory bowel disease. *Baillieres Clin Gastroenterol.* 1998 Dec;12(4):719-38.

4   Gupta S, Aggarwal S, Rashanravan B, Lee T. Th1- and Th2-like cytokines in CD4+ and CD8+ T cells in autism. *J Neuroimmunol.* 1998 May 1;85(1):106-9.

5   van Gent T, Heijnen CJ, Treffers PD. Autism and the immune system. *J Child Psychol Psychiatry.* 1997 Mar;38(3):337-49.

6   Warren RP, Singh VK, Averett RE, Odell JD, Maciulis A, Burger RA, Daniels WW, Warren WL. Immunogenetic studies in autism and related disorders. *Mol Chem Neuropathol.* 1996 May-Aug;28(1-3):77-81.

7   Yonk LJ, Warren RP, Burger RA, Cole P, Odell JD, Warren WL, White E, Singh VK. CD4+ helper T cell depression in autism. *Immunol Lett.* 1990 Sep;25(4):341-5.

8   Ferrante P, Saresella M, Guerini FR, Marzorati M, Musetti MC, Cazzullo AG. Significant association of HLA A2-DR11 with CD4 naive decrease in autistic children. *Biomed Pharmacother.* 2003 Oct;57(8):372-4.

9   Fiumara A, Sciotto A, Barone R, D'Asero G, Munda S, Parano E, Pavone L. Peripheral lymphocyte subsets and other immune aspects in Rett syndrome. *Pediatr Neurol.* 1999 Sep;21(3):619-21.

10   Warren RP, Foster A, Margaretten NC. Reduced natural killer cell activity in autism. *J Am Acad Child Adolesc Psychiatry.* 1987 May;26(3):333-5.

11   Ashwood P, Anthony A, Pellicer AA, Torrente F, Walker-Smith JA, Wakefield AJ. Intestinal lymphocyte populations in children with regressive autism: evidence for extensive mucosal immunopathology. *J Clin Immunol.* 2003 Nov;23(6):504-17.

12   Sweeten TL, Posey DJ, McDougle CJ. High blood monocyte counts and neopterin levels in children with autistic disorder. *Am J Psychiatry.* 2003 Sep;160(9):1691-3.

13   Ashwood P, Anthony A, Pellicer AA, Torrente F, Walker-Smith JA, Wakefield AJ. Intestinal lymphocyte populations in children with regressive autism: evidence for extensive mucosal immunopathology. *J Clin Immunol.* 2003 Nov;23(6):504-17.

14   Croonenberghs J, Wauters A, Devreese K, Verkerk R, Scharpe S, Bosmans E, Egyed B, Deboutte D, Maes M. Increased serum albumin, gamma globulin, immunoglobulin IgG, and IgG2 and IgG4 in autism. *Psychol Med.* 2002 Nov;32(8):1457-63.

15   Krause I, He XS, Gershwin ME, Shoenfeld Y. Brief report: immune factors in autism: a critical review. *J Autism Dev Disord.* 2002 Aug;32(4):337-45.

16   Trajkovski V, Ajdinski L, Spiroski M. Plasma concentration of immunoglobulin classes and subclasses in children with autism in the Republic of Macedonia: retrospective study. *Croat Med J.* 2004 Dec;45(6):746-9.

17   Furlano RI, Anthony A, Day R, Brown A, McGavery L, Thomson MA, Davies SE, Berelowitz M, Forbes A, Wakefield AJ, Walker-Smith JA, Murch SH. Colonic CD8 and gamma delta T-cell infiltration with epithelial damage in children with autism. *Pediatrics* 2001;138:366-72.

18   Ashwood P, Anthony A, Pellicer AA, Torrente F, Walker-Smith JA, Wakefield AJ. Intestinal lymphocyte populations in children with regressive autism: evidence for extensive mucosal immunopathology. *J Clin Immunol.* 2003 Nov;23(6):504-17.

19   Stubbs EG, Crawford ML. Depressed lymphocyte responsiveness in autistic children. *J Autism Child Schizophr.* 1977 Mar;7(1):49-55.

20   Warren RP, Margaretten NC, Pace NC, Foster A. Immune abnormalities in patients with autism. *J Autism Dev Disord.* 1986 Jun;16(2):189-97.

21   Plioplys AV. Autism: electroencephalogram abnormalities and clinical improvement with valproic acid. *Arch Pediatr Adolesc Med.* 1994 Feb;148(2):220-2.

22   Denney DR, Frei BW, Gaffney GR. Lymphocyte subsets and interleukin-2 receptors in autistic children. *J Autism Dev Disord.* 1996 Feb;26(1):87-97.

23   Fiumara A, Sciotto A, Barone R, D'Asero G, Munda S, Parano E, Pavone L. Peripheral lymphocyte subsets and other immune aspects in Rett syndrome. *Pediatr Neurol.* 1999 Sep;21(3):619-21.

24   Warren RP, Foster A, Margaretten NC. Reduced natural killer cell activity in autism. *J Am Acad Child Adolesc Psychiatry.* 1987 May;26(3):333-5.

25   Engstrom HA, Ohlson S, Stubbs EG, Maciulis A, Caldwell V, Odell JD, Torres A.R. Decreased Expression of CD95 (FAS/APO-1) on CD4+ T-lymphocytes from Participants with Autism. *J Dev Phys Disabil.* 2003 Jun 15;2:155-163(9).

26   Korvatska E, Van de Water J, Anders TF, Gershwin ME. Genetic and immunologic considerations in autism. *Neurobiol Dis.* 2002 Mar;9(2):107-25.

27   Singh VK. Plasma increase of interleukin-12 and interferon-gamma. Pathological significance in autism. *J Neuroimmunol.* 1996 May;66(1-2):143-5.

28   Gupta S, Aggarwal S, Rashanravan B, Lee T. Th1- and Th2-like cytokines in CD4+ and CD8+ T cells in autism. *J Neuroimmunol.* 1998 May 1;85(1):106-9.

29   Molloy C, Morrow A, Meinzen-Derr J, Schleifer K, Dienger K, Manning-Courtney P, Altaye M, Wills-Karp M. Elevated cytokine levels in children with autism spectrum disorder. *J Neuroimmunology.* 2006;172:198-205.

30   Singh VK. Th1- and Th2-like cytokines in CD4+ and CD8+ T cells in autism. *J Neuroimmunol.* 1998 May 1;85(1):106-9.

31 Sweeten TL, Posey DJ, McDougle CJ. High blood monocyte counts and neopterin levels in children with autistic disorder. *Am J Psychiatry.* 2003 Sep;160(9):1691-3.

32 Zimmerman AW, Jyonouchi H, Comi AM, Connors SL, Milstien S, Varsou A, Heyes MP. Cerebrospinal fluid and serum markers of inflammation in autism. *Pediatr Neurol.* 2005 Sep;33(3):195-201.

33 Jyonouchi H, Sun S, Le H. Proinflammatory and regulatory cytokine production associated with innate and adaptive immune responses in children with autism spectrum disorders and developmental regression. *J Neuroimmunol.* 2001 Nov 1; 120(1-2):170-9.

34 Ashwood P, Anthony A, Pellicer AA, Torrente F, Walker-Smith JA, Wakefield AJ. Intestinal lymphocyte populations in children with regressive autism: evidence for extensive mucosal immunopathology. *J Clin Immunol.* 2003 Nov;23(6):504-17.

35 Sweeten TL, Posey DJ, Shankar S, McDougle CJ. High nitric oxide production in autistic disorder: a possible role for interferon-gamma. *Bio Psychiatry.* 2004 Feb 15:55(4):434-7.

36 Ashwood P, Anthony A, Torrente F, Wakefield AJ. Spontaneous mucosal lymphocyte cytokine profiles in children with autism and gastrointestinal symptoms: mucosal immune activation and reduced counter regulatory interleukin-10. *J Clin Immunol.* 2004 Nov;24(6):664-73.

37 Jyonouchi H, Geng L, Ruby A, Reddy C, Zimmerman-Bier B. Evaluation of an association between gastrointestinal symptoms and cytokine production against common dietary proteins in children with autism spectrum disorders. *J Pediatr.* 2005 May;146(5):605-10.

38 Okada K, Hashimoto K, Iwata Y, Nakamura K, Tsujii M, Tsuchiya KJ, Sekine Y, Suda S, Suzuki K, Sugihara GI, Matsuzaki H, Sugiyama T, Kawai M, Minabe Y Takei N, Mori N. Decreased serum levels of transforming growth factor-beta1 in patients with autism. *Prog Neuropsychopharmacol Biol Psychiatry.* 2006 Oct 5; [Epub ahead of print].

39 Vargas DL, Nascimbene C, Krishnan C, Zimmerman AW, Pardo CA. Neuroglial activation and neuroinflammation in the brain of patients with autism. *Ann Neurol.* 2005 Jan;57(1)67-81.

40 Pardo CA, Vargas DL, Zimmerman AW. Immunity, neuroglia and neuroinflammation in autism. *Int Rev Psychiatry.* 2005 Dec;17(6):485-95.

41 Comi AM, Zimmerman AW, Frye VH, Law PA, Peeden JN. Familial clustering of autoimmune disorders and evaluation of medical risk factors in autism. *J Child Neurol.* 1999 Jun;14(6):388-94.

42 Sweeten TL, Bowyer SL, Posey DJ, Halberstadt GM, McDougle CJ. Increased prevalence of familial autoimmunity in probands with pervasive developmental disorders. *Pediatrics.* 2003 Nov;112(5):e420.

43 Ashwood P, Van de Water J. Is autism an autoimmune disease? *Autoimmun Rev.* 2004 Nov;3(7-8):557-62.

44   Todd RD, Hickok JM, Anderson GM, Cohen DJ. Antibrain antibodies in infantile autism. *Biol Psychiatry*. 1988 Mar 15;23(6):644-7.

45   Silva SC, Correia C, Fesel C, Barreto M, Coutinho AM, Marques C, Miguel TS, Ataide A, Bento C, Borges L, Oliveira G, Vicente AM. Autoantibody repertoires to brain tissue in autism nuclear families. *J Neuroimmunol*. 2004 Jul;152(1-2):176-82.

46   Singh VK, Warren R, Averett R, Ghaziuddin M. Circulating autoantibodies to neuronal and glial filament proteins in autism. *Pediatr Neurol*. 1997 Jul;17(1):88-90.

47   Singh VK, Warren RP, Odell JD, Warren WL, Cole P. Antibodies to myelin basic protein in children with autistic behavior. *Brain Behav Immun*. 1993 Mar;7(1): 97-103.

48   Singh VK, Singh EA, Warren RP. Hyperserotoninemia and serotonin receptor antibodies in children with autism but not mental retardation. *Biol Psychiatry*. 1997 Mar 15;41(6):753-5.

49   Singh VK, Rivas WH. Prevalence of serum antibodies to caudate nucleus in autistic children. *Neurosci Lett*. 2004 Jan 23;355(1-2):53-6.

50   Singer HS, Morris CM, Williams PN, Yoon DY, Hong JJ, Zimmerman AW. Antibrain antibodies in children with autism and their unaffected siblings. *J Neuroimmunol*. 2006 Sep;178(1-2):149-155.

51   Ibid.

52   Ibid.

53   Ibid.

54   Singh VK, Warren R, Averett R, Ghaziuddin M. Circulating autoantibodies to neuronal and glial filament proteins in autism. *Pediatr Neurol*. 1997 Jul;17(1):88-90.

55   Singer HS, Morris CM, Williams PN, Yoon DY, Hong JJ, Zimmerman AW. Antibrain antibodies in children with autism and their unaffected siblings. *J Neuroimmunol*. 2006 Sep;178(1-2):149-155.

56   Plioplys AV, Greaves A. Yoshida W. Anti-CNS antibodies in childhood neurologic diseases. *Neuropediatrics*. 1989;20:93.

57   Connolly AM, Chez MG, Pestronk A, Arnold ST, Mehta S, Deuel RK. Serum autoantibodies to brain in Landau-Kleffner variant, autism, and other neurologic disorders. *J Pediatr*. 1999 May;134(5):607-13.

58   Tuchman RF, Rapin I, Shinnar S. Autistic and dysphasic children. I: Clinical characteristics. *Pediatrics*. 1991 Dec;88(6):1211-8.

59   Todd RD, Hickok JM, Anderson GM, Cohen DJ. Antibrain antibodies in infantile autism. *Biol Psychiatry*. 1988 Mar 15;23(6):644-7.

60   Silva SC, Correia C, Fesel C, Barreto M, Coutinho AM, Marques C, Miguel TS, Ataide A, Bento C, Borges L, Oliveira G, Vicente AM. Autoantibody repertoires to brain tissue in autism nuclear families. *J Neuroimmunol*. 2004 Jul;152(1-2):176-82.

61   Ahlsen G, Rosengren L, Belfrage M, Palm A, Haglid K, Hamberger A, Gillberg C. Glial fibrillary acidic protein in the cerebrospinal fluid of children with autism and other neuropsychiatric disorders. *Biol Psychiatry*. 1993 May 15;33(10):734-43.

62   Rumsey JM, Ernst M. Functional neuroimaging of autistic disorders. *Ment Retard Dev Disabil Res Rev.* 2000;6(3):171-9.

63   Torrente F, Ashwood P, Day R, Machado N, Furlano RI, Anthony A, Davies SE, Wakefield AJ, Thomson MA, Walker-Smith JA, Murch SH. Small intestinal enteropathy with epithelial IgG and complement deposition in children with regressive autism. *Mol Psychiatry.* 2002;7(4):375-82, 334.

64   Mehler MF, Kessler JA. Cytokines in brain development and function. *Adv Protein Chem.* 1998;52:223-51.

65   Dalton P, Deacon R, Blamire A, Pike M, McKinlay I, Stein J, Styles P, Vincent A. Maternal neuronal antibodies associated with autism and a language disorder. *Ann Neurol.* 2003 Apr;53(4):533-7.

66   Zimmerman AW, Connors SL, Matteson KJ, Lee LC, Singer HS, Castaneda JA, Pearce DA. Maternal antibrain antibodies in autism. *Brain Behav Immun.* 2006 Oct 5;[Epub ahead of print].

67   Warren RP, Cole P, Odell JD, Pingree CB, Warren WL, White E, Yonk J, Singh VK. Detection of maternal antibodies in infantile autism. *J Am Acad Child Adolesc Psychiatry.* 1990 Nov;29(6):873-7.

68   Meyer U, Nyffeler M, Engler A, Urwyler A, Schedlowski M, Knuesel I, Yee BK, Feldon J. The time of prenatal immune challenge determines the specificity of inflammation-mediated brain and behavioral pathology. *J Neurosci.* 2006 May 3; 26(18):4752-62.

69   Lucarelli S, Frediani T, Zingoni AM, Ferruzzi F, Giardini O, Quintieri F, Barbato M, D'Eufemia P, Cardi E. Food allergy and infantile autism. *Panminerva Med.* 1995 Sep;37(3):137-41.

70   Jyonouchi H, Sun S, Itokazu N. Innate immunity associated with inflammatory responses and cytokine production against common dietary proteins in patients with autism spectrum disorder. *Neuropsychobiology.* 2002;46(2):76-84.

71   Jyonouchi H, Geng L, Ruby A, Reddy C, Zimmerman-Bier B. Evaluation of an association between gastrointestinal symptoms and cytokine production against common dietary proteins in children with autism spectrum disorders. *J Pediatr.* 2005 May;146(5):605-10.

72   Jyonouchi H, Geng L, Ruby A, Zimmerman-Bier B. Dysregulated innate immune responses in young children with autism spectrum disorders: their relationship to gastrointestinal symptoms and dietary intervention. *Neuropsychobiology.* 2005;51(2):77-85.

73   Campbell DB, Sutcliffe JS, Ebert PJ, Militerni R, Bravaccio C, Trillo S, Elia M, Schneider C, Melmed R, Sacco R, Persico AM, Levitt P. A genetic variant that disrupts MET transcription is associated with autism. *Proc Natl Acad Sci U S A.* 2006 Oct 19.

74   Vojdani A, Campbell AW, Anyanwu E, Kashanian A, Bock K, Vojdani E. Antibodies to neuron-specific antigens in children with autism: possible cross-reaction with encephalitogenic proteins from milk, Chlamydia pneumoniae and Streptococcus group A. *J Neuroimmunol.* 2002 Aug;129(1-2):168-77.

75 James SJ, Cutler P, Melnyk S, Jernigan S, Janak L, Gaylor DW, Neubrander JA. Metabolic biomarkers of increased oxidative stress and impaired methylation capacity in children with autism. *Am J Clin Nutr.* 2004 Dec;80(6):1611-7.

76 Libbey JE, Sweeten TL, McMahon WM, Fujinami RS. Autistic disorder and viral infections. *J Neurovirol.* 2005 Feb;11(1):1-10.

77 Lopez-Pison J, Rubio-Rubio R, Urena-Hornos T, Omenaca-Teres M, Sans A, Cabrerizo de Diago R, Pena-Segura JL. Retrospective diagnosis of congenital infection by cytomegalovirus in the case of one infant. *Rev Neurol.* 2005 Jun 16-30; 40(12):733-6.

78 Pletnikov MV, Jones ML, Rubin SA, Moran TH, Carbone KM. Rat model of autism spectrum disorders. Genetic background effects on Borna disease virus-induced developmental brain damage. *Ann N Y Acad Sci.* 2001 Jun;939:318-9.

79 Chess S, Fernandez P, Korn S. Behavioral consequences of congenital rubella. *J Pediatr.* 1978 Oct;93(4):699-703.

80 Swisher CN, Swisher L. Letter: Congenital rubella and autistic behavior. *N Engl J Med.* 1975 Jul 24;293(4):198.

81 DeLong GR, Bean SC, Brown FR 3rd. Acquired reversible autistic syndrome in acute encephalopathic illness in children. *Arch Neurol.* 1981 Mar;38(3):191-4.

82 Sweeten TL, Posey DJ, McDougle CJ. Brief report: autistic disorder in three children with cytomegalovirus infection. *J Autism Dev Disord.* 2004 Oct;34(5): 583-6.

83 Bach JF. Infections and autoimmune diseases. *J Autoimmun.* 2005;25 Suppl:74-80.

84 Gurney JG, McPheeters ML, Davis MM. Parental report of health conditions and health care use among children with and without autism: National Survey of Children's Health. *Arch Pediatr Adolesc Med.* 2006 Aug;160(8):825-30.

85 Croen LA, Najjar DV, Ray GT, Lotspeich L, Bernal P. A comparison of health care utilization and costs of children with and without autism spectrum disorders in a large group-model health plan. *Pediatrics.* 2006 Oct;118(4):e1203-11.

86 Niehus R, Lord C. Early medical history of children with autism spectrum disorders. *J Dev Behav Pediatr.* 2006 Apr;27(2 Suppl):S120-7.

87 Fallon J. Could one of the most widely prescribed antibiotics amoxicillin/clavulanate "augmentin" be a risk factor for autism? *Med Hypotheses.* 2005;64(2): 312-5.

88 Konstantareas MM, Homatidis S. Ear infections in autistic and normal children. *J Autism Dev Disord.* 1987 Dec;17(4):585-94.

CHAPTER 8

1 Wakefield AJ, Murch SH, Anthony A, Linn ell J, Caisson DM, Mali M, Berelowitz M, Dhillon AP, Thomson MA, Harvey P, Valentine A, Davies SE, Walker-Smith JA: Ileal-lymphoid-nodular hyperplasia, non-specific colitis, and pervasive developmental disorder in children. *Lancet* 1998 Feb 28;351(9103): 637-41.

2   Taylor B, Miller E, Farrington CP, Petropoulos MC, Favot-Mayaud I, Li J,Waight P. Autism and measles, mumps, and rubella vaccine: no epidemiological evidence for a causal association. *Lancet.* 1999;353:2026-2029.

3   Madsen KM, Hviid A, Vestergaard M, Schendel D,Wohlfahrt J, Thorsen P, Olsen J, Melbye M. A population-based study of measles, mumps, and rubella vaccination and autism. *N Engl J Med.* 2002 Nov 7;347(19):1477-82.

4   Wakefield AJ. MMR vaccination and autism. *Lancet.* 1999;354:949-50.

5   Altmann D. Autism and measles, mumps, and rubella vaccine. *Lancet* 2000;355:409.

6   Stott C, Blaxill M,Wakefield A. MMR and Autism in Perspective: the Denmark story. *J Am Phys Surg.* 2004;9 (3): 89-91.

7   Goin-Kochel RP, Mackintosh VH, Myers BJ. How many doctors does it take to make an autism spectrum diagnosis? *Autism.* 2006 Sep;10(5):439-51.

8   Madsen KM, Hviid A, Vestergaard M, Schendel D,Wohlfahrt J, Thorsen P, Olsen J, Melbye M. A population-based study of measles, mumps, and rubella vaccination and autism. *N Engl J Med.* 2002 Nov 7;347(19):1477-82.

9   Goldman GS, Yazbak FE. An investigation of the association between MMR vaccination and autism in Denmark. *J Am Phys Surg.* 2004;9:70-75.

10   Lauritsen MB, Pedersen CB, Mortensen PB. The incidence and prevalence of pervasive developmental disorders: a Danish population-based study. *Psychol Med.* 2004;34:1339-1346.

11   Wilson K, Mills E, Ross C, McGowan J, Jadad A. Association of autistic spectrum disorder and the measles, mumps, and rubella vaccine: a systematic review of current epidemiological evidence. *Arch Pediatr Adolesc Med.* 2003 Jul;157(7):628-34.

12   Gillberg C, Heijbel H. MMR and autism. *Autism.* 1998;2:423-24.

13   Kaye JA, del Mar Melero-Montes M, Jick H. Mumps, Measles, and rubella vaccine and the incidence of autism recorded by general practitioners: a time trend analysis. *BMJ* 2001;322:460-3.

14   Dales L, Hammer SJ, Smith NJ.Time trends in autism and MMR immunization coverage in California. *JAMA.* 2001;285:1183-1185.

15   Fombonne E, Chakrabarti S. No evidence for a new variant of measles-mumps-rubella- induced autism. *Pediatrics.* 2001;108:991.

16   Taylor B, Miller E, Lingam R, Andrews N, Simmons A, Stowe J. Measles, mumps, and rubella vaccination and bowel problems or developmental regression in children with autism: population study. *BMJ.* 2002 Feb 16;324(7334):393-6.

17   Patja A, Davidkin I, Kurki T, Kallio M, Valle M, Peltola H. Serious adverse events after measles-mumps-rubella vaccination during a fourteen-year prospective followup. *Pediatr Infect Dis J.* 2000;19:1127-34.

18   Farrington CP, Miller E,Taylor B. MMR and autism: further evidence against a causal association. *Vaccine.* 2001 Jun 14;19(27):3632-5.

19   DeWilde S, Carey IM, Richards N, Hilton SR, Cook DG. Do children who become autistic consult more often after MMR vaccination? *Br J Gen Pract.* 2001 Mar;51(464):226-7.

20 Fombonne E, Chakrabarti S. No evidence for a new variant of measles-mumps-rubella-induced autism. *Pediatrics.* 2001;108:991.

21 Makela A, Nuorti JP, Peltola H. Neurologic disorders after measles-mumps-rubella vaccination. *Pediatrics.* 2002 Nov;110(5):957-63.

22 Chen W, Landau S, Sham P, Fombonne E. No evidence for links between autism, MMR and measles virus. *Psychol Med.* 2004 Apr;34(3):543-53.

23 Taylor B, Miller E, Lingam R, Andrews N, Simmons A, Stowe J. Measles, mumps, and rubella vaccination and bowel problems or developmental regression in children with autism: population study. *BMJ.* 2002 Feb 16;324(7334):393-6.

24 Fombonne E, Chakrabarti S. No evidence for a new variant of measles-mumps-rubella-induced autism. *Pediatrics.* 2001;108:991.

25 Peltola H, Patja A, Leinikki P, Valle M, Davidkin I, Paunio M. No evidence for measles, mumps, and rubella vaccine-associated inflammatory bowel disease or autism in a 14-year prospective study. *The Lancet.* 1998; 351:1327-1328.

26 Makela A, Nuorti JP, Peltola H. Neurologic disorders after measles-mumps-rubella vaccination. *Pediatrics.* 2002 Nov;110(5):957-63.

27 Smeeth L. Measles, mumps, and rubella (MMR) vaccine and autism: ecological studies cannot answer main question. *BMJ* 2001 Jul;323(7305):163.

28 Edwardes M, Baltzan M. Measles, mumps, and rubella (MMR) vaccine and autism. Argument is too simplistic. *BMJ.* 2001 Jul 21;323(7305):163; author reply 164.

29 Yazbak FE. Measles, mumps, and rubella (MMR) vaccine and autism. MMR cannot be exonerated without explaining increased incidence of autism. *BMJ.* 2001 Jul 21;323(7305):163-4.

30 Edwardes M, Baltzan M. MMR Immunization and Autism. *JAMA* 2001;285: 2852- 3.

31 Spitzer WO. Measles, mumps, and rubella vaccination and autism. *N Engl J Med.* 2003 Mar 6;348(10):951-4; author reply 951-4.

32 Wakefield AJ. Measles, mumps, and rubella vaccination and autism. *N Engl J Med.* 2003 Mar 6;348(10):951-4; author reply 951-4.

33 Wakefield AJ. MMR vaccination and autism. *Lancet.* 1999;354:949-50.

34 Richler J, Luyster R, Risi S, Hsu WL, Dawson G, Bernier R, Dunn M, Hepburn S, Hyman SL, McMahon WM, Goudie-Nice J, Minshew N, Rogers S, Sigman M, Spence MA, Goldberg WA,Tager-Flusberg H, Volkmar FR, Lord C. Is There a 'Regressive Phenotype' of Autism Spectrum Disorder Associated with the Measles-Mumps-Rubella Vaccine? A CPEA Study. *J Autism Dev Disord.* 2006 Apr;36(3):299-316.

35 Stott C. Phenotypic features of pervasive developmental disorder (PDD) following exposure to polyvalent measles containing vaccine data from a UK litigation cohort. IMFAR presentation, 2005.

36 Honda H, Shimizu Y, Rutter M. No effect of MMR withdrawal on the incidence of autism: a total population study. *J Child Psychol Psychiatry.* 2005 Jun;46(6):572-9.

37   Wakefield AJ and Montgomery SM. Measles, mumps, rubella vaccine: through a glass, darkly. *Adverse Drug React Toxicol Rev.* 2000:19(4): 265–83.

38   Wakefield AJ, Stott C. No effect of MMR withdrawal on the incidence of autism: a total population study. www.thoughtfulhouse.org/pr/pr_030805072428.htm.

39   Takahashi H, Suzumura S, Shirakizawa F,Wada N,Tanaka-Taya K, Arai S, Okabe N, Ichikawa H, Sato T. An epidemiological study on Japanese autism concerning routine childhood immunization history. *Jpn J Infect Dis.* 2003 Jun;56(3):114-7.

40   Geier M, Geier D. Pediatric MMR Vaccination Safety. *Int Pediatr.* 2003:18/(2); 203- 208.

41   Zhou W, Pool V, Iskander JK, English-Bullard R, Ball R,Wise RP, Haber P, Pless RP, Mootrey G, Ellenberg SS, Braun MM, Chen RT. Surveillance for safety after immunization: Vaccine Adverse Event Reporting System (VAERS)—United States, 1991-2001. *MMWR Surveill Summ.* 2003 Jan 24;52(1):1-24.

42   Richler J Luyster R, Risi S, Hsu WL, Dawson G, Bernier R, Dunn M, Hepburn S, Hyman SL, McMahon WM, Goudie-Nice J, Minshew N, Rogers S, Sigman M, Spence MA, Goldberg WA,Tager-Flusberg H, Volkmar FR, Lord C. Is There a 'Regressive Phenotype' of Autism Spectrum Disorder Associated with the Measles-Mumps-Rubella Vaccine? A CPEA Study. *J Autism Dev Disord.* 2006 Apr;36(3): 299-316.

43   Rima BK, Duprex WP. Morbilliviruses and human disease. *J Pathol.* 2006 Jan; 208(2):199-214.

44   Wakefield AJ and Montgomery SM. *Adverse Drug React Toxicol Rev.* 2000:19(4): 265–83.

45   Wakefield AJ., Puleston J. Montgomery SM., Anthony A., O'Leary J.J., Murch SH Entero-colonic encephalopathy, autism and opioid receptor ligands. *Aliment Pharmacol Ther.* 2002;16:663-674.

46   Wakefield AJ. Enterocolitis, Autism and Measles Virus. *Mol Psychiatry.* 2002; 7 Suppl 2:S44-6.

47   Wakefield AJ and Montgomery SM. *Adverse Drug React Toxicol Rev.* 2000:19(4): 265–83.

48   Ibid.

49   Connolly J, Allen I, Hurwitz L, Millar JHD. Measles antibody and antigen in SSPE. *Lancet* 1967;i:542

50   Freeman JM, Magoffin RL, Lennette EH, Herndon RM. Additional evidence of relation between subacute inclusion body encephalitis and measles virus. *Lancet* 1967;ii:129-131.

51   Montgomery SM, Morris DL, Pounder RE,Wakefield AJ. Paramyxovirus infections in childhood and subsequent inflammatory bowel disease. *Gastroenterology.* 1999 Apr;116(4):796-803.

52   Jirapinyo P, Thakernpol K, Chaichanwatanakul K. Cytopathic effects of measles virus on the human intestinal mucosa. *J. Paed. Gastroenterol. Nutrit.*1990;10:550-554.

53 Landrigan PJ,Witte JJ. Neurologic disorders following live measles-virus vaccination. *JAMA.* 1973;223:1459-1462.

54 Plesner A-M, Hansen FJ,Taadon K, Nielson LH, Larsen CB, Pedersen E. Gait disturbance interpreted as cerebellar ataxia after MMR vaccination at 15 months of age: a follow-up study. *Acta Paediatrica* 2000;89:58-63.

55 Weibel RE, Caserta V, Benor DE. Acute encephalopathy followed by permanent brain injury or death associated with further attenuated measles vaccines: a review of claims submitted to the National Vaccine Injury Compensation Programme. *Paediatrics* 1998;101:383-387.

56 Garenne M, Leroy O, Bean J-P, Sene I, Child mortality after high titre measles vaccines: prospective study in Senegal. *Lancet* 1991;2:903-907.

57 Montgomery SM, Morris DL, Pounder RE,Wakefield AJ. Paramyxovirus infections in childhood and subsequent inflammatory bowel disease. *Gastroenterology.* 1999 Apr;116(4):796-803.

58 Ki M, Park T, Gon Yi S, Kyoung Oh J, Youl Chi B. Risk Analysis of Aseptic Meningitis after Measles-Mumps-Rubella Vaccination in Korean Children by Using a Case-Crossover Design. *Am J Epidemiol* 2003; 157:158-165.

59 Miller E, Goldacre M, Pugh S, Colville A, Farrington P, Flower A, Nash J, MacFarlane L,Tettmar R. Risk of aseptic meningitis after measles, mumps, and rubella vaccine in UK children. *Lancet.* 1993 Apr 17;341(8851):979-82.

60 Uhlmann V, Martin CM, Sheils O, Pilkington L, Silva I, Killalea A, Murch SB, Walker-Smith J, Thomson M,Wakefield AJ, O'Leary JJ. Potential viral pathogenic mechanism for new variant inflammatory bowel disease.*Mol Pathol.* 2002 Apr;55(2):84-90.

61 Ashwood P. Detection of Measles virus antigen in children with autistic enterocolitis. Publication pending.

62 Kawashima H, Mori T, Kashiwagi Y,Takekuma K, Hoshika A,Wakefield A. Detection and sequencing of measles virus from peripheral mononuclear cells from patients with inflammatory bowel disease and autism. *Dig Dis Sci.* 2000 Apr;45(4):723-9.

63 Uhlmann V, Martin CM, Sheils O, Pilkington L, Silva I, Killalea A, Murch SB, Walker-Smith J, Thomson M,Wakefield AJ, O'Leary JJ. Potential viral pathogenic mechanism for new variant inflammatory bowel disease.*Mol Pathol.* 2002 Apr;55(2):84-90.

64 Walker SJ, Hepner K, Segal J, Krigsman A. Persistent ileal measles virus in a large cohort of regressive autistic children with ileocolitis and lymphonodular hyperplasia: revisitation of an earlier study. IMFAR.

65 Immunization Safety Review Committee, Institute of Medicine. *Measles-Mumps-Rubella Vaccine and Autism.*Washington, DC: National Academy Press; 2001.

66 Wakefield A, Stott C, Limb K. Gastrointestinal comorbidity, autistic regression and Measles-containing vaccines: positive re-challenge and biological gradient. *Medical Veritas:* 3 (2006) 796–802.

67   Singh VK, Lin SX, Yang V. Serological association of measles virus and human herpesvirus- 6 with brain autoantibodies in autism. *Clin Immun Immunopathol.* 1998 Oct:89(1):105-108.

68   Singh VK, Lin SX, Newell E, Nelson C. Abnormal measles-mumps-rubella antibodies and CNS autoimmunity in children with autism. *J Biomed Sci.* 2002; 9:359-364.

69   Singh VK, Jensen RL. Elevated levels of measles antibodies in children with autism. *Pediatr Neurol.* 2003 Apr;28(4):292-4.

70   Bradstreet J, El Dahr J, Anthony A, Kartzinel J,Wakefield, A. Detection of Measles Virus Genomic RNA in Cerebrospinal Fluid of Children with Regressive Autism: a Report of Three Cases. *J Am Phys Surg,* Vol 9 No 2, 2004.

71   Bradstreet J, El Dahr J,Walker S, Montgomery S.M, Kartzinel J,Wakefield A, Sheils O, O'Leary J. TaqMan RT-PCR Detection of Measles Virus Genomic RNA in Cerebrospinal Fluid in Children with Regressive Autism. Presented IMFAR, MIND Institute May 2004.

CHAPTER 9

1   D'Souza Y, Fombonne E,Ward BJ. No evidence of persisting measles virus in peripheral blood mononuclear cells from children with autism spectrum disorder. *Pediatrics.* 2006 Oct;118(4):1664-75.

2   Valicenti-McDermott M, McVicar K, Rapin I,Wershil BK, Cohen H, Shinnar S. Frequency of gastrointestinal symptoms in children with autistic spectrum disorders and association with family history of autoimmune disease. *J Dev Behav Pediatr.* 2006 Apr;27(2 Suppl):S128-36.

3   Melmed RD, Schneider CK, Fabes RA. Metabolic markers and gastrointestinal symptoms in children with autism and related disorders. *J Pediatr Gastroenterol Nutr* 2000:31(suppl 2)S31-32.

4   Levy S, Souders MC,Wray J, Jawad AF, Gallagher PR, Coplan J, Belchic JK, Gerdes M, Mitchell R, Mulberg AE. Children with autistic spectrum disorders. I: Comparison of placebo and single dose of human synthetic secretin. *Arch. Dis. Child.* 2003;88;731-736.

5   Horvath K, Perman JA. Autistic disorder and gastrointestinal disease. *Curr Opin Pediatr.* 2002 Oct;14(5):583-7.

6   Fombonne E, Chakrabarti S. No evidence for a new variant of measles-mumps-rubella-induced autism. *Pediatrics.* 2001 Oct;108(4):E58.

7   Taylor B, Miller E, Lingam R, Andrews N, Simmons A, Stowe J. Measles, mumps, and rubella vaccination and bowel problems or developmental regression in children with autism: population study. *BMJ.* 2002 Feb 16;324(7334):393-6.

8   Black C, Kaye JA, Jick H. Relation of childhood gastrointestinal disorders to autism: nested case-control study using data from the UK General Practice Research Database. *BMJ.* 2002 Aug 24;325(7361):419-21.

9   Kuddo T, Nelson KB. How common are gastrointestinal disorders in children with autism. *Curr Opin Pediatr* 2003: 15(3); 339-343.

10   Horvath K, Papadimitriou JC, Rabazlan A. Gastrointestinal abnormalities in children with autistic disorder. *J Pediatr* 1999, 135:559-563.

11   Wakefield A. Commentary. Autistic Enterocolitis: is it a Histopathological Entity?—not yet published.

12   Krigsman A, Boris M, Goldblatt A. Frequency of histologic enterocolitis and lymphonodular hyperplasia in autistic children presenting for ileocolonoscopy. IMFAR. May 7th, 2004.

13   Afzal N, Murch S, Thirrupathy K, Berger L, Fagbemi A, Heuschkel R. Constipation with acquired megarectum in children with autism. *Pediatrics.* 2003 Oct;112(4):939-42.

14   Wakefield AJ, Murch SH, Anthony A et al. Ileal-lymphoid nodular hyperplasia non-specific colitis and pervasive developmental disorder in children. *Lancet.* 1998;351:637-41.

15   Wakefield AJ, Anthony A, Murch SH, Thomson M, Montgomery SM, Davies S, O'Leary JJ, Berelowitz M, Walker-Smith JA. Enterocolitis in children with developmental disorders. *Am J Gastroenterol.* 2000 Sep;95(9):2285-95.

16   Wakefield AJ, Ashwood P, Limb K, Anthony A. The significance of ileo-colonic lymphoid nodular hyperplasia in children with autistic spectrum disorder. *Eur J Gastroenterol Hepatol.* 2005 Aug;17(8):827-36.

17   Walker SJ, Hepner K, Segal J, Krigsman A. Persistent ileal measles virus in a large cohort of regressive autistic children with ileocolitis and lymphonodular hyperplasia: revisitation of an earlier study. IMFAR. June 1, 2006.

18   Kushak R, Winter H, Farber N, Buie T. Gastrointestinal symptoms and intestinal disaccharidase activities in children with autism. Abstract of presentation to the North American Society of Pediatric Gastroenterology, Hepatology, and Nutrition, Annual Meeting, October 20-22, 2005, Salt Lake City, Utah.

19   Balzola F, Barbon V, Repici A, Rizzetto M. Panenteric IBD-like disease in a patient with regressive autism shown for the first time by the wireless capsule enteroscopy: another piece in the jigsaw of this gut-brain syndrome? *Am J Gastro.* 2005; 979-981.

20   Balzola F, Daniela C, Repici A, Barbon V, Sapino A, Barbera C, Calvo PL, Gandione M, Rigardetto R, Rizzetto M. Autistic enterocolitis: confirmation of a new inflammatory bowel disease in an Italian cohort of patients. *Gastroenterology.* 2005;128:Suppl.2;A-303.

21   Gonzalez L, Lopez K, Navarro D, Negron L, Flores L, Rodriguez R, Martinez M, Sabra A. Endoscopic and Histological Characteristics of the digestive mucosa in autistic children with gastrointestinal symptoms. *Arch Venez Pueric Pediatr* 69; 1:19-25.

22   Balzola F, Barbon V, Repici A, Rizzetto M. Panenteric IBD-like disease in a patient with regressive autism shown for the first time by the wireless capsule enteroscopy: another piece in the jigsaw of this gut-brain syndrome? *Am J Gastro* 2005; 979-981.

23   Furlano RI, Anthony A, Day R, Brown A, McGavery L, Thomson MA, Davies SE, Berelowitz M, Forbes A, Wakefield AJ, Walker-Smith JA, Murch SH. Colonic

CD8 and gamma delta T-cell infiltration with epithelial damage in children with autism. *Pediatrics* 2001;138:366-72.

24 Torrente F, Machado N, Perez-Machado M, Furlano R, Thomson M, Davies S, Wakefield AJ, Walker-Smith JA, Murch SH. Enteropathy with T cell infiltration and epithelial IgG deposition in autism. *Mol Psychiatry.* 2002;7:375-382.

25 Torrente F, Anthony A. Focal-enhanced gastritis in regressive autism with features distinct from Crohn's disease and helicobacter Pylori gastritis. *Am J Gastroenterol* 2004 Apr;99(4):598-605.

26 Ashwood P, Wakefield AJ. Immune activation of peripheral blood and mucosal CD3+ lymphocyte cytokine profiles in children with autism and gastrointestinal symptoms. *J Neuroimmunol.* 2006 Apr;173(1-2):126-34.

27 Wakefield AJ, Puleston JM, Montgomery SM, Anthony A, O'Leary JJ, Murch SH. Review article: the concept of entero-colonic encephalopathy, autism and opioid receptor ligands. *Aliment Pharmacol Ther.* 2002 Apr;16(4):663-74.

28 D'Eufemia P, Celli M, Finocchiaro R, Pacifico L, Viozzi L, Zaccagnini M, Cardi E, Giardini O. Abnormal intestinal permeability in children with autism. *Acta Paediatr.* 1996 Sep;85(9):1076-9.

29 Horvath K, Perman JA. Autistic disorder and gastrointestinal disease. *Curr Opin Pediatr* 2002:14:583-7.

30 Alberti A, Pirrone P, Elia M, Waring R, Romano C. Sulphation deficit in "low-functioning" autistic children: a pilot study. *Biol Psychiatry* 1999; 46 (3), 420-424.

31 Owens S. Mechanisms Behind the Leaky Gut. Autism One. www.autismone.org/uploads/Owens %20Susan.doc.

32 Goodwin MS, Cowen MA, Goodwin TC. Malabsorption and cerebral dysfunction. *J Autism Child Schizophr.* 1971;1:48-62.

33 Reichelt KL, Saelid G, Lindback T, Boler JB. Childhood autism: a complex disorder. *Biol Psychiatry.* 1986 Nov;21(13):1279-90.

34 Shattock P, Kennedy A, Rowell F, Berney T. Role of neuropeptides in autism and their relationship with classical neurotransmitters. *Brain Dysfunction* 1990:3: 328-345.

35 Shattock P, Lowdon G. Proteins, peptides and autism: Part 2: Implications for the education and care of people with autism. *Brain Dysfunction.* 1991;4: 323-334.

36 Reichelt KL, Knivsberg AM, Lind G, Nodland M: Probable Etiology and Possible Treatment of Childhood Autism. *Brain Dysfuntion* 1991; 4: 308-319.

37 Knivsberg AM, Reichelt KL, Nodland M, Hoein T: Autistic Syndromes and Diet: a follow-up study. *Scandinavian Journal of Educational Research* 1995; 39: 223-236.

38 Cade R, Privette M, Fregly M, Rowland N, Sun Z, Zele V, Wagemaker H, Edelstein C. Autism and schizophrenia: Intestinal disorders. *Nutr Neurosci.* 2000; 3, 57–72.

39 Knivsberg AM, Reichelt KL, Nodland M. Reports on dietary intervention in autistic disorders. *Nutr Neurosci.* 2001;4(1):25-37.

40 Knivsberg AM, Reichelt KL, Hoien T, Nodland M. A randomised, controlled study of dietary intervention in autistic syndromes. *Nutr Neurosci.* 2002 Sep; 5(4):251-61.

41 Reichelt KL, Knivsberg AM. Can the pathophysiology of autism be explained by the nature of the discovered urine peptides? *Nutr Neurosci.* 2003 Feb;6(1):19-28.

42 Bolte ER. Autism and Clostridium tetani. *Med Hypotheses.* 1998 Aug;51(2):133-44.

43 Song Y, Liu C, Finegold SM. Real-time PCR quantitation of clostridia in feces of autistic children. *Appl Environ Microbiol.* 2004 Nov;70(11):6459-65.

44 Parracho HM, Bingham MO, Gibson GR, McCartney AL. Differences between the gut microflora of children with autistic spectrum disorders and that of healthy children. *J Med Microbiol.* 2005 Oct;54(Pt 10):987-91.

45 Finegold SM, Molitoris D, Song Y, Liu C, Vaisanen ML, Bolte E, McTeague M, Sandler R, Wexler H, Marlowe EM, Collins MD, Lawson PA, Summanen P, Baysallar M, Tomzynski TJ, Read E, Johnson E, Rolfe R, Nasir P, Shah H, Haake DA, Manning P, Kaul A. Gastrointestinal microflora studies in late-onset autism. *Clin Infect Dis.* 2002 Sep 1;35(Suppl 1):S6-S16.

46 Rosseneu S. DAN! Conference presentation. April 16, 2004.

47 Sandler RH, Finegold SM, Bolte ER, Buchanan CP, Maxwell AP, Vaisanen ML, Nelson MN, Wexler HM. Short-term benefit from oral vancomycin treatment of regressive-onset autism. *J Child Neurol.* 2000 Jul;15(7):429-35.

48 Shaw W, Kassen E, Chaves E. Increased urinary excretion of analogs of Krebs cycle metabolites and arabinose in two brothers with autistic features. *Clin Chem.* 1995 Aug;41(8 Pt 1):1094-104.

49 Baker S, Pangborn J. *Autism: Effective Biomedical Treatments (Have We Done Everything We Can For This Child? Individuality In An Epidemic).* San Diego: Autism Research Institute; 2nd Edition Sept. 2005.

50 Parent Ratings of Behavioral Effects of Biomedical Interventions. Autism Research Institute. www.autismwebsite.com/ari/treatment/form34q.htm.

CHAPTER 10

1 James J. DAN! Conference presentation. April 6-9, 2006.

2 Deth R. DAN! Conference presentation. Spring 2005.

3 Waly M, Olteanu H, Banerjee R, Choi SW, Mason JB, Parker BS, Sukumar S, Shim S, Sharma A, Benzecry JM, Power Charnitsky VA, Deth RC. Activation of methionine synthase by insulin-like growth factor-1 and dopamine: a target for neurodevelopmental toxins and thimerosal. *Mol Psychiatry.* 2004 Apr;9(4):358-70.

4 Aschner M, Syversen T, Souza DO, Rocha JB. Metallothioneins: mercury species-specific induction and their potential role in attenuating neurotoxicity. *Exp Biol Med (Maywood).* 2006 Oct;231(9):1468-73.

5 James SJ, Cutler P, Melnyk S, Jernigan S, Janak L, Gaylor DW, Neubrander JA. Metabolic biomarkers of increased oxidative stress and impaired methylation capacity in children with autism. *Am J Clin Nutr.* 2004 Dec;80(6):1611-7.

6 Kern JK, Jones AM. Evidence of toxicity, oxidative stress, and neuronal insult in autism. *J Toxicol Environ Health B Crit Rev.* 2006 Nov-Dec;9(6):485-99.

7   Cai J, Chen Y, Seth S, Furukawa S, Compans RW, Jones DP. Inhibition of influenza infection by glutathione. *Free Radic Biol Med.* 2003 Apr 1;34(7):928-36.

8   Sido B, Hack V, Hochlehnert A, Lipps H, Herfarth C, Droge W. Impairment of intestinal glutathione synthesis in patients with inflammatory bowel disease. *Gut.* 1998 Apr;42(4):485-92.

9   Aw TY. Intestinal glutathione: determinant of mucosal peroxide transport, metabolism, and oxidative susceptibility. *Toxicol Appl Pharmacol.* 2005 May 1; 204(3):320-8.

10 James SJ, Cutler P, Melnyk S, Jernigan S, Janak L, Gaylor DW, Neubrander JA. Metabolic biomarkers of increased oxidative stress and impaired methylation capacity in children with autism. *Am J Clin Nutr.* 2004 Dec;80(6):1611-7.

11 James SJ, Melnyk S, Jernigan S, Cleves MA, Halsted CH, Wong DH, Cutler P, Bock K, Boris M, Bradstreet JJ, Baker SM, Gaylor DW. Metabolic endophenotype and related genotypes are associated with oxidative stress in children with autism. *Am J Med Genet B Neuropsychiatr Genet.* 2006 Aug 17; [Epub ahead of print].

12 Stubbs EG, Budden SS, Burger DR, Vandenbark AA. Transfer factor immunotherapy of an autistic child with congenital cytomegalovirus. *J Autism Dev Disord.* 1980 Dec;10(4):451-8.

13 James SJ, Cutler P, Melnyk S, Jernigan S, Janak L, Gaylor DW, Neubrander JA. Metabolic biomarkers of increased oxidative stress and impaired methylation capacity in children with autism. *Am J Clin Nutr.* 2004 Dec;80(6):1611-7.

14 James SJ, Melnyk S, Jernigan S, Cleves MA, Halsted CH, Wong DH, Cutler P, Bock K, Boris M, Bradstreet JJ, Baker SM, Gaylor DW. Metabolic endophenotype and related genotypes are associated with oxidative stress in children with autism. *Am J Med Genet B Neuropsychiatr Genet.* 2006 Aug 17; [Epub ahead of print].

15 Boris M, Goldblatt A, Galanko J, James SJ. Association of MTHFR gene variants with autism. *J Am Phys Surg.* 2004: 9(4):106-108.

16 Parent Ratings of Behavioral Effects of Biomedical Interventions. Autism Research Institute. www.autismwebsite.com/ari/treatment/form34q.htm.

17 Rimland B. Vitamin B6 (and magnesium) in the treatment of autism. *Autism Research Review International,* 1987, Vol. 1, No. 4, page 3.

18 Adams, J. Nutritional Abnormalities in Children with Autism. ASA conference. June 23-24, 2006.

CHAPTER 11

1   Grandjean P, Landrigan PJ. Developmental neurotoxicity of industrial chemicals. *Lancet.* 2006 Dec 16;368(9553):2167-78.

2   Davidson PW, Myers GJ, Weiss B. Mercury exposure and child development outcomes. *Pediatrics.* 2004;113(4 Suppl):1023-9.

3   Dally A. The rise and fall of pink disease. *Soc Hist Med.* 1997 Aug;10(2):291-304.

4   Sanfeliu C, Sebastia J, Cristofol R, Rodriguez-Farre E. Neurotoxicity of organomercurial compounds. *Neurotox Res.* 2003;5(4):283-305.

5   Ibid.

6   Davidson PW, Myers GJ, Cox C, Axtell C, Shamlaye C, Sloane-Reeves J, Cernichiari E, Needham L, Choi A, Wang Y, Berlin M, Clarkson TW. Effects of prenatal and postnatal methylmercury exposure from fish consumption on neurodevelopment: outcomes at 66 months of age in the Seychelles Child Development Study. *JAMA.* 1998 Aug 26;280(8):701-7.

7   Myers GJ, Davidson PW, Cox C, Shamlaye CF, Palumbo D, Cernichiari E, Sloane-Reeves J, Wilding GE, Kost J, Huang LS, Clarkson TW. Prenatal methylmercury exposure from ocean fish consumption in the Seychelles child development study. *Lancet.* 2003 May 17;361(9370):1686-92.

8   Grandjean P, Weihe P, White RF, Debes F, Araki S, Yokoyama K, Murata K, Sorensen N, Dahl R, Jorgensen PJ. Cognitive deficit in 7-year-old children with prenatal exposure to methylmercury. *Neurotoxicol Teratol.* 1997 Nov-Dec; 19(6):417-28.

9   Davidson PW, Myers GJ, Weiss B. Mercury exposure and child development outcomes. *Pediatrics.* 2004;113(4 Suppl):1023-9.

10   Ellefsen A, Kampmann H, Billstedt E, Gillberg IC, Gillberg C. Autism in the Faroe Islands. An Epidemiological Study. *J Autism Dev Disord.* 2006 Oct 7; [Epub ahead of print].

11   Black J. The puzzle of pink disease. *J R Soc Med.* 1999 Sep;92(9):478-81.

12   Autism A.L.A.R.M. Centers for Disease Control and Prevention. www.medicalhomeinfo.org/health/Autism%20downloads/AutismAlarm.pdf

13   Bernard S, Enayati A, Redwood L, Roger H, Binstock T. Autism: a novel form of mercury poisoning. *Med Hypotheses.* 2001 Apr;56(4):462-71.

14   Ball LK, Ball R, Pratt RD. An assessment of thimerosal use in childhood vaccines. *Pediatrics.* 2001 May;107(5):1147-54.

15   David Kirby. *Evidence of Harm.* St. Martin's Press: 2005. P. 207.

16   Mukhtarova ND. Late sequelae of nervous system pathology caused by the action of low concentrations of ethyl mercury chloride. *Gig Tr Prof Zabol.* 1977 Mar(3):4-7.

17   David Kirby. *Evidence of Harm.* New York: St. Martin's Press: 2005. Pg. 208.

18   Letter of July 22, 1935 from Director, Biological Laboratories of Pitman-Moore Company to W.A. Jamieson, Director, Biological Division, Eli Lilly & Company. Subcommittee on Human Rights and Wellness, Government Reform Committee. Mercury in Medicine Report, Washington, D.C. Congressional Record, May 21, 2003: E1011- 30.

19   Engley FB Jr. Evaluation of mercurial compounds as antiseptics. *Ann N Y Acad Sci.* 1950 Aug;53(1):197-206.

20   Nelson EA, Gottshall RY. Enhanced toxicity for mice of pertussis vaccines when preserved with Merthiolate. *Appl Microbiol.* 1967 May;15(3):590-3.

21   Eli Lilly memo from J.W. Smith to Dr. M. Michael Sigel. September 7, 1971.

22   David Kirby. *Evidence of Harm.* New York: St. Martin's Press: 2005. P. 208.

23   Andrea Rock, "Toxic Tipping Point: Are the CDC, the FDA, and other health agencies covering up evidence that a mercury preservative in children's vaccines caused a rise in autism?" *Mother Jones.* March/April, 2004.

24 E-mail from Peter Patriarca to Martin G. Meyers, June 29, 1999.

25 Madsen KM, Lauritsen MB, Pedersen CB, Thorsen P, Plesner AM, Andersen PH, Mortensen PB. Thimerosal and the occurrence of autism: negative ecological evidence from Danish population-based data. *Pediatrics.* 2003p;112(3 Pt 1):604-6.

26 Blaxill M. Danish Thimerosal-Autism Study in *Pediatrics*: Misleading and Uninformative on Autism-Mercury Link. Sep 2, 2003. www.safeminds.org/research/docs/Blaxill-DenmarkAutismThimerosalPediatrics.pdf

27 Hviid A, Stellfeld M, Wohlfahrt J, Melbye M. Association between thimerosal-containing vaccine and autism. *JAMA.* 2003 Oct 1;290(13):1763-6.

28 Bernard S. Analysis of the Danish Autism Registry Data Base in Response to the Hviid *et al.* Paper on Thimerosal in *JAMA.* October, 2003. www.safeminds.org/research/docs/Hviid_et_alJAMA-SafeMindsAnalysis.pdf

29 Verstraeten T, Davis RL, DeStefano F, Lieu TA, Rhodes PH, Black SB, Shinefield H, Chen RT; Vaccine Safety Datalink Team. Safety of thimerosal-containing vaccines: a two-phased study of computerized health maintenance organization databases. *Pediatrics.* 2003 Nov;112(5):1039-48.

30 SafeMinds. *Generation Zero.* www.safeminds.org/Generation%20Zero%20Syn.pdf

31 Transcript, "Scientific Review of Vaccine Safety Datalink Information," Simpsonwood Retreat Center, Norcross, Georgia, June 7-8, 2000, at 31. Accessed online June 15, 2005 at www.nomercury.org/science/documents/Simpsonwood_Transcript.pdf, p.40

32 Rhodes P. Simpsonwood. www.safeminds.org/legislation/foia/Simpsonwood_Transcript.pdf

33 SafeMinds. *Generation Zero.* www.safeminds.org/Generation%20Zero%20Syn.pdf.

34 Verstraeten T. Thimerosal, the Centers for Disease Control and Prevention, and GlaxoSmithKline. *Pediatrics.* 2004;113;932.

35 Fombonne E, Zakarian R, Bennett A, Meng L, McLean-Heywood D. Pervasive developmental disorders in Montreal, Quebec, Canada: prevalence and links with immunizations. *Pediatrics.* 2006 Jul;118(1):e139-50.

36 Geier MR, Geier DA. An assessment of the impact of thimerosal on childhood neurodevelopmental disorders. *Pediatr Rehabil.* 2003 Apr-Jun;6(2):97-102.

37 Geier DA, Geier MR. A comparative evaluation of the effects of MMR immunization and mercury doses from thimerosal-containing childhood vaccines on the population prevalence of autism. *Med Sci Monit.* 2004 Mar;10(3):PI33-9.

CHAPTER 12

1 Magos L. Review on the toxicity of ethylmercury, including its presence as a preservative in biological and pharmaceutical products. *J Appl Toxicol.* 2001 Jan-Feb; 21(1):1-5.

2 Stajich GV, Lopez GP, Harry SW, Sexson WR. Iatrogenic exposure to mercury after hepatitis B vaccination in preterm infants. *J Pediatr.* 2000 May;136(5):679-81.

3 Robert Kennedy Jr. "Deadly Immunity." *salon.com* June 16th, 2005.

4   Pichichero ME, Cernichiari E, Lopreiato J, Treanor J. Mercury concentrations and metabolism in infants receiving vaccines containing thiomersal: a descriptive study. *Lancet*. 2002 Nov 30;360(9347):1737-41.

5   Blair AMJN, Clark B, Clarke AJ, Wood P. Tissue concentrations of mercury after chronic dosing of squirrel monkeys with thiomersal. *Toxicology*. 1975;3(2):171-6.

6   Magos L, Brown AW, Sparrow S, Bailey E, Snowden RT, Skipp WR. The comparative toxicology of ethyl- and methylmercury. *Arch Toxicol*. 1985 Sep; 57(4):260-7.

7   Magos L. Neurotoxic character of thimerosal and the allometric extrapolation of adult clearance half-time to infants. *J Appl Toxicol*. 2003 Jul-Aug;23(4):263-9.

8   Burbacher TM, Shen DD, Liberato N, Grant KS, Cernichiari E, Clarkson T. Comparison of blood and brain mercury levels in infant monkeys exposed to methylmercury or vaccines containing thimerosal. *Environ Health Perspect*. 2005 Aug;113(8):1015-21.

9   Vargas DL, Nascimbene C, Krishnan C, Zimmerman AW, Pardo CA. Neuroglial activation and neuroinflammation in the brain of patients with autism. *Ann Neurol*. 2005 Jan;57(1):67-81.

10 Baskin DS, Ngo H, Didenko VV. Thimerosal induces DNA breaks, caspase-3 activation, membrane damage, and cell death in cultured human neurons and fibroblasts. *Toxicol Sci*. 2003 Aug;74(2):361-8.

11 Makani S, Gollapudi S, Yel L, Chiplunkar S, Gupta S. Biochemical and molecular basis of thimerosal-induced apoptosis in T cells: a major role of mitochondrial pathway. *Genes Immun*. 2002 Aug;3(5):270-8.

12 Mutkus L, Aschner JL, Syversen T, Shanker G, Sonnewald U, Aschner M. In vitro uptake of glutamate in GLAST- and GLT-1-transfected mutant CHO-K1 cells is inhibited by the ethylmercury-containing preservative thimerosal. *Biol Trace Elem Res*. 2005 Summer;105(1-3):71-86.

13 Parran DK, Barker A, Ehrich M. Effects of thimerosal on NGF signal transduction and cell death in neuroblastoma cells. *Toxicol Sci*. 2005 Jul;86(1):132-40.

14 Hornig M, Chian D, Lipkin WI. Neurotoxic effects of postnatal thimerosal are mouse strain dependent. *Mol Psychiatry*. 2004 Sep;9(9):833-45.

15 Havarinasab S, Hultman P. Organic mercury compounds and autoimmunity. *Autoimmunity Rev* 2005;4:270-275.

16 Havarinasab S, Haggqvist B, Bjorn E, Pollard KM, Hultman P. Immunosuppressive and autoimmune effects of thimerosal in mice. *Toxicol Appl Pharmacol*. 2005 Apr 15; 204(2):109-21.

17 Goth SR, Chu RA, Gregg JP, Cherednichenko G, Pessah IN. Uncoupling of ATP-Mediated Calcium Signaling and Dysregulated Interleukin-6 Secretion in Dendritic Cells by Nanomolar Thimerosal. *Environ Health Perspect*. 2006 Jul;114(7):1083-91.

18 Waly M, Olteanu H, Banerjee R, Choi SW, Mason JB, Parker BS, Sukumar S, Shim S, Sharma A, Benzecry JM, Power-Charnitsky VA, Deth RC. Activation of methionine synthase by insulin-like growth factor-1 and dopamine: a target for neurodevelopmental toxins and thimerosal. *Mol Psychiatry*. 2004 Apr;9(4):358-70.

19   James SJ, Slikker W 3rd, Melnyk S, New E, Pogribna M, Jernigan S. Thimerosal neurotoxicity is associated with glutathione depletion: protection with glutathione precursors. *Neurotoxicology.* 2005 Jan;26(1):1-8.

20   Ueha-Ishibashi T, Tatsuishi T, Iwase K, Nakao H, Umebayashi C, Nishizaki Y, Nishimura Y, Oyama Y, Hirama S, Okano Y. Property of thimerosal-induced decrease in cellular content of glutathione in rat thymocytes: a flow cytometric study with 5-chloromethylfluorescein diacetate. *Toxicol In Vitro.* 2004 Oct;18(5):563-9.

21   Ueha-Ishibashi T, Oyama Y, Nakao H, Umebayashi C, Nishizaki Y, Tatsuishi T, Iwase K, Murao K, Seo H. Effect of thimerosal, a preservative in vaccines, on intracellular Ca2+ concentration of rat cerebellar neurons. *Toxicology.* 2004 Jan 15; 195(1):77-84.

22   Alexandre H, Delsinne V, Goval JJ, Van Cauwenberge A. Effect of taxol and okadaic acid on microtubule dynamics in thimerosal-arrested primary mouse oocytes: a confocal study. *Biol Cell.* 2003 Sep;95(6):407-14.

23   Westphal GA, Asgari S, Schulz TG, Bunger J, Muller M, Hallier E. Thimerosal induces micronuclei in the cytochalasin B block micronucleus test with human lymphocytes. *Arch Toxicol.* 2003 Jan;77(1):50-5. Epub 2002 Nov 6.

24   Holmes AS, Blaxill MF, Haley BE. Reduced levels of mercury in first baby haircuts of autistic children. *Int J Toxicol.* 2003 Jul-Aug;22(4):277-85.

25   Bradstreet J, Geier DA, Kartzinel JJ, Adams JB, Geier MR. A case control study of mercury burden in children with autistic spectrum disorders. *J Am Phys Surg.* 2003;8(3):76.

26   Palmer RF, Blanchard S, Stein Z, Mandell D, Miller C. Environmental mercury release, special education rates, and autism disorder: an ecological study of Texas. *Health Place.* 2006 Jun;12(2):203-9.

27   Windham G, Zhang L, Gunier R, Croen L, Grether J. Autism Spectrum Disorders in Relation to Distribution of Hazardous Air Pollutants in the San Francisco Bay Area. *Environ Health Perspect.* 2006 Sep;114(9):1438-44.

28   Institute of Medicine, Immunization Safety Review Committee, Thimerosal-containing vaccines and Neurodevelopmental Disorders, Oct. 1, 2001

29   Institute of Medicine, Immunization Safety Review: Vaccines and Autism. May 17, 2004.

30   Rock, Andrea. The Toxic Tipping Point: Are the CDC, the FDA, and other health agencies covering up evidence that a mercury preservative in children's vaccines caused a rise in autism? *Mother Jones.* March/April 2004.

CHAPTER 13

1   Redcay E, Courchesne E. When is the brain enlarged in autism? A meta-analysis of all brain size reports. *Biol Psychiatry.* 2005 Jul 1;58(1):1-9.

2   Courchesne E, Karns CM, Davis HR, Ziccardi R, Carper RA, Tigue ZD, Chisum HJ, Moses P, PierceK, Lord C, Lincoln AJ, Pizzo S, Schreibman L, Haas RH,

Akshoomoff NA, Courchesne RY. Unusual brain growth patterns in early life in patients with autistic disorder: an MRI study. *Neurology.* 2001 Jul 24;57(2):245-54.

3   Courchesne E, Pierce K. Brain overgrowth in autism during a critical time in development: implications for frontal pyramidal neuron and interneuron development and connectivity. *Int J Dev Neurosci.* 2005 Apr-May;23(2-3):153-70.

4   Hazlett HC, Poe MD, Gerig G, Smith RG, Piven J. Cortical gray and white brain tissue volume in adolescents and adults with autism. *Biol Psychiatry.* 2006 Jan 1; 59(1):1-6.

5   Piven J, Arndt S, Bailey J, Andreasen N. Regional brain enlargement in autism: a magnetic resonance imaging study. *J Am Acad Child Adolesc Psychiatry.* 1996 Apr;35(4):530-6.

6   Acosta MT, Pearl PL. Imaging data in autism: from structure to malfunction. *Semin Pediatr Neurol.* 2004 Sep;11(3):205-13.

7   Courchesne E, Townsend J, Saitoh O. The brain in infantile autism: posterior fossa structures are abnormal. *Neurology.* 1994 Feb;44(2):214-23.

8   Courchesne E. Neuroanatomic imaging in autism. *Pediatrics.* 1991 May;87(5 Pt 2): 781-90.

9   Ashwood P, Wills S, Van de Water J. The immune response in autism: a new frontier for autism research. *J Leukoc Biol.* 2006 Jul;80(1):1-15.

10 Courchesne E. Neuroanatomic imaging in autism. *Pediatrics.* 1991 May;87 (5 Pt 2):781-90.

11 Palmen SJ, van Engeland H, Hof PR, Schmitz C. Neuropathological findings in autism. *Brain.* 2004 Dec;127(Pt 12):2572-83.

12 Kern JK, Jones AM. Evidence of toxicity, oxidative stress, and neuronal insult in autism. *J Toxicol Environ Health B Crit Rev.* 2006 Nov-Dec;9(6):485-99.

13 Trottier G, Srivastava L, Walker CD. Etiology of infantile autism: a review of recent advances in genetic and neurobiological research. *J Psychiatry Neurosci.* 1999 Mar;24(2):103-15.

14 Courchesne E, Townsend J, Akshoomoff NA, Saitoh O, Yeung-Courchesne R, Lincoln AJ, James HE, Haas RH, Schreibman L, Lau L. Impairment in shifting attention in autistic and cerebellar patients. *Behav Neurosci.* 1994 Oct;108(5): 848-65.

15 Palmen SJ, van Engeland H, Hof PR, Schmitz C. Neuropathological findings in autism. *Brain.* 2004 Dec;127(Pt 12):2572-83.

16 Ibid.

17 Zilbovicius M, Garreau B, Samson Y, Remy P, Barthelemy C, Syrota A, Lelord G. Delayed maturation of the frontal cortex in childhood autism. *Am J Psychiatry.* 1995 Feb;152(2):248-52.

18 Acosta MT, Pearl PL. Imaging data in autism: from structure to malfunction. *Semin Pediatr Neurol.* 2004 Sep;11(3):205-13.

19 Courchesne E, Pierce K. Brain overgrowth in autism during a critical time in development: implications for frontal pyramidal neuron and interneuron development and connectivity. *Int J Dev Neurosci.* 2005 Apr-May;23(2-3):153-70.

20 Akshoomoff N, Pierce K, Courchesne E. The neurobiological basis of autism from a developmental perspective. *Dev Psychopathol.* 2002 Summer;14(3):613-34.

21 Courchesne E, Pierce K. Brain overgrowth in autism during a critical time in development: implications for frontal pyramidal neuron and interneuron development and connectivity. *Int J Dev Neurosci.* 2005 Apr-May;23(2-3):153-70.

22 Gershon, Michael. *The Second Brain: A Groundbreaking New Understanding of Nervous Disorders of the Stomach and Intestine.* Harper paperbacks, 1999. P. xii.

23 Wilson CJ, Finch CE, Cohen HJ. Cytokines and cognition—the case for a head-to-toe inflammatory paradigm. *J Am Geriatr Soc.* 2002 Dec;50(12):2041-56.

24 Zhao B, Schwartz JP. Involvement of cytokines in normal CNS development and neurological diseases: recent progress and perspectives. *J Neurosci Res.* 1998 Apr 1; 52(1):7-16.

25 Larson SJ. Behavioral and motivational effects of immune-system activation. *J Gen Psychol.* 2002 Oct;129(4):401-14.

26 Ashwood P, Wills S, Van de Water J. The immune response in autism: a new frontier for autism research. *J Leukoc Biol.* 2006 Jul;80(1):1-15.

27 Mignini F, Streccioni V, Amenta F. Autonomic innervation of immune organs and neuroimmune modulation. *Auton Autacoid Pharmacol.* 2003 Feb;23(1):1-25.

28 Vega JA, Garcia-Suarez O, Hannestad J, Perez-Perez M, Germana A. Neurotrophins and the immune system. *J Anat.* 2003 Jul;203(1):1-19.

29 Nelson KB, Grether JK, Croen LA, Dambrosia JM, Dickens BF, Jelliffe LL, Hansen RL, Phillips TM. Neuropeptides and neurotrophins in neonatal blood of children with autism or mental retardation. *Ann Neurol.* 2001 May;49(5):597-606.

30 Dunzendorfer S, Kaser A, Meierhofer C, Tilg H, Wiedermann CJ. Cutting edge: peripheral neuropeptides attract immature and arrest mature blood-derived dendritic cells. *J Immunol.* 2001 Feb 15;166(4):2167-72.

31 Pashenkov M, Teleshova N, Link H. Inflammation in the central nervous system: the role for dendritic cells. *Brain Pathol.* 2003 Jan;13(1):23-33.

32 Cook EH. Autism: review of neurochemical investigation. *Synapse.* 1990;6(3): 292-308.

33 Lam KS, Aman MG, Arnold LE. Neurochemical correlates of autistic disorder: a review of the literature. *Res Dev Disabil.* 2006 May-Jun;27(3):254-89.

34 Gershon, Michael. *The Second Brain: A Groundbreaking New Understanding of Nervous Disorders of the Stomach and Intestine.* Harper paperbacks, 1999. P. xii.

35 Jarskog LF, Xiao H, Wilkie MB, Lauder JM, Gilmore JH. Cytokine regulation of embryonic rat dopamine and serotonin neuronal survival in vitro. *Int J Dev Neurosci.* 1997 Oct;15(6):711-6.

36 Coutinho AM, Oliveira G, Morgadinho T, Fesel C, Macedo TR, Bento C, Marques C, Ataide A, Miguel T, Borges L, Vicente AM. Variants of the serotonin transporter gene (SLC6A4) significantly contribute to hyperserotonemia in autism. *Mol Psychiatry.* 2004 Mar;9(3):264-71.

37 Conroy J, Meally E, Kearney G, Fitzgerald M, Gill M, Gallagher L. Serotonin transporter gene and autism: a haplotype analysis in an Irish autistic population. *Mol Psychiatry.* 2004 Jun;9(6):587-93.

38 Lam KS, Aman MG, Arnold LE. Neurochemical correlates of autistic disorder: a review of the literature. *Res Dev Disabil.* 2006 May-Jun;27(3):254-89.

39 Martineau J, Barthelemy C, Jouve J, Muh JP, Lelord G. Monoamines (serotonin and catecholamines) and their derivatives in infantile autism: age-related changes and drug effects. *Dev Med Child Neurol.* 1992 Jul;34(7):593-603.

40 Narayan M, Srinath S, Anderson GM, Meundi DB. Cerebrospinal fluid levels of homovanillic acid and 5-hydroxyindoleacetic acid in autism. *Biol Psychiatry.* 1993 Apr 15-May 1;33(8-9):630-5.

41 Todd RD, Ciaranello RD. Demonstration of inter- and intraspecies differences in serotonin binding sites by antibodies from an autistic child. *Proc Natl Acad Sci U S A.* 1985 Jan;82(2):612-6.

42 Cook EH Jr, Perry BD, Dawson G, Wainwright MS, Leventhal BL. Receptor inhibition by immunoglobulins: specific inhibition by autistic children, their relatives, and control subjects. *J Autism Dev Disord.* 1993 Mar;23(1):67-78.

43 Chugani DC, Muzik O, Rothermel R, Behen M, Chakraborty P, Mangner T, da Silva EA, Chugani HT. Altered serotonin synthesis in the dentatothalamocortical pathway in autistic boys. *Ann Neurol.* 1997 Oct;42(4):666-9.

44 Ibid.

45 Lam KS, Aman MG, Arnold LE. Neurochemical correlates of autistic disorder: a review of the literature. *Res Dev Disabil.* 2006 May-Jun;27(3):254-89.

46 McDougle CJ, Naylor ST, Cohen DJ, Volkmar FR, Heninger GR, Price LH. A double-blind, placebo-controlled study of fluvoxamine in adults with autistic disorder. *Arch Gen Psychiatry.* 1996 Nov;53(11):1001-8.

47 Fukuda T, Sugie H, Ito M, Sugie Y. Clinical evaluation of treatment with fluvoxamine, a selective serotonin reuptake inhibitor in children with autistic disorder. *No To Hattatsu.* 2001 Jul;33(4):314-8.

48 Lam KS, Aman MG, Arnold LE. Neurochemical correlates of autistic disorder: a review of the literature. *Res Dev Disabil.* 2006 May-Jun;27(3):254-89.

49 Pandina GJ, Bossie CA, Youssef E, Zhu Y, Dunbar F. Risperidone Improves Behavioral Symptoms in Children with Autism in a Randomized, Double-Blind, Placebo-Controlled Trial. *J Autism Dev Disord.* 2006 Oct 4; [Epub ahead of print].

50 Pandina GJ, Aman MG, Findling RL. Risperidone in the management of disruptive behavior disorders. *J Child Adolesc Psychopharmacol.* 2006 Aug;16(4):379-92.

51 Findling RL, Aman MG, Eerdekens M, Derivan A, Lyons B. Risperidone Disruptive Behavior Study Group. Long-term, open-label study of risperidone in children with severe disruptive behaviors and below-average IQ. *Am J Psychiatry.* 2004 Apr;161(4):677-84.

52 Turgay A, Binder C, Snyder R, Fisman S. Long-term safety and efficacy of risperidone for the treatment of disruptive behavior disorders in children with subaverage IQs. *Pediatrics.* 2002 Sep;110(3):e34.

53 Croonenberghs J, Fegert JM, Findling RL, De Smedt G, Van Dongen S; Risperidone Disruptive Behavior Study Group. Risperidone in children with disruptive behavior disorders and subaverage intelligence: a 1-year, open-label study of 504 patients. *J Am Acad Child Adolesc Psychiatry.* 2005 Jan;44(1):64-72.

54 Lam KS, Aman MG, Arnold LE. Neurochemical correlates of autistic disorder: a review of the literature. *Res Dev Disabil.* 2006 May-Jun;27(3):254-89.

55 Martineau J, Barthelemy C, Jouve J, Muh JP, Lelord G. Monoamines (serotonin and catecholamines) and their derivatives in infantile autism: age-related changes and drug effects. *Dev Med Child Neurol.* 1992 Jul;34(7):593-603.

56 Narayan M, Srinath S, Anderson GM, Meundi DB. Cerebrospinal fluid levels of homovanillic acid and 5-hydroxyindoleacetic acid in autism. *Biol Psychiatry.* 1993 Apr 15-May 1;33(8-9):630-5.

57 Lam KS, Aman MG, Arnold LE. Neurochemical correlates of autistic disorder: a review of the literature. *Res Dev Disabil.* 2006 May-Jun;27(3):254-89.

58 Axelrod FB, Chelimsky GG, Weese-Mayer DE. Pediatric autonomic disorders. *Pediatrics.* 2006 Jul;118(1):309-21.

59 Lam KS, Aman MG, Arnold LE. Neurochemical correlates of autistic disorder: a review of the literature. *Res Dev Disabil.* 2006 May-Jun;27(3):254-89.

60 Lee M, Martin-Ruiz C, Graham A, Court J, Jaros E, Perry R, Iversen P, Bauman M, Perry E. Nicotinic receptor abnormalities in the cerebellar cortex in autism. *Brain.* 2002 Jul;125(Pt 7):1483-95.

61 Modahl C, Green L, Fein D, Morris M, Waterhouse L, Feinstein C, Levin H. Plasma oxytocin levels in autistic children. *Biol Psychiatry.* 1998 Feb 15;43(4):270-7.

62 Green L, Fein D, Modahl C, Feinstein C, Waterhouse L, Morris M. Oxytocin and autistic disorder: alterations in peptide forms. *Biol Psychiatry.* 2001 Oct 15; 50(8):609-13.

63 Young LJ, Pitkow LJ, Ferguson JN. Neuropeptides and social behavior: animal models relevant to autism. *Mol Psychiatry.* 2002;7 Suppl 2:S38-9.

64 Gimpl G, Fahrenholz F. The oxytocin receptor system: structure, function, and regulation. *Physiol Rev.* 2001 Apr;81(2):629-83.

65 Bittigau P, Ikonomidou C. Glutamate in neurologic diseases. *J Child Neurol.* 1997 Nov;12(8):471-85.

66 Fatemi SH, Halt AR, Stary JM, Kanodia R, Schulz SC, Realmuto GR. Glutamic acid decarboxylase 65 and 67 kDa proteins are reduced in autistic parietal and cerebellar cortices. *Biol Psychiatry.* 2002 Oct 15;52(8):805-10.

67 Lam KS, Aman MG, Arnold LE. Neurochemical correlates of autistic disorder: a review of the literature. *Res Dev Disabil.* 2006 May-Jun;27(3):254-89.

68 Bradl M, Hohlfeld R. Molecular pathogenesis of neuroinflammation. *J Neurol Neurosurg Psychiatry.* 2003 Oct;74(10):1364-70.

69   Zagon IS, McLaughlin PJ. Identification of opioid peptides regulating proliferation of neurons and glia in the developing nervous system. *Brain Res.* 1991 Mar 1;542(2): 318-23.

70   Peterson PK, Molitor TW, Chao CC. The opioid-cytokine connection. *J Neuroimmunol.* 1998 Mar 15;83(1-2):63-9.

71   Shattock P, Kennedy A, Rowell F, Berney T. Role of neuropeptides in autism and their relationship with classical neurotransmitters. *Brain Dysfunction* 1990:3: 328-345.

72   Reichelt KL, Knivsberg AM. Can the pathophysiology of autism be explained by the nature of the discovered urine peptides? *Nutr Neurosci.* 2003 Feb;6(1):19-28.

73   Shattock P, Lowdon G. Proteins, peptides and autism: Part 2: Implications for the education and care of people with autism. *Brain Dysfunction.* 1991;4:323-334.

74   Knivsberg AM, Reichelt KL, Nodland M. Reports on dietary intervention in autistic disorders. *Nutr Neurosci.* 2001;4(1):25-37.

75   Symons FJ, Thompson A, Rodriguez MC. Self-injurious behavior and the efficacy of naltrexone treatment: a quantitative synthesis. *Ment Retard Dev Disabil Res Rev.* 2004;10(3):193-200.

76   Trevathan E. Seizures and epilepsy among children with language regression and autistic spectrum disorders. *J Child Neurol.* 2004 Aug;19 Suppl 1:S49-57.

77   Tuchman R, Rapin I. Epilepsy in autism. *Lancet Neurol.* 2002 Oct;1(6):352-8.

78   Ballaban-Gil K, Tuchman R. Epilepsy and epileptiform EEG: association with autism and language disorders. *Ment Retard Dev Disabil Res Rev.* 2000;6(4):300-8.

79   Tuchman RF. Language disorders: is EEG clinically useful? *Rev Neurol.* 1997 May;25(141):744-9.

80   Kawasaki Y, Yokota K, Shinomiya M, Shimizu Y, Niwa S. Brief report: electroencephalographic paroxysmal activities in the frontal area emerged in middle childhood and during adolescence in a follow-up study of autism. *J Autism Dev Disord.* 1997 Oct;27(5):605-20.

81   Tuchman R. Autism and Epilepsy: What Has Regression got to do with it? *Epilepsy Currents.* 6(4) 2006:107-111.

82   Trevathan E. Seizures and epilepsy among children with language regression and autistic spectrum disorders. *J Child Neurol.* 2004 Aug;19 Suppl 1:S49-57.

83   Jan JE, O'Donnell ME. Use of melatonin in the treatment of paediatric sleep disorders. *J Pineal Res.* 1996 Nov;21(4):193-9.

84   Ishizaki A, Sugama M, Takeuchi N. Usefulness of melatonin for developmental sleep and emotional/behavior disorders—studies of melatonin trial on 50 patients with developmental disorders. *No To Hattatsu.* 1999 Sep;31(5):428-37.

85   Malow BA. Sleep disorders, epilepsy, and autism. *Ment Retard Dev Disabil Res Rev.* 2004;10(2):122-5.

CHAPTER 16

1   Raiten DJ, Massaro T. Perspectives on the nutritional ecology of autistic children. *J Autism Dev Disord.* 1986 Jun;16(2):133-43.

2   Kushak R, Winter W, Farber N, Buie T. Gastrointestinal symptoms and intestinal disaccharidase activities in children with autism. *J Pediatr Gastroenterol Nutr.* 2005 Oct: 41(4):508.

3   Horvath K, Perman JA. Autistic disorder and gastrointestinal disease. *Curr Opin Pediatr.* 2002 Oct;14(5):583-7

4   Adams JB, George F, Audhya T. Abnormally high plasma levels of vitamin B6 in children with autism not taking supplements compared to controls not taking supplements. *J Altern Complement Med.* 2006 Jan-Feb;12(1):59-63.

5   Ames BN, Elson-Schwab I, Silver EA. High-dose vitamin therapy stimulates variant enzymes with decreased coenzyme binding affinity (increased K (m)): relevance to genetic disease and polymorphisms. *Am J Clin Nutr.* 2002 Apr;75(4):616-58.

6   Rimland B. Controversies in the treatment of autistic children: vitamin and drug therapy. *J Child Neurol.* 1988;3 Suppl:S68-72.

7   Rimland B, Callaway E, Dreyfus P. The effect of high doses of vitamin B6 on autistic children: a double-blind crossover study. *Am J Psychiatry.* 1978 Apr; 135(4):472-5.

8   Kidd PM. Autism, an extreme challenge to integrative medicine. Part 2: medical management. *Altern Med Rev.* 2002 Dec;7(6):472-99.

9   Levy J. Immunonutrition: the pediatric experience. *Nutrition.* 1998 Jul-Aug;14 (7-8):641-7.

10 Megson MN. Is autism a G-alpha protein defect reversible with natural vitamin A? *Med Hypotheses.* 2000 Jun;54(6):979-83.

11 Calingasan NY, Huang PL, Chun HS, Fabian A, Gibson GE. Vascular factors are critical in selective neuronal loss in an animal model of impaired oxidative metabolism. *J Neuropathol Exp Neurol.* 2000 Mar;59(3):207-17.

12 Kornreich L, Bron-Harlev E, Hoffmann C, Schwarz M, Konen O, Schoenfeld T, Straussberg R, Nahum E, Ibrahim AK, Eshel G, Horev G. Thiamine deficiency in infants: MR findings in the brain. *Am J Neuroradiol.* 2005 Aug;26(7):1668-74.

13 Dhawan M, Kachru DN, Tandon SK. Influence of thiamine and ascorbic acid supplementation on the antidotal efficacy of thiol chelators in experimental lead intoxication. *Arch Toxicol.* 1988;62(4):301-4.

14 Lonsdale D, Shamberger RJ, Audhya T. Treatment of autism spectrum children with thiamine tetrahydrofurfuryl disulfide: a pilot study. *Neuro Endocrinol Lett.* 2002 Aug;23(4):303-8.

15 Boris M, Goldblatt A, Galanko J, James SJ. Association of MTHFR gene variants with autism. *J Am Phys Surg.* 2004: 9(4):106-108.

16 Ueland PM, Hustad S, Schneede J, Refsum H, Vollset SE. Biological and clinical implications of the MTHFR C677T polymorphism. *Trends Pharmacol Sci.* 2001 Apr;22(4):195-201.

17 Kleijnen J, Knipschild P. Niacin and vitamin B6 in mental functioning: a review of controlled trials in humans. *Biol Psychiatry.* 1991 May 1;29(9):931-41.

18 Chugani DC, Sundram BS, Behen M, Lee ML, Moore GJ. Evidence of altered energy metabolism in autistic children. *Prog Neuropsychopharmacol Biol Psychiatry.* 1999 May;23(4):635-41.

19 Martineau J, Barthelemy C, Garreau B, Lelord G. Vitamin B6, magnesium, and combined B6-Mg: therapeutic effects in childhood autism. *Biol Psychiatry.* 1985 May;20(5):467-78.

20 Kleijnen J, Knipschild P. Niacin and vitamin B6 in mental functioning: a review of controlled trials in humans. *Biol Psychiatry.* 1991 May 1;29(9):931-41.

21 Ibid.

22 Rimland, B. High dosage levels of certain vitamins in the treatment of children with severe mental disorders. In D. Hawkins & L. Pauling (Eds.), *Orthomolecular Psychiatry*. 1973 (pp. 513-538).

23 Rimland B, Callaway E, Dreyfus P. The effect of high doses of vitamin B6 on autistic children: a double-blind crossover study. *Am J Psychiatry.* 1978 Apr; 135(4):472-5.

24 Barthelemy C, Garreau B, Leddet I, Sauvage D, Domenech J, Muh JP, Lelord G. Biological and clinical effects of oral magnesium and associated magnesium-vitamin B6 administration on certain disorders observed in infantile autism. *Therapie.* 1980 Sep-Oct;35(5):627-32.

25 Jonas C, Etienne T, Barthelemy C, Jouve J, Mariotte N. Clinical and biochemical value of Magnesium + vitamin B6 combination in the treatment of residual autism in adults. *Therapie.* 1984 Nov-Dec;39(6):661-9.

26 Martineau J, Barthelemy C, Garreau B, Lelord G. Vitamin B6, magnesium, and combined B6-Mg: therapeutic effects in childhood autism. *Biol Psychiatry.* 1985 May;20(5):467-78.

27 Lelord G, Muh JP, Barthelemy C, Martineau J, Garreau B, Callaway E. Effects of pyridoxine and magnesium on autistic symptoms—initial observations. *J Autism Dev Disord.* 1981 Jun;11(2):219-30.

28 Lelord G, Callaway E, Muh JP. Clinical and biological effects of high doses of vitamin B6 and magnesium on autistic children. *Acta Vitaminol Enzymol.* 1982;4(1-2):27-44.

29 Mousain-Bosc M, Roche M, Polge A, Pradal-Prat D, Rapin J, Bali JP. Improvement of neurobehavioral disorders in children supplemented with magnesium-vitamin B6. II. Pervasive developmental disorder-autism. *Magnes Res.* 2006 Mar;19(1):53-62.

30 Rimland, B. High dosage levels of certain vitamins in the treatment of children with severe mental disorders. In D. Hawkins & L. Pauling (Eds.), *Orthomolecular Psychiatry.* 1973 (pp. 513-538). New York: W.H. Freeman.

31 Kleijnen J, Knipschild P. Niacin and vitamin B6 in mental functioning: a review of controlled trials in humans. *Biol Psychiatry.* 1991 May 1;29(9):931-41.

32   Adams JB, Holloway C. Pilot study of a moderate dose multivitamin/mineral supplement for children with autistic spectrum disorder. *J Altern Complement Med.* 2004 Dec;10(6):1033-9.

33   Adams JB, George F, Audhya T. Abnormally high plasma levels of vitamin B6 in children with autism not taking supplements compared to controls not taking supplements. *J Altern Complement Med.* 2006 Jan-Feb;12(1):59-63.

34   Moretti R, Torre P, Antonello RM, Cattaruzza T, Cazzato G, Bava A. Vitamin B12 and folate depletion in cognition: a review. *Neurol India.* 2004 Sep;52(3):310-8.

35. Grattan-Smith PJ, Wilcken B, Procopis PG, Wise GA. The neurological syndrome of infantile cobalamin deficiency: developmental regression and involuntary movements. *Mov Disord.* 1997 Jan;12(1):39-46.

36. Moretti R, Torre P, Antonello RM, Cattaruzza T, Cazzato G, Bava A. Vitamin B12 and folate depletion in cognition: a review. *Neurol India.* 2004 Sep;52(3):310-8.

37   James SJ, Cutler P, Melnyk S, Jernigan S, Janak L, Gaylor DW, Neubrander JA. Metabolic biomarkers of increased oxidative stress and impaired methylation capacity in children with autism. *Am J Clin Nutr.* 2004 Dec;80(6):1611-7.

38   Wakefield AJ, Murch SH, Anthony A, Linnell J, Casson DM, Malik M, Berelowitz M, Dhillon AP, Thomson MA, Harvey P, Valentine A, Davies SE, Walker-Smith JA. Ileal-lymphoid-nodular hyperplasia, non-specific colitis, and pervasive developmental disorder in children. *Lancet.* 1998 Feb 28;351(9103):637-41.

39   White JF. Intestinal pathophysiology in autism. *Exp Biol Med* (Maywood). 2003 Jun;228(6):639-49.

40   Litov RE, Combs GF Jr. Selenium in pediatric nutrition. *Pediatrics.* 1991 Mar; 87(3):339-51.

41   Mahadik SP, Scheffer RE. Oxidative injury and potential use of antioxidants in schizophrenia. *Prostaglandins Leukot Essent Fatty Acids.* 1996 Aug;55(1-2):45-54.

42   Dhawan M, Kachru DN, Tandon SK. Influence of thiamine and ascorbic acid supplementation on the antidotal efficacy of thiol chelators in experimental lead intoxication. *Arch Toxicol.* 1988;62(4):301-4.

43   Goebel L, Driscoll H. Scurvy. www.emedicine.com. 7-15-05.

44   Johnston CS, Thompson LL. Vitamin C status of an outpatient population. *J Am Coll Nutr.* 1998, 17(4)366-370.

45   Schectman G, Byrd JC, Hoffmann R. Ascorbic acid requirements for smokers: analysis of a population survey. *Am J Clin Nutr.* 1991 Jun;53(6):1466-70.

46   Dickinson VA, Block G, Russek-Cohen E. Supplement use, other dietary and demographic variables, and serum vitamin C in NHANES II. *J Am Coll Nutr.* 1994 Feb;13(1):22-32.

47   Hunt C, Chakravorty NK, Annan G, Habibzadeh N, Schorah CJ. The clinical effects of vitamin C supplementation in elderly hospitalised patients with acute respiratory infections. *Int J Vitam Nutr Res.* 1994;64(3):212-9.

48 Schorah CJ, Downing C, Piripitsi A, Gallivan L, Al-Hazaa AH, Sanderson MJ, Bodenham A. Total vitamin C, ascorbic acid, and dehydroascorbic acid concentrations in plasma of critically ill patients. *Am J Clin Nutr.* 1996 May;63(5): 760-5.

49 Singh RB, Niaz MA, Agarwal P, Begom R, Rastogi SS. Effect of antioxidant-rich foods on plasma ascorbic acid, cardiac enzyme, and lipid peroxide levels in patients hospitalized with acute myocardial infarction. *J Am Diet Assoc.* 1995 Jul;95(7): 775-80.

50 Adams JB, Holloway C. Pilot study of a moderate dose multivitamin/mineral supplement for children with autistic spectrum disorder. *J Altern Complement Med.* 2004 Dec;10(6):1033-9.

51 Dolske MC, Spollen J, McKay S, Lancashire E, Tolbert L. A preliminary trial of ascorbic acid as supplemental therapy for autism. *Prog Neuropsychopharmacol Biol Psychiatry.* 1993 Sep;17(5):765-74.

52 Whiting SJ, Calvo MS. Dietary recommendations for vitamin D: a critical need for functional end points to establish an estimated average requirement. *J Nutr.* 2005 Feb;135(2):304-9.

53 Bronner F. Extracellular and intracellular regulation of calcium homeostasis. *ScientificWorldJournal.* 2001 Dec 22;1:919-25.

54 Baker SB, Worthley LI. The essentials of calcium, magnesium and phosphate metabolism: part I. Physiology. *Crit Care Resusc.* 2002 Dec;4(4):301-6.

55 Deluca HF. The vitamin D system: a view from basic science to the clinic. *Clin Biochem.* 1981 Oct;14(5):213-22.

56 Whiting SJ, Calvo MS. Dietary recommendations for vitamin D: a critical need for functional end points to establish an estimated average requirement. *J Nutr.* 2005 Feb;135(2):304-9.

57 Moon J. The role of vitamin D in toxic metal absorption: a review. *J Am Coll Nutr.* 1994 Dec;13(6):559-64.

58 Litov RE, Combs GF Jr. Selenium in pediatric nutrition. *Pediatrics.* 1991Mar; 87(3):339-51.

59 Levy J. Immunonutrition: the pediatric experience. *Nutrition.* 1998 Jul-Aug; 14(7-8):641-7.

60 Mahadik SP, Scheffer RE. Oxidative injury and potential use of antioxidants in schizophrenia. *Prostaglandins Leukot Essent Fatty Acids.* 1996 Aug;55(1-2):45-54.

61 Tchantchou F, Graves M, Shea TB. Expression and activity of methionine cycle genes are altered following folate and vitamin E deficiency under oxidative challenge: modulation by apolipoprotein E-deficiency. *Nutr Neurosci.* 2006 Feb-Apr; 9(1-2):17-24.

62 Fernstrom JD. Can nutrient supplements modify brain function? *Am J Clin Nutr.* 2000 Jun;71(6 Suppl):1669S-75S.

63 Moretti R, Torre P, Antonello RM, Cattaruzza T, Cazzato G, Bava A. Vitamin B12 and folate depletion in cognition: a review. *Neurol India.* 2004 Sep;52(3):310-8.

64   Grattan-Smith PJ, Wilcken B, Procopis PG, Wise GA. The neurological syndrome of infantile cobalamin deficiency: developmental regression and involuntary movements. *Mov Disord.* 1997 Jan;12(1):39-46.

65   Rosenberg IH. Folic acid and neural-tube defects—time for action? *N Engl J Med.* 1992 Dec 24;327(26):1875-7.

66   James SJ, Cutler P, Melnyk S, Jernigan S, Janak L, Gaylor DW, Neubrander JA. Metabolic biomarkers of increased oxidative stress and impaired methylation capacity in children with autism. *Am J Clin Nutr.* 2004 Dec;80(6):1611-7.

67   Sugiura I, Furie B, Walsh CT, Furie BC. Propeptide and glutamate-containing substrates bound to the vitamin K-dependent carboxylase convert its vitamin K epoxidase function from an inactive to an active state. *Proc Natl Acad Sci U S A.* 1997 Aug 19;94(17):9069-74.

68   Zitterman A. Effects of vitamin K on calcium and bone metabolism. *Curr Opin Clin Nutr Metab Care.* 2001 Nov 4(6):483-487.

69   Vervoort LM, Ronden JE, Thijssen HH. The potent antioxidant activity of the vitamin K cycle in microsomal lipid peroxidation. *Biochem Pharmacol.* 1997 Oct 15; 54(8):871-6.

70   Li J, Lin JC, Wang H, Peterson JW, Furie BC, Furie B, Booth SL, Volpe JJ, Rosenberg PA. Novel role of vitamin K in preventing oxidative injury to developing oligodendrocytes and neurons. *J Neuroscience.* 2003 Jul: 23(13):5816-5826.

71   Reddi K, Henderson B, Meghji S, Wilson M, Poole S, Hopper C, Harris M, Hodges SJ. Interleukin 6 production by lipopolysaccharide-stimulated human fibroblasts is potently inhibited by naphthoquinone (vitamin K) compounds. *Cytokine.* 1995 Apr;7(3):287-90.

72. Ohsaki Y, Shirakawa H, Hiwatashi K, Furukawa Y, Mizutani T, Komai M. Vitamin K suppresses lipopolysaccharide-induced inflammation in the rat. *Biosci Biotechnol Biochem.* 2006 Apr;70(4):926-32.

73   Schoon EJ, Muller MC, Vermeer C, Schurgers LJ, Brummer RJ, Stockbrugger RW. Low serum and bone vitamin K status in patients with longstanding Crohn's disease: another pathogenetic factor of osteoporosis in Crohn's disease? *Gut.* 2001 Apr; 48(4):473-7.

74   Kidd PM. Autism, an extreme challenge to integrative medicine. Part 2: medical management. *Altern Med Rev.* 2002 Dec;7(6):472-99.

75   Pfeiffer CC, Braverman ER. Zinc, the brain and behavior. *Biol Psychiatry.* 1982 Apr; 17(4):513-32.

76   Walsh WJ, Glab LB, Haakenson ML. Reduced violent behavior following biochemical therapy. *Physiol Behav.* 2004 Oct 15;82(5):835-9.

77   Levy J. Immunonutrition: the pediatric experience. *Nutrition.* 1998 Jul-Aug;14(7-8): 641-7.

78   Johnson S. Micronutrient accumulation and depletion in schizophrenia, epilepsy, autism and Parkinson's disease? *Med Hypotheses.* 2001 May;56(5):641-5.

79 Walsh WJ, Usman A, Tarpey J. Disordered metal metabolism in a large autism population. Presented at the APA Annual Meeting, New Orleans, 5-2001.

80 Levy J. Immunonutrition: the pediatric experience. *Nutrition.* 1998 Jul-Aug; 14(7-8):641-7.

81 William J. Walsh. Zinc deficiency, metal metabolism, and behavior disorders. Unpublished monograph. Health Research Institute, March 1995.

82 Baker SB, Worthley LI. The essentials of calcium, magnesium and phosphate metabolism: part I. Physiology. *Crit Care Resusc.* 2002 Dec;4(4):301-6.

83 Martineau J, Barthelemy C, Garreau B, Lelord G. Vitamin B6, magnesium, and combined B6-Mg: therapeutic effects in childhood autism. *Biol Psychiatry.* 1985 May;20(5):467-78.

84 Mousain-Bosc M, Roche M, Polge A, Pradal-Prat D, Rapin J, Bali JP. Improvement of neurobehavioral disorders in children supplemented with magnesium-vitamin B6. II. Pervasive developmental disorder-autism. *Magnes Res.* 2006 Mar;19(1):53-62.

85 Kozielec T, Starobrat-Hermelin B. Assessment of magnesium levels in children with attention deficit hyperactivity disorder (ADHD). *Magnes Res.* 1997 Jun;10(2):143-8.

86 Starobrat-Hermelin B, Kozielec T. The effects of magnesium physiological supplementation on hyperactivity in children with attention deficit hyperactivity disorder (ADHD). Positive response to magnesium oral loading test. *Magnes Res.* 1997 Jun;10(2):149-56.

87 Mousain-Bosc M, Roche M, Polge A, Pradal-Prat D, Rapin J, Bali JP. Improvement of neurobehavioral disorders in children supplemented with magnesium-vitamin B6. II. Pervasive developmental disorder-autism. *Magnes Res.* 2006 Mar;19(1):53-62.

88 Mousain-Bosc M, Roche M, Rapin J, Bali JP. Magnesium VitB6 intake reduces central nervous system hyperexcitability in children. *J Am Coll Nutr.* 2004 Oct;23(5):545S-548S.

89 Liebscher DH, Liebscher DE. About the misdiagnosis of magnesium deficiency. *J Am Coll Nutr.* 2004 Dec;23(6):730S-1S.

90 Bronner F. Extracellular and intracellular regulation of calcium homeostasis. *ScientificWorldJournal.* 2001 Dec 22;1:919-25.

91 Baker SB, Worthley LI. The essentials of calcium, magnesium and phosphate metabolism: part I. Physiology. *Crit Care Resusc.* 2002 Dec;4(4):301-6.

92 Litov RE, Combs GF Jr. Selenium in pediatric nutrition. *Pediatrics.* 1991 Mar; 87(3):339-51.

93 Levy J. Immunonutrition: the pediatric experience. *Nutrition.* 1998 Jul-Aug; 14(7-8):641-7.

94 Olmez A, Yalcin S, Yurdakok K, Coskun T. Serum selenium levels in acute gastroenteritis of possible viral origin. *J Trop Pediatr.* 2004 Apr;50(2):78-81.

95 Geoghegan M, McAuley D, Eaton S, Powell-Tuck J. Selenium in critical illness. *Curr Opin Crit Care.* 2006 Apr;12(2):136-41.

96 Litov RE, Combs GF Jr. Selenium in pediatric nutrition. *Pediatrics.* 1991 Mar; 87(3):339-51.

97   Geoghegan M, McAuley D, Eaton S, Powell-Tuck J. Selenium in critical illness. *Curr Opin Crit Care.* 2006 Apr;12(2):136-41.

98   Waring RH, Klovrza LV. Sulphur metabolism in autism. *J Nutr Env Med.* 2000:10:25-35.

99   Fernstrom JD. Can nutrient supplements modify brain function? *Am J Clin Nutr.* 2000 Jun;71(6 Suppl):1669S-75S.

100 Richardson AJ. Omega-3 fatty acids in ADHD and related neurodevelopmental disorders. *Int Rev Psychiatry.* 2006 Apr;18(2):155-72.

101 Bell JG, Sargent JR, Tocher DR, Dick JR. Red blood cell fatty acid compositions in a patient with autistic spectrum disorder: a characteristic abnormality in neurodevelopmental disorders? *Prostaglandins Leukot Essent Fatty Acids.* 2000 Jul-Aug;63(1-2):21-5.

102 Vancassel S, Durand G, Barthelemy C, Lejeune B, Martineau J, Guilloteau D, Andres C, Chalon S. Plasma fatty acid levels in autistic children. *Prostaglandins Leukot Essent Fatty Acids.* 2001 Jul;65(1):1-7.

103 Bu B, Ashwood P, Harvey D, King IB, Water JV, Jin LW. Fatty acid compositions of red blood cell phospholipids in children with autism. *Prostaglandins Leukot Essent Fatty Acids.* 2006 Apr;74(4):215-21.

104 Amminger GP, Berger GE, Schafer MR, Klier C, Friedrich MH, Feucht M. Omega-3 Fatty Acids Supplementation in Children with Autism: A Double-blind Randomized, Placebo-controlled Pilot Study. *Biol Psychiatry.* 2006 Aug 22; [Epub ahead of print].

105 Young G, Conquer J. Omega-3 fatty acids and neuropsychiatric disorders. *Reprod Nutr Dev.* 2005 Jan-Feb;45(1):1-28.

106 Richardson AJ. Omega-3 fatty acids in ADHD and related neurodevelopmental disorders. *Int Rev Psychiatry.* 2006 Apr;18(2):155-72.

107 Imura K, Okada A. Amino acid metabolism in pediatric patients. *Nutrition.* 1998 Jan;14(1):143-8.

108 Aldred S, Moore KM, Fitzgerald M, Waring RH. Plasma amino acid levels in children with autism and their families. *J Autism Dev Disord.* 2003 Feb;33(1):93-7.

109 Arnold GL, Hyman SL, Mooney RA, Kirby RS. Plasma amino acids profiles in children with autism: potential risk of nutritional deficiencies. *J Autism Dev Disord.* 2003 Aug;33(4):449-54.

110 Imura K, Okada A. Amino acid metabolism in pediatric patients. *Nutrition.* 1998 Jan;14(1):143-8.

111 Kidd PM. Autism, an extreme challenge to integrative medicine. Part 2: medical management. *Altern Med Rev.* 2002 Dec;7(6):472-99.

112 Sturman JA, Chesney RW. Taurine in pediatric nutrition. *Pediatr Clin North Am.* 1995 Aug;42(4):879-97.

113 Gaull GE. Taurine in pediatric nutrition: review and update. *Pediatrics.* 1989 Mar;83(3):433-42.

114 Van Gelder NM, Sherwin AL, Sacks C, Anderman F. Biochemical observations following administration of taurine to patients with epilepsy. *Brain Res.* 1975 Aug 29; 94(2):297-306.

115 James SJ, Cutler P, Melnyk S, Jernigan S, Janak L, Gaylor DW, Neubrander JA. Metabolic biomarkers of increased oxidative stress and impaired methylation capacity in children with autism. *Am J Clin Nutr.* 2004 Dec;80(6):1611-7.

116 Pangborn J, Baker SM. *Autism: Effective Biomedical Treatments (Have We Done Everything We Can For This Child? Individuality In An Epidemic).* San Diego: Autism Research Institute; 2nd Edition Sept. 2005:232-235.

117 Imura K, Okada A. Amino acid metabolism in pediatric patients. *Nutrition.* 1998 Jan;14(1):143-8.

118 Kidd PM. Autism, an extreme challenge to integrative medicine. Part 2: medical management. *Altern Med Rev.* 2002 Dec;7(6):472-99.

119 Levy J. Immunonutrition: the pediatric experience. *Nutrition.* 1998 Jul-Aug; 14(7-8):641-7.

120 Ibid.

121 Sogut S, Zoroglu SS, Ozyurt H, Yilmaz HR, Ozugurlu F, Sivasli E, Yetkin O, Yanik M, Tutkun H, Savas HA, Tarakcioglu M, Akyol O. Changes in nitric oxide levels and antioxidant enzyme activities may have a role in the pathophysiological mechanisms involved in autism. *Clin Chim Acta.* 2003 May;331(1-2):111-7.

122 Zoroglu SS, Yurekli M, Meram I, Sogut S, Tutkun H, Yetkin O, Sivasli E, Savas HA, Yanik M, Herken H, Akyol O. Pathophysiological role of nitric oxide and adrenomedullin in autism. *Cell Biochem Funct.* 2003 Mar;21(1):55-60.

123 Pangborn J, Baker SM. *Autism: Effective Biomedical Treatments (Have We Done Everything We Can For This Child? Individuality In An Epidemic).* San Diego: Autism Research Institute; 2nd Edition Sept. 2005: 280.

124 Ibid, p. 279-284.

125 Whiteley P, Waring R, Williams L, Klovrza L, Nolan F, Smith S, Farrow M, Dodou K, Lough WJ, Shattock P. Spot urinary creatinine excretion in pervasive developmental disorders. *Pediatr Int.* 2006 Jun;48(3):292-7.

126 Friedman SD, Shaw DW, Artru AA, Richards TL, Gardner J, Dawson G, Posse S, Dager SR. Regional brain chemical alterations in young children with autism spectrum disorder. *Neurology.* 2003 Jan 14;60(1):100-7.

127 Filipek PA, Juranek J, Nguyen MT, Cummings C, Gargus JJ. Relative carnitine deficiency in autism. *J Autism Dev Disord.* 2004 Dec;34(6):615-23.

128 Chez MG, Buchanan CP, Aimonovitch MC, Becker M, Schaefer K, Black C, Komen J. Double-blind, placebo-controlled study of L-carnosine supplementation in children with autistic spectrum disorders. *J Child Neurol.* 2002 Nov;17(11):833-7.

129 Chugani DC, Sundram BS, Behen M, Lee ML, Moore GJ. Evidence of altered energy metabolism in autistic children. *Prog Neuropsychopharmacol Biol Psychiatry.* 1999 May;23(4):635-41.

130 Coleman M, Steinberg G, Tippett J, Bhagavan HN, Coursin DB, Gross M, Lewis C, DeVeau L. A preliminary study of the effect of pyridoxine administration in a subgroup of hyperkinetic children: a double-blind crossover comparison with methylphenidate. *Biol Psychiatry.* 1979 Oct;14(5):741-51.

Chapter 17

1 Kaila M, Isolauri E, Soppi E, Virtanen E, Laine S, Arvilommi H. Enhancement of the circulating antibody secreting cell response in human diarrhea by a human Lactobacillus strain. *Pediatr Res.* 1992 Aug;32(2):141-4.

2 Itoh T, Fujimoto Y, Kawai Y, Toba T, Saito T. Inhibition of food-borne pathogenic bacteria by bacteriocins from Lactobacillus gasseri. *Lett Appl Microbiol.* 1995 Sep; 21(3):137-41.

3 Levy J. Immunonutrition: the pediatric experience. *Nutrition.* 1998 Jul-Aug; 14(7-8):641-7.

4 Buts JP, De Keyser N, De Raedemaeker L. Saccharomyces boulardii enhances rat intestinal enzyme expression by endoluminal release of polyamines. *Pediatr Res.* 1994 Oct;36(4):522-7.

5 Haskey N, Dahl WJ. Synbiotic therapy: a promising new adjunctive therapy for ulcerative colitis. *Nutr Rev.* 2006 Mar;64(3):132-8.

6 Buts JP, De Keyser N. Effects of Saccharomyces boulardii on intestinal mucosa. *Dig Dis Sci.* 2006 Aug;51(8):1485-92.

7 Buts JP, De Keyser N, Marandi S, Hermans D, Sokal EM, Chae YH, Lambotte L, Chanteux H, Tulkens PM. Saccharomyces boulardii upgrades cellular adaptation after proximal enterectomy in rats. *Gut.* 1999 Jul;45(1):89-96.

8 Sougioultzis S, Simeonidis S, Bhaskar KR, Chen X, Anton PM, Keates S, Pothoulakis C, Kelly CP. Saccharomyces boulardii produces a soluble anti-inflammatory factor that inhibits NF-kappaB-mediated IL-8 gene expression. *Biochem Biophys Res Commun.* 2006 Apr 28;343(1):69-76.

9 Isolauri E, Juntunen M, Rautanen T, Sillanaukee P, Koivula T. A human Lactobacillus strain (Lactobacillus casei sp strain GG) promotes recovery from acute diarrhea in children. *Pediatrics.* 1991 Jul;88(1):90-7.

10 Biller JA, Katz AJ, Flores AF, Buie TM, Gorbach SL. Treatment of recurrent Clostridium difficile colitis with Lactobacillus GG. *J Pediatr Gastroenterol Nutr.* 1995 Aug;21(2):224-6.

11 Saavedra JM, Bauman NA, Oung I, Perman JA, Yolken RH. Feeding of Bifidobacterium bifidum and Streptococcus thermophilus to infants in hospital for prevention of diarrhoea and shedding of rotavirus. *Lancet.* 1994 Oct 15;344(8929):1046-9.

12 Majamaa H, Isolauri E, Saxelin M, Vesikari T. Lactic acid bacteria in the treatment of acute rotavirus gastroenteritis. *J Pediatr Gastroenterol Nutr.* 1995 Apr;20(3):333-8.

13 Lin MY, Savaiano D, Harlander S. Influence of nonfermented dairy products containing bacterial starter cultures on lactose maldigestion in humans. *J Dairy Sci.* 1991 Jan;74(1):87-95.

14 Shermak MA, Saavedra JM, Jackson TL, Huang SS, Bayless TM, Perman JA. Effect of yogurt on symptoms and kinetics of hydrogen production in lactose-malabsorbing children. *Am J Clin Nutr.* 1995 Nov;62(5):1003-6.

15 Sutas Y, Hurme M, Isolauri E. Down-regulation of anti-CD3 antibody-induced IL-4 production by bovine caseins hydrolysed with Lactobacillus GG-derived enzymes. *Scand J Immunol.* 1996 Jun;43(6):687-9.

16 Majamaa H, Isolauri E, Saxelin M, Vesikari T. Lactic acid bacteria in the treatment of acute rotavirus gastroenteritis. *J Pediatr Gastroenterol Nutr.* 1995 Apr;20(3):333-8.

17 Haskey N, Dahl WJ. Synbiotic therapy: a promising new adjunctive therapy for ulcerative colitis. *Nutr Rev.* 2006 Mar;64(3):132-8.

18 Gottschall, Elaine G. *Breaking the Vicious Cycle: Intestinal Health Through Diet.* Ontario: Kirkton Press. 1994.

19 Kushak R, Winter H, Farber N, Buie T. Gastrointestinal symptoms and intestinal disaccharidase activities in children with autism. *J Pediatr Gastroenterol Nutr.* 2005 Oct;41(4).

20 Horvath K, Papadimitriou JC, Rabsztyn A, Drachenberg C, Tildon JT. Gastrointestinal abnormalities in children with autistic disorder. *J Pediatr.* 1999 Nov; 135(5):559-63.

21 Ibid.

22 Reichelt KL, Knivsberg AM. Can the pathophysiology of autism be explained by the nature of the discovered urine peptides? *Nutr Neurosci.* 2003 Feb;6(1):19-28.

23 Aldred S, Moore KM, Fitzgerald M, Waring RH. Plasma amino acid levels in children with autism and their families. *J Autism Dev Disord.* 2003 Feb;33(1):93-7.

24 Brudnak MA, Rimland B, Pangborn JB, Buchholz I. Beneficial effects of enzyme-based therapy for autism spectrum disorders. www.list.feat.org/wa.exe?A2=ind0112 &L=featnews&P=1643

25 Liu Z, Li N, Neu J. Tight junctions, leaky intestines, and pediatric diseases. *Acta Paediatr.* 2005 Apr;94(4):386-93.

26 Waring RH, Klovrza LV. Sulphur metabolism in autism. *J Nutr Env Med.* 2000; 10,25-32.

27 Afzal N, Murch S, Thirrupathy K, Berger L, Fagbemi A, Heuschkel R. Constipation with acquired megarectum in children with autism. *Pediatrics.* 2003 Oct;112(4):939-42.

28 North American Society for Pediatric Gastroenterology, Hepatology and Nutrition. Evaluation and treatment of constipation in children: summary of updated recommendations of the North American Society for Pediatric Gastroenterology, Hepatology and Nutrition. *J Pediatr Gastroenterol Nutr.* 2006 Sep;43(3):405-7.

29   Horvath KD, Jobe BA, Herron DM, Swanstrom LL. Laparoscopic Toupet fundoplication is an inadequate procedure for patients with severe reflux disease. *J Gastrointest Surg.* 1999 Nov-Dec;3(6):583-91.

30   Torrente F, Ashwood P, Day R, Machado N, Furlano RI, Anthony A, Davies SE, Wakefield AJ, Thomson MA, Walker-Smith JA, Murch SH. Small intestinal enteropathy with epithelial IgG and complement deposition in children with regressive autism. *Mol Psychiatry.* 2002;7(4):375-82, 334.

31   Torrente F, Anthony A, Heuschkel RB, Thomson MA, Ashwood P, Murch SH. Focal-enhanced gastritis in regressive autism with features distinct from Crohn's and Helicobacter pylori gastritis. *Am J Gastroenterol.* 2004 Apr;99(4):598-605.

32   Hassall E. Decisions in diagnosing and managing chronic gastroesophageal reflux disease in children. *J Pediatr.* 2005 Mar;146(3 Suppl):S3-12.

33   Bousvaros A, Sylvester F, Kugathasan S, Szigethy E, Fiocchi C, Colletti R, Otley A, Amre D, Ferry G, Czinn SJ, Splawski JB, Oliva-Hemker M, Hyams JS, Faubion WA, Kirschner BS, Dubinsky MC; and the Members of the Challenges in Pediatric IBD Study Groups. Challenges in pediatric inflammatory bowel disease. *Inflamm Bowel Dis.* 2006 Sep;12(9):885-913.

34   Ueland PM, Hustad S, Schneede J, Refsum H, Vollset SE. Biological and clinical implications of the MTHFR C677T polymorphism. *Trends Pharmacol Sci.* 2001 Apr;22(4):195-201.

35   Homan M, Baldassano RN, Mamula P. Managing complicated Crohn's disease in children and adolescents. *Nat Clin Pract Gastroenterol Hepatol.* 2005 Dec;2(12):572-9.

36   Ibid.

37   Macdonald A. Omega-3 fatty acids as adjunctive therapy in Crohns disease. *Gastroenterol Nurs.* 2006 Jul-Aug;29(4):295-301.

38   Working Group of the Japanese Society for Pediatric Gastroenterology, Hepatology and Nutrition; Konno M, Kobayashi A, Tomomasa T, Kaneko H, Toyoda S, Nakazato Y, Nezu R, Maisawa S, Miki K. Guidelines for the treatment of Crohn's disease in children. *Pediatr Int.* 2006 Jun;48(3):349-52.

39   Macdonald A. Omega-3 fatty acids as adjunctive therapy in Crohns disease. *Gastroenterol Nurs.* 2006 Jul-Aug;29(4):295-301; quiz 302-3.

40   Belluzzi A, Brignola C, Campieri M, Pera A, Boschi S, Miglioli M. Effect of an enteric-coated fish-oil preparation on relapses in Crohn's disease. *N Engl J Med.* 1996 Jun 13;334(24):1557-60.

41   Romano C, Cucchiara S, Barabino A, Annese V, Sferlazzas C. Usefulness of omega-3 fatty acid supplementation in addition to mesalazine in maintaining remission in pediatric Crohn's disease: a double-blind, randomized, placebo-controlled study. *World J Gastroenterol.* 2005 Dec 7;11(45):7118-21.

42   Schneider CK, Melmed RD, Barstow LE, Enriquez FJ, Ranger-Moore J, Ostrem JA. Oral Human Immunoglobulin for Children with Autism and Gastrointestinal Dysfunction: A Prospective, Open-Label Study. *J Autism Dev Disord.* 2006 Jul 15; [Epub ahead of print].

CHAPTER 18

1   Chauhan V, Chauhan A. Oxidative stress in Alzheimer's disease. *Pathophysiology.* 2006 Aug;13(3):195-208.

2   Yorbik O, Sayal A, Akay C, Akbiyik DI, Sohmen T. Investigation of antioxidant enzymes in children with autistic disorder. *Prostaglandins Leukot Essent Fatty Acids.* 2002 Nov;67(5):341-3.

3   Chauhan V, Chauhan A. Oxidative stress in Alzheimer's disease. *Pathophysiology.* 2006 Aug;13(3):195-208.

4   Chauhan A, Chauhan V, Brown WT, Cohen I. Oxidative stress in autism: increased lipid peroxidation and reduced serum levels of ceruloplasmin and transferrin—the antioxidant proteins. *Life Sci.* 2004 Oct 8;75(21):2539-49.

5   Zoroglu SS, Armutcu F, Ozen S, Gurel A, Sivasli E, Yetkin O, Meram I. Increased oxidative stress and altered activities of erythrocyte free radical scavenging enzymes in autism. *Eur Arch Psychiatry Clin Neurosci.* 2004 Jun;254(3):143-7.

6   Ming X, Stein TP, Brimacombe M, Johnson WG, Lambert GH, Wagner GC. Increased excretion of a lipid peroxidation biomarker in autism. *Prostaglandins Leukot Essent Fatty Acids.* 2005 Nov;73(5):379-84.

7   Sogut S, Zoroglu SS, Ozyurt H, Yilmaz HR, Ozugurlu F, Sivasli E, Yetkin O, Yanik M, Tutkun H, Savas HA, Tarakcioglu M, Akyol O. Changes in nitric oxide levels and antioxidant enzyme activities may have a role in the pathophysiological mechanisms involved in autism. *Clin Chim Acta.* 2003 May;331(1-2):111-7.

8   Zoroglu SS, Yurekli M, Meram I, Sogut S, Tutkun H, Yetkin O, Sivasli E, Savas HA, Yanik M, Herken H, Akyol O. Pathophysiological role of nitric oxide and adrenomedullin in autism. *Cell Biochem Funct.* 2003 Mar;21(1):55-60.

9   McGuiness W. Oxidative stress in autism. *Alternative Therapies.* 2004;10(6):22-37.

10 James SJ, Melnyk S, Jernigan S, Cleves MA, Halsted CH, Wong DH, Cutler P, Bock K, Boris M, Bradstreet JJ, Baker SM, Gaylor DW. Metabolic endophenotype and related genotypes are associated with oxidative stress in children with autism. *Am J Med Genet B Neuropsychiatr Genet.* 2006 Aug 17; [Epub ahead of print].

11 Yorbik O, Sayal A, Akay C, Akbiyik DI, Sohmen T. Investigation of antioxidant enzymes in children with autistic disorder. *Prostaglandins Leukot Essent Fatty Acids.* 2002 Nov;67(5):341-3.

12 Pasca SP, Nemes B, Vlase L, Gagyi CE, Dronca E, Miu AC, Dronca M. High levels of homocysteine and low serum paraoxonase 1 arylesterase activity in children with autism. *Life Sci.* 2006 Apr 4;78(19):2244-8.

13 Golse B, Debray-Ritzen P, Durosay P, Puget K, Michelson AM. Alterations in two enzymes: superoxide dismutase and glutathione peroxidase in developmental infantile psychosis (infantile autism). *Rev Neurol (Paris).* 1978 Nov;134(11): 699-705.

14 Sogut S, Zoroglu SS, Ozyurt H, Yilmaz HR, Ozugurlu F, Sivasli E, Yetkin O, Yanik M, Tutkun H, Savas HA, Tarakcioglu M, Akyol O. Changes in nitric oxide

levels and antioxidant enzyme activities may have a role in the pathophysiological mechanisms involved in autism. *Clin Chim Acta.* 2003 May;331(1-2):111-7.

15 James SJ, Cutler P, Melnyk S, Jernigan S, Janak L, Gaylor DW, Neubrander JA. Metabolic biomarkers of increased oxidative stress and impaired methylation capacity in children with autism. *Am J Clin Nutr.* 2004 Dec;80(6):1611-7.

16 Zoroglu SS, Armutcu F, Ozen S, Gurel A, Sivasli E, Yetkin O, Meram I. Increased oxidative stress and altered activities of erythrocyte free radical scavenging enzymes in autism. *Eur Arch Psychiatry Clin Neurosci.* 2004 Jun;254(3):143-7.

17 Yorbik O, Sayal A, Akay C, Akbiyik DI, Sohmen T. Investigation of antioxidant enzymes in children with autistic disorder. *Prostaglandins Leukot Essent Fatty Acids.* 2002 Nov;67(5):341-3.

18 Golse B, Debray-Ritzen P, Durosay P, Puget K, Michelson AM. Alterations in two enzymes: superoxide dismutase and glutathione peroxidase in developmental infantile psychosis (infantile autism). *Rev Neurol (Paris).* 1978 Nov;134(11):699-705.

19 Chauhan A, Chauhan V, Brown WT, Cohen I. Oxidative stress in autism: increased lipid peroxidation and reduced serum levels of ceruloplasmin and transferrin—the antioxidant proteins. *Life Sci.* 2004 Oct 8;75(21):2539-49.

20 Ibid.

21 James SJ, Cutler P, Melnyk S, Jernigan S, Janak L, Gaylor DW, Neubrander JA. Metabolic biomarkers of increased oxidative stress and impaired methylation capacity in children with autism. *Am J Clin Nutr.* 2004 Dec;80(6):1611-7.

22 Ibid.

23 James SJ, Melnyk S, Jernigan S, Cleves MA, Halsted CH, Wong DH, Cutler P, Bock K, Boris M, Bradstreet JJ, Baker SM, Gaylor DW. Metabolic endophenotype and related genotypes are associated with oxidative stress in children with autism. *Am J Med Genet B Neuropsychiatr Genet.* 2006 Aug 17; [Epub ahead of print]

24 Chauhan V, Chauhan A. Oxidative stress in Alzheimer's disease. *Pathophysiology.* 2006 Aug;13(3):195-208.

25 Boris M, Goldblatt A, Galanko J, James J. Association of MTHFR gene variants with autism. *J Am Phys Surg.* 2004;9(4)106-8.

26 James SJ, Cutler P, Melnyk S, Jernigan S, Janak L, Gaylor DW, Neubrander JA. Metabolic biomarkers of increased oxidative stress and impaired methylation capacity in children with autism. *Am J Clin Nutr.* 2004 Dec;80(6):1611-7.

27 Walsh WJ, Glab LB, Haakenson ML. Reduced violent behavior following biochemical therapy. *Physiol Behav.* 2004 Oct 15;82(5):835-9.

28 Waring RH, Klovrza LV. Sulphur metabolism in autism. *J Nutr Env Med.* 2000;10:25-32.

29 James SJ, Cutler P, Melnyk S, Jernigan S, Janak L, Gaylor DW, Neubrander JA. Metabolic biomarkers of increased oxidative stress and impaired methylation capacity in children with autism. *Am J Clin Nutr.* 2004 Dec;80(6):1611-7.

30 Neubrander, James. Methyl B12. Autism One presentation. Chicago, Il, 5/29/05.

CHAPTER 19

1   Kidd PM. Autism, an extreme challenge to integrative medicine. Part 2: medical management. *Altern Med Rev.* 2002 Dec;7(6):472-99.

2   Ebina T, Sato A, Umezu K, Aso H, Ishida N, Seki H, Tsukamoto T, Takase S, Hoshi S, Ohta M. Treatment of multiple sclerosis with anti-measles cow colostrum. *Med Microbiol Immunol (Berl).* 1984;173(2):87-93.

3   Kelly GS. Bovine colostrums: a review of clinical uses. *Altern Med Rev.* 2003 Nov;8(4):378-94.

4   Zimecki M, Artym J. Therapeutic properties of proteins and peptides from colostrum and milk. *Postepy Hig Med Dosw.* 2005;59:309-23.

5   Pizza G, Amadori M, Ablashi D, De Vinci C, Viza D. Cell mediated immunity to meet the avian influenza A (H5N1) challenge. *Med Hypotheses.* 2006;67(3):601-8.

6   Flores Sandoval G, Gomez Vera J, Orea Solano M, Lopez Tiro J, Serrano E, Rodriguez A, Rodriguez A, Estrada Parra S, Jimenez Saab N. Transfer factor as specific immunomodulator in the treatment of moderate-severe atopic dermatitis. *Rev Alerg Mex.* 2005 Nov-Dec;52(6):215-20.

7   Estrada-Parra S, Nagaya A, Serrano E, Rodriguez O, Santamaria V, Ondarza R, Chavez R, Correa B, Monges A, Cabezas R, Calva C, Estrada-Garcia I. Comparative study of transfer factor and acyclovir in the treatment of herpes zoster. *Int J Immunopharmacol.* 1998 Oct;20(10):521-35.

8   Gupta S. Immunological treatments for autism. *J Autism Dev Disord.* 2000 Oct; 30(5):475-9.

9   Fudenberg HH. Dialysable lymphocyte extract (DLyE) in infantile onset autism: a pilot study. *Biotherapy.* 1996;9(1-3):143-7.

10 Stubbs EG, Budden SS, Burger DR, Vandenbark AA. Transfer factor immunotherapy of an autistic child with congenital cytomegalovirus. *J Autism Dev Disord.* 1980 Dec;10(4):451-8.

11 Schneider CK, Melmed RD, Barstow LE, Enriquez FJ, Ranger-Moore J, Ostrem JA. Oral Human Immunoglobulin for Children with Autism and Gastrointestinal Dysfunction: A Prospective, Open-Label Study. *J Autism Dev Disord.* 2006 Jul 15; [Epub ahead of print].

12 Bayary J, Dasgupta S, Misra N, Ephrem A, Van Huyen JP, Delignat S, Hassan G, Caligiuri G, Nicoletti A, Lacroix-Desmazes S, Kazatchkine MD, Kaveri S. Intravenous immunoglobulin in autoimmune disorders: an insight into the immunoregulatory mechanisms. *Int Immunopharmacol.* 2006 Apr;6(4):528-34.

13 Siragam V, Crow AR, Brinc D, Song S, Freedman J, Lazarus AH. Intravenous immunoglobulin ameliorates ITP via activating Fc gamma receptors on dendritic cells. *Nat Med.* 2006 Jun;12(6):688-92.

14 Koski CL, Patterson JV. Intravenous immunoglobulin use for neurologic diseases. *J Infus Nurs.* 2006 May-Jun;29(3 Suppl):S21-8.

15 Bayary J, Dasgupta S, Misra N, Ephrem A, Van Huyen JP, Delignat S, Hassan G, Caligiuri G, Nicoletti A, Lacroix-Desmazes S, Kazatchkine MD, Kaveri S. Intravenous immunoglobulin in autoimmune disorders: an insight into the immunoregulatory mechanisms. *Int Immunopharmacol.* 2006 Apr;6(4):528-34.

16 Gupta S, Aggarwal S, Heads C. Dysregulated immune system in children with autism: beneficial effects of intravenous immune globulin on autistic characteristics. *J Autism Dev Disord.* 1996 Aug;26(4):439-52.

17 DelGiudice-Asch G, Simon L, Schmeidler J, Cunningham-Rundles C, Hollander E. Brief report: A pilot open clinical trial of intravenous immunoglobulin in childhood autism. *J Autism Dev Disord.* 1999:29(2):157-60.

18 Plioplys AV. Intravenous immunoglobulin treatment of children with autism. *J Child Neurol.* 1998 Feb;13(2):79-82.

19 Boris M, Goldblatt A, Edelson S. Improvement in children treated with intravenous gamma globulin. *J Nutr Environmental Med.* Dec 2006; 15(4):1-8.

20 Swedo SE, Leonard HL, Garvey M, Mittleman B, Allen AJ, Perlmutter S, Lougee L, Dow S, Zamkoff J, Dubbert BK. Pediatric autoimmune neuropsychiatric disorders associated with streptococcal infections: clinical description of the first 50 cases. *Am J Psychiatry.* 1998 Feb;155(2):264-71.

21 Swedo SE, Leonard HL, Rapoport JL. The pediatric autoimmune neuropsychiatric disorders associated with streptococcal infection (PANDAS) subgroup: separating fact from fiction. *Pediatrics.* 2004 Apr;113(4):907-11.

22 Swedo SE, Grant PJ. Annotation: PANDAS: a model for human autoimmune disease. *J Child Psychol Psychiatry.* 2005 Mar;46(3):227-34.

23 Walker SJ, Hepner K, Segal J, Krigsman A. Persistent ileal measles virus in a large cohort of regressive autistic children with ileocolitis and lymphonodular hyperplasia: revisitation of an earlier study. IMFAR.

24 Bradstreet JJ, El Dahr JM, Anthony A, Kartzinel JJ, Wakefield AJ. Detection of measles virus genomic RNA in cerebrospinal fluid of children with regressive autism: a report of three cases. *J Am Phys Surg.* 2004:9(2):38-45.

25 Keating MR. Antiviral agents for non-human immunodeficiency virus infections. *Mayo Clin Proc.* 1999 Dec;74(12):1266-83.

26 James SJ, Cutler P, Melnyk S, Jernigan S, Janak L, Gaylor DW, Neubrander JA. Metabolic biomarkers of increased oxidative stress and impaired methylation capacity in children with autism. *Am J Clin Nutr.* 2004 Dec;80(6):1611-7.

27 Rea WJ, Didriksen N, Simon TR, Pan Y, Fenyves EJ, Griffiths B. Effects of toxic exposure to molds and mycotoxins in building-related illnesses. *Arch Environ Health.* 2003 Jul;58(7):399-405.

28 Rea WJ, Ross GH. Food and chemicals as environmental incitants. *Nurse Pract.* 1989 Sep;14(9):17-8, 28, 30 passim.

29 Rea WJ, Podell RN, Williams ML, Fenyves E, Sprague DE, Johnson AR. Elimination of oral food challenge reaction by injection of food extracts. A double-blind evaluation. *Arch Otolaryngol.* 1984 Apr;110(4):248-52.

30 Weiner JM. Allergen injection immunotherapy. *Med J Aust.* 2006 Aug 21; 185(4):234.

31 Werner-Klein M, Kalkbrenner F, Erb KJ. Sublingual immunotherapy of allergic diseases. *Expert Opin Drug Deliv.* 2006 Sep;3(5):599-612.

32 Sicherer SH, Leung DY. Advances in allergic skin disease, anaphylaxis, and hypersensitivity reactions to foods, drugs, and insects. *J Allergy Clin Immunol.* 2006 Jul;118(1):170-7.

33 Penagos M, Compalati E, Tarantini F, Baena-Cagnani R, Huerta J, Passalacqua G, Canonica GW. Efficacy of sublingual immunotherapy in the treatment of allergic rhinitis in pediatric patients 3 to 18 years of age: a meta-analysis of randomized, placebo-controlled, double-blind trials. *Ann Allergy Asthma Immunol.* 2006 Aug;97(2):141-8.

34 Douglass JA, O'Hehir RE. 1. Diagnosis, treatment and prevention of allergic disease: the basics. *Med J Aust.* 2006 Aug 21;185(4):228-33.

35 Lewis JD, Lichtenstein GR, Stein RB, Deren JJ, Judge TA, Fogt F, Furth EE, Demissie EJ, Hurd LB, Su CG, Keilbaugh SA, Lazar MA, Wu GD. An open-label trial of the PPAR-gamma ligand rosiglitazone for active ulcerative colitis. *Am J Gastroenterol.* 2001 Dec;96(12):3323-8.

36 Rios-Vazquez R, Marzoa-Rivas R, Gil-Ortega I, Kaski JC. Peroxisome proliferator-activated receptor-gamma agonists for management and prevention of vascular disease in patients with and without diabetes mellitus. *Am J Cardiovasc Drugs.* 2006;6(4):231-42.

37 Youseff S, Steinman L. At once harmful and beneficial: the dual properties of NFKB. *Nature Immunology.* 2006; 7(9):901-902

38 Chinetti G, Fruchart JC, Staels B. Peroxisome proliferators-activated receptors (PPAR): nuclear receptors at the crossroads between lipid metabolism and inflammation. *Inflamm Res* 2000;49:497-505.

39 Vargas DL, Nascimbene C, Krishnan C, Zimmerman AW, Pardo CA. Neuroglial activation and neuroinflammation in the brain of patients with autism. *Ann Neurol.* 2005 Jan;57(1):67-81.

40 Meffert M, Baltimore D. Physiological Functions of brain NF-KB. *Trends in Neurosciences.* 2005;28(1):37-43.

41 Pershadsingh HA. Peroxisome proliferator-activated receptor-gamma: therapeutic target for diseases beyond diabetes: quo vadis? *Expert Opin Investig Drugs.* 2004 Mar;13(3):215-28.

42 Storer PD, Xu J, Chavis J, Drew PD. Peroxisome proliferator-activated receptor-gamma agonists inhibit the activation of microglia and astrocytes: implications for multiple sclerosis. *J Neuroimmunol.* 2005 Apr;161(1-2):113-22.

43 Schmidt S, Moric E, Schmidt M, Sastre M, Feinstein DL, Heneka MT. Anti-inflammatory and antiproliferative actions of PPAR-gamma agonists on T lymphocytes derived from MS patients. *J Leukoc Biol.* 2004 Mar;75(3):478-85.

44 Feinstein DL. Therapeutic potential of peroxisome proliferator-activated receptor agonists for neurological disease. *Diabetes Technol Ther.* 2003;5(1):67-73.

45 Inestrosa NC, Godoy JA, Quintanilla RA, Koenig CS, Bronfman M. Peroxisome proliferator-activated receptor gamma is expressed in hippocampal neurons and its activation prevents beta-amyloid neurodegeneration: role of Wnt signaling. *Exp Cell Res.* 2005 Mar 10;304(1):91-104.

46 Boris M, Kaiser C, Goldblatt A, Elice MW, Edelson SM, Feinstein DL. Effect of Pioglitazone treatment on behavioral symptoms in autistic children.

47 Boris M. DAN conference report. Oct 2006.

48 Geier DA, Geier MR. A Clinical and Laboratory Evaluation of Methionine Cycle-Transsulfuration and Androgen Pathway Markers in Children with Autistic Disorders. *Horm Res.* 2006 Jul 5;66(4):182-188.

49 Knickmeyer R, Baron-Cohen S, Raggatt P, Taylor K. Foetal testosterone, social relationships, and restricted interests in children. *J Child Psychol Psychiatry.* 2005 Feb;46(2):198-210.

50 Tordjman S, Ferrari P, Sulmont V, Duyme M, Roubertoux P. Androgenic activity in autism. *Am J Psychiatry.* 1997 Nov;154(11):1626-7.

51 Bradstreet JJ, Smith S, Granpeesheh D, El-Dahr JM, Rossignol D. Spironolactone Might be a Desirable Immunologic and Hormonal Intervention in Autism Spectrum Disorders. *Med Hypotheses.* 2006 Dec 4.

52 Elchaar GM, Maisch NM, Augusto LM, Wehring HJ. Efficacy and safety of naltrexone use in pediatric patients with autistic disorder. *Ann Pharmacother.* 2006 Jun;40(6):1086-95.

53 Agrawal YP. Low dose naltrexone therapy in multiple sclerosis. *Med Hypotheses.* 2005;64(4):721-4.

54 Good P. Low-dose naltrexone for multiple sclerosis and autism: does its benefit reveal a common cause? *Med Hypotheses.* 2006;67(3):671-2.

55 Scifo R, Cioni M, Nicolosi A, Batticane N, Tirolo C, Testa N, Quattropani MC, Morale MC, Gallo F, Marchetti B. Opioid-immune interactions in autism: behavioural and immunological assessment during a double-blind treatment with naltrexone. *Ann Ist Super Sanita.* 1996;32(3):351-9.

CHAPTER 20

1 Ashkenazi A, Levin S, Krasilowsky D. Gluten and autism. *Lancet.* 1980 Jan 19; 1(8160):157.

2 Christison GW, Ivany K. Elimination diets in autism spectrum disorders: any wheat amidst the chaff? *J Dev Behav Pediatr.* 2006 Apr;27(2 Suppl):S162-71.

3 King BH, Bostic JQ. An update on pharmacologic treatments for autism spectrum disorders. *Child Adolesc Psychiatr Clin N Am.* 2006 Jan;15(1):161-75.

4 Kidd PM. Autism, an extreme challenge to integrative medicine. Part 2: medical management. *Altern Med Rev.* 2002 Dec;7(6):472-99.

5 Bolman WM, Richmond JA. A double-blind, placebo-controlled, crossover pilot trial of low dose dimethylglycine in patients with autistic disorder. *J Autism Dev Disord.* 1999 Jun;29(3):191-4.

6   Rimland B. Dimethylglycine, a nontoxic metabolite, and autism. *Autism Research Review International.* 1990;4(2)3.

7   Bolman WM, Richmond JA. A double-blind, placebo-controlled, crossover pilot trial of low dose dimethylglycine in patients with autistic disorder. *J Autism Dev Disord.* 1999 Jun;29(3):191-4.

8   Kern JK, Miller VS, Cauller PL, Kendall PR, Mehta PJ, Dodd M. Effectiveness of N,N-dimethylglycine in autism and pervasive developmental disorder. *J Child Neurol.* 2001 Mar;16(3):169-73.

9   Turner EH, Loftis JM, Blackwell AD. Serotonin a la carte: supplementation with the serotonin precursor 5-hydroxytryptophan. *Pharmacol Ther.* 2006 Mar;109(3):325-38.

10 Bruni O, Ferri R, Miano S, Verrillo E. L -5-Hydroxytryptophan treatment of sleep terrors in children. *Eur J Pediatr.* 2004 Jul;163(7):402-7.

11 Keithahn C, Lerchl A. 5-hydroxytryptophan is a more potent in vitro hydroxyl radical scavenger than melatonin or vitamin C. *J Pineal Res.* 2005 Jan;38(1):62-6.

12 Posey DJ, Puntney JI, Sasher TM, Kem DL, McDougle CJ. Guanfacine treatment of hyperactivity and inattention in pervasive developmental disorders: a retrospective analysis of 80 cases. *J Child Adolesc Psychopharmacol.* 2004 Summer;14(2):233-41.

13 Connor DF, Fletcher KE, Swanson JM.A meta-analysis of clonidine for symptoms of attention-deficit hyperactivity disorder. *J Am Acad Child Adolesc Psychiatry.* 1999 Dec;38(12):1551-9.

14 Megson MN. Is autism a G-alpha protein defect reversible with natural vitamin A? *Med Hypotheses.* 2000 Jun;54(6):979-83.

15 Erickson CA, Posey DJ, Stigler KA, Mullett J, Katschke AR, McDougle CJ. A retrospective study of memantine in children and adolescents with pervasive developmental disorders. *Psychopharmacology (Berl).* 2006 Oct 3; [Epub ahead of print].

16 Ishizaki A, Sugama M, Takeuchi N. Usefulness of melatonin for developmental sleep and emotional/behavior disorders—studies of melatonin trial on 50 patients with developmental disorders. *No To Hattatsu.* 1999 Sep;31(5):428-37.

17 Bubenik GA, Blask DE, Brown GM, Maestroni GJM, Pang SF, Reiter RJ, Viswanathan M, Zisapel N. Propsects of the clinical utilization of melatonin. *Biological Signals and Receptors.* 1998;7:195-219.

18 Kotler M, Rodriguez C, Sainz RM, Antolin I, Menendez-Pelaez A. Melatonin increases gene expression for antioxidant enzymes in rat brain cortex. *J Pineal Res.* 1998 Mar;24(2):83-9.

19 Reiter RJ, Tan DX, Burkhardt S. Reactive oxygen and nitrogen species and cellular and organismal decline: amelioration with melatonin. *Mech Ageing Dev.* 2002 Apr 30; 123(8):1007-19.

20 Bubenik GA, Blask DE, Brown GM, Maestroni GJM, Pang SF, Reiter RJ, Viswanathan M, Zisapel N. Propsects of the clinical utilization of melatonin. *Biological Signals and Receptors* 1998;7:195-219

21   Giannotti F, Cortesi F, Cerquiglini A, Bernabei P. An open-label study of controlled-release melatonin in treatment of sleep disorders in children with autism. *J Autism Dev Disord.* 2006 Aug;36(6):741-52.

22   Hollander E, Bartz J, Chaplin W, Phillips A, Sumner J, Soorya L, Anagnostou E, Wasserman S. Oxytocin Increases Retention of Social Cognition in Autism. *Biol Psychiatry.* 2006 Aug 10; [Epub ahead of print].

23   Williams KW, Wray JJ, Wheeler DM. Intravenous secretin for autism spectrum disorder. *Cochrane Database Syst Rev.* 2005 Jul 20;(3):CD003495.

24   Toda Y, Mori K, Hashimoto T, Miyazaki M, Nozaki S, Watanabe Y, Kuroda Y, Kagami S. Administration of secretin for autism alters dopamine metabolism in the central nervous system. *Brain Dev.* 2006 Mar;28(2):99-103.

25   Welch MG, Ludwig RJ, Opler M, Ruggiero DA. Secretin's role in the cerebellum: a larger biological context and implications for developmental disorders. *Cerebellum.* 2006;5(1):2-6.

26   Ryu YH, Lee JD, Yoon PH, Kim DI, Lee HB, Shin YJ. Perfusion impairments in infantile autism on technetium-99m ethyl cysteinate dimer brain single-photon emission tomography: comparison with findings on magnetic resonance imaging. *Eur J Nucl Med.* 1999 Mar;26(3):253-9.

27   Ohnishi T, Matsuda H, Hashimoto T, Kunihiro T, Nishikawa M, Uema T, Sasaki M. Abnormal regional cerebral blood flow in childhood autism. *Brain.* 2000 Sep; 123 (Pt 9):1838-44.

28   Rossignol DA, Rossignol LW. Hyperbaric oxygen therapy may improve symptoms in autistic children. *Med Hypotheses.* 2006;67(2):216-28. Epub 2006 Mar 22.

29   Abidia A, Laden G, Kuhan G, Johnson BF, Wilkinson AR, Renwick PM, Masson EA, McCollum PT. The role of hyperbaric oxygen therapy in ischaemic diabetic lower extremity ulcers: a double-blind randomised-controlled trial. *Eur J Vasc Endovasc Surg.* 2003 Jun;25(6):513-8.

30   Kessler L, Bilbault P, Ortega F, Grasso C, Passemard R, Stephan D, Pinget M, Schneider F. Hyperbaric oxygenation accelerates the healing rate of nonischemic chronic diabetic foot ulcers: a prospective randomized study. *Diabetes Care.* 2003 Aug;26(8):2378-82.

31   Buchman AL, Fife C, Torres C, Smith L, Aristizibal J. Hyperbaric oxygen therapy for severe ulcerative colitis. *J Clin Gastroenterol.* 2001 Oct;33(4):337-9.

32   Dekleva M, Neskovic A, Vlahovic A, Putnikovic B, Beleslin B, Ostojic M. Adjunctive effect of hyperbaric oxygen treatment after thrombolysis on left ventricular function in patients with acute myocardial infarction. *Am Heart J.* 2004 Oct;148(4):E14.

33   Yildiz S, Kiralp MZ, Akin A, Keskin I, Ay H, Dursun H, Cimsit M. A new treatment modality for fibromyalgia syndrome: hyperbaric oxygen therapy. *J Int Med Res.* 2004 May-Jun;32(3):263-7.

34 Kiralp MZ, Yildiz S, Vural D, Keskin I, Ay H, Dursun H. Effectiveness of hyperbaric oxygen therapy in the treatment of complex regional pain syndrome. *J Int Med Res.* 2004 May-Jun;32(3):258-62.

35 Liptak GS. Complementary and alternative therapies for cerebral palsy. *Ment Retard Dev Disabil Res Rev.* 2005;11(2):156-63.

36 Marois P, Vanasse M. Hyperbaric oxygen therapy and cerebral palsy. *Dev Med Child Neurol.* 2003 Sep;45(9):646-7.

37 Stoller KP. Quantification of neurocognitive changes before, during, and after hyperbaric oxygen therapy in a case of fetal alcohol syndrome. *Pediatrics.* 2005 Oct; 116(4):e586-91.

38 Rockswold GL, Ford SE, Anderson DC, Bergman TA, Sherman RE. Results of a prospective randomized trial for treatment of severely brain-injured patients with hyperbaric oxygen. *J Neurosurg.* 1992 Jun;76(6):929-34.

39 Fischer BH, Marks M, Reich T. Hyperbaric-oxygen treatment of multiple sclerosis. A randomized, placebo-controlled, double-blind study. *N Engl J Med.* 1983 Jan 27; 308(4):181-6.

40 Joiner, JT (Ed.). The Proceedings of the 2nd International Symposium on Hyperbaric Oxygenation for Cerebral Palsy and the Brain-Injured Child. Flagstaff, AZ: Best Publishing Company. (2002).

41 Helms AK,Whelan HT,Torbey MT. Hyperbaric oxygen therapy of cerebral ischemia. *Cerebrovasc Dis.* 2005;20(6):417-26.

42 Sakoda M, Ueno S, Kihara K, Arikawa K, Dogomori H, Nuruki K,Takao S, Aikou T. A potential role of hyperbaric oxygen exposure through intestinal nuclear factorkappaB. *Crit Care Med.* 2004 Aug;32(8):1722-9.

43 Yang Z, Nandi J,Wang J, Bosco G, Gregory M, Chung C, Xie Y, Yang X, Camporesi EM. Hyperbaric oxygenation ameliorates indomethacin-induced enteropathy in rats by modulating TNF-alpha and IL-1beta production. *Dig Dis Sci.* 2006 Aug;51(8):1426-33.

44 Yasar M, Yildiz S, Mas R, Dundar K, Yildirim A, Korkmaz A, Akay C, Kaymakcioglu N, Ozisik T, Sen D. The effect of hyperbaric oxygen treatment on oxidative stress in experimental acute necrotizing pancreatitis. *Physiol Res.* 2003;52(1):111-6.

45 Dennog C, Gedik C,Wood S, Speit G. Analysis of oxidative DNA damage and HPRT mutations in humans after hyperbaric oxygen treatment. *Mutat Res.* 1999 Dec 17;431(2):351-9.

46 Rossignol DA, Rossignol LW. Hyperbaric oxygen therapy may improve symptoms in autistic children. *Med Hypotheses.* 2006;67(2):216-28.

47 Chez MG, Buchanan CP, Aimonovitch MC, Becker M, Schaefer K, Black C, Komen J. Double-blind, placebo-controlled study of L-carnosine supplementation in children with autistic spectrum disorders. J Child Neurol. 2002 Nov;17(11): 833-7.

48   Pangborn, Jon, and Baker, Sidney M. *Autism: Effective Biomedical Treatments (Have We Done Everything We Can For This Child? Individuality In An Epidemic).* San Diego: Autism Research Institute, 2005:299-301.

GLOSSARY

A

acetylcholine: A neurotransmitter that conveys impulses from one nerve cell to another; it's released at the gap (called the synapse) between two cells.

acrodynia: Chronic exposure to mercury compounds as manifested in babies and children, it results in pain, swelling, and pinkish discoloration of the fingers and toes, weakness in the extremities, extreme irritability, alterations in level of consciousness and, sometimes, death. (Also called pink disease.)

adaptive immune response: Enables the immune system to recognize and remember specific pathogens, and to mount stronger attacks in future encounters with the pathogen.

adenosine: A powerful anti-inflammatory present in all living cells.

adenosine deaminase: An enzyme involved in purine metabolism, needed for the breakdown of adenosine from food and for the turnover of nucleic acids in tissues.

adenosine monophosphate (AMP): A nucleotide composed of adenosine and one phosphate group that is reversibly convertible to ADP and ATP in metabolic reactions.

alanine: A simple nonessential amino acid.

amino acids: The building blocks of proteins, synthesized by living cells or derived from food.

anaerobe: An organism that lives without oxygen present.

anaerobic: Living, active, occurring, or existing in the absence of free oxygen.

antibody: A protein produced within the body by specialized B cells, after stimulation by an antigen. They act against the specific antigen in an immune response. (Compare to "cell-mediated" immune response.)

antigen: Anything foreign to the body that causes an immune response.

antigen presenting cells (APCs): Cells that take up an antigen and turn it into a form recognized by and serving to activate a specific helper T cell.

antioxidant: A substance that inhibits oxidation, or reactions promoted by oxygen, peroxides, or free radicals. Beta-carotene and vitamin C are examples.

aphthoid ulcerations: Canker-like sores, found in the intestinal lining.

apoptosis: Normal intended cell death eliminating DNA-damaged, superfluous, or unwanted cells.

Applied Behavioral Analysis (ABA): A program for modifying behavior through the positive and negative reinforcement of targeted behaviors.

arachidonic acid (AA): A liquid unsaturated fatty acid that occurs in most animal fats; it is a precursor of prostaglandins, and is considered essential in nutrition.

arginine: A basic amino acid derived from guanidine.

asparagine: A nonessential amino acid.

Asperger's Syndrome: A developmental disorder related to autism that is characterized by impaired social interaction, by restricted and repetitive behaviors and activities, and by normal language and cognitive development.

ataxia: An inability to control movement, not due to muscle weakness; symptomatic of some central nervous system disorders and injuries.

atopic allergy: Allergic reaction that takes place in a part of the body not in contact with the allergen.

attenuated: Weakened.

autism spectrum disorder (ASD): Characterized by varying degrees of impairment in communication skills, social interactions, and restricted, repetitive, or stereotyped patterns of behavior.

autistic enterocolitis: Lymphoid nodular hyperplasia (cell overgrowth in the lymph nodes) and mild-to-moderate inflammation of the intestine, in association with autism, and lacking the specific diagnostic features of either Crohn's disease or ulcerative colitis.

autoantibody: An antibody active against the body's own tissue.

autoimmune disease: The failure of the body to recognize its own parts as "self", resulting in a destructive immune response against its own cells and tissues.

B

B-cells: Lymphocytes that have surfaces that can bind (disable) antigens. They're essential to the adaptive immune system.

barium small-bowel follow-through radiography: A contrast material called barium is used to make the intestines show up clearly on an X-ray of the small and large intestines.

betaine (trimethylglycine or TMG): A metabolite of choline that participates in the S-adenosylmethionine synthesis pathways.

blood-brain barrier: The cellular envelope or "wall" of tight junctions that block entry to harmful substances from the bloodstream, protecting the central nervous system.

body ecology diet (BED): Promotes the growth of beneficial microorganisms in the digestive tract by adding cultured foods, changing the quality of fats and oils, and drastically reducing the intake of carbohydrates and sugars.

bolus dose: A large dose.

Borna disease virus: Causes movement and behavioral disturbances similar to some neuro-psychiatric syndromes.

bronchospasm: Constriction of the air passages of the lung (as in asthma) by spasmodic contraction of the bronchial muscles.

C

Candida albicans: One of the many organisms that live in the mouth and GI tract, ordinarily with no harmful effects. Overgrowth results in candidiasis, which is common in immuno-compromised individuals.

capryllic acid: A fatty acid occurring in fats and oils, known to have anti-fungal effects.

carnitine: A compound derived from the amino acid lysine, responsible for the transport of fatty acids from the fluid inside the cells into the mitochondria (cellular "power plants").

carnosine: Highly concentrated in muscle and brain tissues, it's proven to scavenge ROS (radical oxygen species) as well as alpha-beta unsaturated aldehydes formed from per-oxidation of cell membrane fatty acids during oxidative stress.

carotenoids: Organic pigments in organisms that use photosynthesis to make food.

casein: A protein in dairy (milk-based) products.

casomorphine: A peptide chain from a protein found in milk called casein; it can cause an opiate effect and be addictive to humans.

catabolism: The metabolic process that breaks down complex food materials (such as proteins or lipids) into smaller units, releasing energy within the organism.

catalase: An enzyme that catalyzes the breakdown of hydrogen peroxide into water and oxygen.

catecholamines: Any of various amines (epinephrine, norepinephrine, and dopamine) that function as hormones or neurotransmitters, or both.

caudate nucleus: Located within the basal ganglia in the brain, the caudate is now known to be an important part of the brain's learning and memory system.

CDER status 1 or 2 autism: Equates to full DSM-IV criteria autism.

cell-mediated: The term used to describe immune response mediated primarily by T cells.

cellular metabolism: How living cells process nutrient molecules. Metabolism has two parts: anabolism, in which a cell uses energy and reducing power to construct complex molecules and perform other life functions such as creating cellular structure; and catabolism, in which a cell breaks down complex molecules to yield energy and produce power.

Centers for Disease Control and Prevention (CDC): An agency of the US Department of Health and Human Services, charged with the responsibility for protecting the public health and safety.

central nervous system (CNS): The largest part of the nervous system, it includes the brain and the spinal cord. (The peripheral nervous system is the part of the whole that resides outside the CNS.) The CNS governs conscious behavior.

cerebrospinal fluid (CSF): A clear fluid found between the skull and the cerebral cortex, the ventricular system of the brain, and in and around the spinal cord. A prime indication of the separation of brain function from the rest of the body, all CSF is generated locally in the brain. It can be tested for the diagnosis of some neurological diseases.

ceruloplasmin: A copper-binding transport protein synthesized in the liver.

chelators: Substances that bond to metal atoms; they are used medically to remove unwanted metals from the body, such as lead and mercury.

chemokines: Substances that can attract immune cells to sites of infection or damage.

choline: Choline maintains structural integrity and signaling roles for cell membranes, helps make acetylcholine, and is a major source for methyl groups needed in the S-adenosylmethionine synthesis pathways.

cholinergic: Releasing, activated by, or involving acetylcholine.

circadian rhythm: The roughly-24-hour cycle in the physiological processes of living beings.

clonidine: An adrenergic agonist originally prescribed for high blood pressure, it's increasingly used to help moderate impulsive and oppositional behavior, and may reduce tics.

Clostridium difficile: A bacterium that causes colitis due to a severe colon infection that can occur after normal gut flora is eradicated by the use of antibiotics.

coenzyme: A molecule that carries chemical groups between enzymes.

coenzyme Q10 (CoQ10): A powerful antioxidant because of its ability to transfer electrons.

cohort: A group of individuals having a statistical factor (like age) in common in a demographic study.

colitis: Inflammation of the colon.

colonoscopy: Examination of the colon (and possibly the ileum) with insertion of a fiber optic camera on a flexible tube.

colostrum: Milk precursor containing high protein and antibody content, secreted for a few days after giving birth.

complement system: Causes an immune biochemical cascade that helps clear pathogens from the body.

computerized tomography (CT) scan: A medical imaging method that generates a three-dimensional image of the inside of the body from a large series of X-rays.

confidence interval: In statistics, a confidence interval is an interval between two numbers with an associated probability which is generated from a random sample of an underlying population, such that if the sampling were repeated numerous times and the confidence interval recalculated from each sample according to the same method, a proportion of the confidence intervals would contain the population parameter in question. Confidence intervals are the most prevalent form of interval estimation.

confounding factor: A hidden variable in a statistical or research model that affects the variables in question but is not known or acknowledged, thus potentially distorting the resulting data.

conjunctival: Refers to the mucous membrane that lines the inner surface of the eyelids and is continued over the front part of the eyeball.

control: A group used for comparison to the subject cohort in an experiment; it is as parallel as possible except for the procedure or agent under test.

creatine: A substance from amino acids that helps to supply energy to muscle cells.

Crohn's disease: A chronic inflammatory disease of the GI tract characterized by cramping and diarrhea.

cysteine: Amino acid found in small amounts in most proteins. When it is exposed to air, cysteine oxidizes to form cystine. Both forms are key in the formation of the critically important anti-oxidant glutathione.

cytokine: Any of a class of proteins (like interleukin or interferon) that regulate immune function.

cytomegalovirus (CMV): A virus that can cause mononucleosis and hepatitis.

cytoskeleton: The network of protein filaments and microtubules that controls cell shape.

cytosol: The internal fluid of cells.

D

Defeat Autism Now (DAN!): The Autism Research Institute (ARI) convened a think tank of about thirty physicians and scientists in 1995 in order to share information and find medical treatment options. Since then DAN! has become a biannual conference that has been attended by hundreds of physicians and thousands of parents.

Diagnostic and Statistical Manual of Mental Disorders (DSM): The handbook used most often in diagnosing mental disorders in the US.

2,3-dimercaptopropane-1-sulphonic acid (DMPS): A chelating agent that forms complexes with heavy metals.

dimethylglycine (DMG): An amino acid produced in cells as an intermediate in the metabolism of choline to glycine.

Dipeptidyl peptidase IV (DPP-IV): An enzyme that influences glucose metabolism and various biochemical messengers in the body.

dimercaptosuccinic acid (DMSA): A chelating agent.

docosahexaenoic acid (DHA): An omega-3 essential fatty acid.

dopamine: Functions in the brain as a neurotransmitter, activating dopamine receptors. It is also a neurohormone released by the hypothalamus. It acts on the sympathetic nervous system, producing effects such as increased heart rate and blood pressure.

double-blind: A way of keeping test results objective by preventing both the subjects and the experimenters from knowing which subjects are in the test and in the control groups during the course of the experiment.

DTwcP: Combined diphtheria, tetanus, and whole cell pertussis vaccine.

dysarthria: Difficulty in articulating words due to disease of the central nervous system.

dysbiosis: Overgrowth of pathogenic bacteria, parasites, or fungus in the gut, causing dysfunction, discomfort, or disease.

E

echolalia: The repetition or echoing of verbal utterances made by another person.

electroencephalogram (EEG): A test for detecting and recording brain waves.

encephalitis: Inflammation of the brain.

endoscope: An illuminated tubular instrument for viewing the interior of a hollow organ or part (like the colon) for diagnostic purposes.

endothelium: A thin, slick layer of flat cells that lines lymph and blood vessels and the inside of some body cavities, serving both as a barrier and a modulator of diffusion for water and other small molecules. (Contrasted with epithelium, the outside layer of cells comprising skin and mucous membranes.)

endotoxin: A natural compound toxic to humans found in pathogens such as bacteria.

enteral/enteric: Of, relating to, or affecting the intestines.

enterocytes: Absorptive cells in the small intestine.

enzymes: Proteins that accelerate biochemical reactions.

epidemic: A disease affecting a disproportionately large number of people within a population, community, or region at the same time.

epidemiological study: A statistical study on human populations that attempts to link human health effects to a specified cause.

epidemiology: The branch of medical science that deals with the incidence, distribution, and control of disease in a population.

epinephrine: A hormone that is the principal blood pressure-raising hormone secreted by the adrenal medulla, a.k.a. *adrenaline.*

epithelium: Both the outside skin and the internal mucous linings that enclose and protect the other parts of the body, produce secretions and excretions, and in the GI tract function in assimilation of food.

esophagogastroduodenoscopy (EGD): A diagnostic endoscopic procedure that visualizes the upper part of the gastrointestinal tract down to the duodenum.

et al. (*et alia* in Latin): "And others"

ethylenediaminetetraacetic acid (EDTA): A chelating agent.

ethylmercury (EtHg): A group of positively charged atoms composed of an ethyl group and a mercury atom. Like all forms of mercury, it's toxic.

etiological: Refers to the cause of a disease.

extracellular: Situated or occurring outside a cell(s).

F

febrile: Marked or caused by fever.

Feingold diet: A diet developed by Dr. Ben Feingold to treat hyperactivity. It eliminates a number of artificial colors and artificial flavors, aspartame, preservatives, and certain salicylates.

5-Hydroxytryptophan (5-HTP): A precursor to serotonin, and an intermediate in tryptophan metabolism. It's marketed as a dietary supplement for use as an antidepressant and as a sleep aid.

free radical: An especially reactive atom produced in the body by natural biological processes or introduced from an outside source (like tobacco smoke, toxins, or pollutants); it can damage cells, proteins, and DNA by altering their chemical structure.

frontal lobes: The part behind the forehead of the left and right brain hemispheres, they play a part in impulse control, judgment, language, memory, motor function, problem solving, sexual behavior, socialization, and spontaneity.

G

gamma-aminobutyric acid (GABA): An amino acid that is an inhibitory neurotransmitter.

gastroenteritis: Inflammation of the lining of the stomach and the intestines, characterized especially by nausea, vomiting, diarrhea, and cramps.

gliadomorphine: A peptide chain derived from a protein found in wheat, rye, oats, and barley called gluten, which can cause an opiate effect, and be addictive to humans. A healthy GI tract prevents its entry into the bloodstream.

glucose-6-phosphate dehydrogenase: An enzyme in a metabolic pathway that maintains the level of the co-enzyme nicotinamide adenine dinucleotide phosphate (NADPH). The NADPH in turn maintains the level of the all-important glutathione in these cells that helps protect the red blood cells against oxidative damage.

glucuronidation: A major inactivating pathway for a huge variety of exogenous and endogenous molecules, including drugs, pollutants, bilirubin, androgens, estrogens, mineralocorticoids, glucocorticoids, fatty acid derivatives, retinoids, and bile acids.

glutamate: A substance that functions as an excitatory neurotransmitter.

glutamic acid: An amino acid widely distributed in plant and animal proteins.

glutamine: One of the twenty amino acids encoded by the standard human genetic code.

glutathione (GSH): An antioxidant, it protects cells from toxins such as free radicals.

glutathione peroxidase (GPx): An enzyme that helps prevent lipid peroxidation of the cell membrane.

gluten: The protein in wheat, rye, oats, spelt, triticale, and barley. It's what makes bread and pasta chewy, and is developed by kneading the dough.

glycogen: The storage form of glucose in human cells.

gray matter: A major component of the central nervous system, consisting of nerve cell bodies, glial cells (astroglia and oligodendrocytes), capillaries, and short nerve cell extensions/processes (axons and dendrites). (Contrasted with white matter, so called because it's covered with a whitish protective layer called myelin.)

guanfacine: An agent that lowers blood pressure.

H

hepatic encephalopathy: A complication of cirrhosis of the liver; toxic substances accumulate in the blood and impair the function of brain cells. Signs can include impaired cognition, a flapping tremor (asterixis), and a decreased level of consciousness.

histamine: A tissue compound that causes dilation of capillaries, contraction of smooth muscle, and stimulation of gastric acid secretion, released during allergic reactions.

homocysteine: Formed from S-adenosyl methionine by a two-step reaction pathway, it can be converted back to methionine, or converted to cysteine or taurine via the transsulfuration pathway.

hormone: A cell product that circulates in body fluids and produces a specific, often stimulatory effect on the activity of cells that are usually remote from its point of origin.

Hunter-Russell syndrome: Severe methylmercury poisoning, resulting in sensory nerve, movement, and visual dysfunction.

hyperbaric oxygen treatment (HBOT): The medical use of oxygen at a higher than atmospheric pressure. The patient spends time in a special chamber that's pressurized in order to make more oxygen available to all body tissues.

I

ileum: The last part of the small intestine, it extends between the jejunum and the large intestine.

immunoglobulins (IgG, IgM, IgA, IgE, IgD): Protein substances produced by specialized B cells after stimulation by an invading antigen; they act against that specific antigen in an immune response.

immunohistochemistry: The scientific process of localizing and identifying proteins in cells of a tissue section. It's used in diagnosis and research, and is based on our knowledge of how antibodies attach to antigens, which are revealed with staining techniques.

incidence: The annual diagnosis rate of a disease; for our purposes, the number of new cases of autism diagnosed each year (i.e. "getting" autism).

Individuals with Disabilities Education Act (IDEA): A law meant to ensure a free public education for students with disabilities, designed to address their individual needs in the least restrictive environment possible.

inflammation: A response to cellular injury, marked by capillary dilatation, leukocytic infiltration, redness, heat, and pain; it starts the removal of noxious agents and of damaged tissue.

inflammatory bowel disease (IBD): Inflammatory condition of the large intestine and, in some cases, the small intestine. Classically defined by two diseases: Crohn's disease and ulcerative colitis; autistic enterocolitis has been described more recently.

innate immune system: Comprising the cells and mechanisms that defend the host from infection by other organisms in a non-specific manner. This means that the cells of the innate system recognize and respond to pathogens in a generic way. The innate system does not provide long-lasting or protective immunity to the host.

intercellular: Between, among, or in the midst of cells.

interferon-gamma (IFN-γ): Produced by T cells, IFN-γ regulates the immune response.

interleukins: Molecules that signal immune responses (cytokines); they are produced by lymphocytes, macrophages, and monocytes.

International Statistical Classification of Diseases and Related Health Problems (ICD): A commonly used international alternative to the American DSM.

intracellular: Existing, occurring, or functioning within a cell.

intravenous immunoglobulin (IVIG): Contains the pooled IgG immunoglobulins (antibodies) extracted from the plasma of over a thousand blood donors. Mainly used as a treatment for inflammatory and autoimmune diseases.

J

K

L

leaky gut syndrome: Damage to the bowel lining caused by antibiotics, toxins, poor diet, parasites, or infection can lead to increased permeability of the gut wall to toxins, microbes, undigested food, waste, or larger than normal macromolecules, all of which can therefore enter the bloodstream, where they decidedly do not belong.

leucine: The most common amino acid found in proteins, essential for optimal growth in infancy and childhood.

limbic system: Includes structures in the human brain involved in emotion, motivation, and emotional association with memory.

lipids: What we think of as "fats" are in fact members of a lipid subgroup. Among their many functions, lipids are used for energy storage, others serve as structural components of cell membranes, and some comprise important hormones or vitamins.

longitudinal study: A research study that involves observations of the same items over long periods of time, often many decades, so that information might emerge that wouldn't be evident in a short-term survey.

low oxalate diet (LOD): Designed around foods that have a lower content of oxalates, which are known to be irritating to body tissues, thus causing inflammation.

lumbar puncture: Collection of a sample of cerebrospinal fluid (CSF) for biochemical, microbiological, and cytological analysis. A.k.a. a spinal tap.

lumen: The interior of a vessel within the body, for this book's purposes the GI tract.

lymph nodes: Parts of a filtering system in the body that collects and destroys bacteria and viruses. When the body is fighting an infection, lymphocytes in the nodes multiply rapidly and produce a characteristic swelling. Humans have approximately 500-600 lymph nodes distributed throughout the body, with clusters found in the underarms, groin, neck, chest, and abdomen.

lymphonodular hyperplasia (LNH): An overgrowth of the cells in the lymph nodes.

lyse: To break up; in the context of this book, disintegration or dissolution of cells.

lysine: An essential amino acid.

M

macrophage: An immune cell that engulfs and digests pathogens and bits of cellular debris, and also stimulates other immune cells to respond to the pathogen.

magnetic resonance imaging (MRI): A noninvasive diagnostic technique that produces computerized images of internal body parts. It can show soft tissue, whereas x-ray shows hard tissue (bone).

maldigestion: What happens when food is poorly digested.

melatonin: A hormone that governs sleep-wake cycles, it is also useful as an anti-oxidant; unlike certain other anti-oxidants, it does not undergo redox cycling, which can paradoxically promote free radicals, and it can cross the blood-brain barrier. The body makes it from the amino acid tryptophan, via serotonin synthesis.

mesenteric adenitis: Inflammation of the lymph nodes in the mesentery (the double layer of peritoneum that connects a part of the small intestine to the posterior wall of the abdomen).

metabolic disease: A medical disorder that affects energy production within individual cells.

metabolism: The chemical changes in living cells by which energy is provided for vital processes and activities, and by which new material is assimilated.

metabolite: A product of metabolism.

metallothioneins (MTs): Proteins that metabolize and regulate metals, synthesized primarily in the liver and kidneys. Their production is dependent on zinc and selenium, and the amino acids histidine and cysteine. They offer protection from the effects of heavy metals in the body.

methionine synthase (MS): An enzyme responsible for the production of methionine from homocysteine, it forms part of the methylation cycle.

methylcobalamin (methyl B12): A coenzyme form of vitamin B12, sometimes prescribed for support of the methylation cycle.

methylenetetrahydrofolate reductase (MTHFR): An enzyme in cells that acts in the folic acid cycle.

methylmercury: an organic form of mercury that humans are most commonly exposed to by ingesting contaminated fish.

microgram (mcg): One millionth of a gram (1 gram = .03 of an ounce).

micromolar: One millionth of a mole.

microorganism: An organism (like a bacterium) of microscopic or ultramicroscopic size.

microtubules: Protein structures found within cells, one of the components of the cytoskeleton.

Minamata Disease: A neurological syndrome caused by severe mercury poisoning. Symptoms include ataxia, numbness in the hands and feet, general muscle weakness, narrowing of the field of vision and damage to hearing and speech. In extreme cases, insanity, paralysis, coma, and death follow within weeks of the onset of symptoms. A congenital form affects fetuses in the womb. Caused by the release of methyl mercury in industrial wastewater from a chemical factory in Japan in 1956, there have been outbreaks elsewhere caused by factors such as treated seed grain in the food supply.

MMR vaccine: A mixture of live attenuated viruses, administered via injection for immunization against measles, mumps, and rubella.

mole: A very small scientific measurement—the International System of Units base unit that measures an amount of substance of a system that contains as many elementary entities as there are atoms in 0.012 kilogram of carbon-12, where the carbon-12 atoms are unbound, at rest, and in their ground state.

monovalent vaccine: One that addresses a single antigen, microorganism, or disease.

mucosal erythema: An abnormal redness of the mucous membrane caused by inflammation.

myelin: An electrically insulating phospholipid layer that surrounds the axons of many neurons. Along *unmyelinated* fibers, impulses move continuously as waves, but in myelinated fibers they take larger jumps along the nerve fiber and are thus able to get to the end quicker. Myelin helps prevent the electrical current from leaving the axon.

myelin basic protein (MBP): A protein believed to be important in producing myelin around the nerves in the central nervous system.

myositis: Inflammation of the muscles.

myringotomy: A surgical procedure in which a tiny incision is created in the eardrum, so as to relieve pressure caused by the excessive buildup of fluid, or to drain pus.

N

N-acetylcysteine (NAC): A medication used as a precursor in the formation of the antioxidant glutathione in the body.

naltrexone: An opioid receptor antagonist used in the management of alcohol and opioid dependence. Low-dose naltrexone (LDN) (in doses approximately one-tenth those used for drug/alcohol rehabilitation purposes) is being used as an off-label treatment for some immune disorders.

nanomolar: A billionth of a mole (see definition for mole).

natural killer (NK) cells: A major component of the innate immune system, NK cells attack cells that have been infected by microbes.

nerve growth factor (NGF): A protein critical for the survival and maintenance of sympathetic and sensory neurons.

neurohormone: Any hormone produced by neurosecretory cells, usually in the brain.

neuron: Electrically excitable cells in the nervous system that process and transmit information. Neurons are the core components of the brain, spinal cord, and peripheral nerves.

neurokines: Neurotrophins that act like cytokines, influencing the development and function of the immune system.

neuron-axon filament protein: Makes up the nerve fibers.

neurotoxin: A substance that acts as a poison to the nervous system.

neurotransmitter: A substance (like norepinephrine or acetylcholine) that transmits nerve impulses across a synapse, the tiny gap between nerve cells.

neurotypical (NT): Developmentally normal.

norepinephrine: Released into the blood as a hormone by the adrenal glands, it is also a neurotransmitter. As a stress hormone, it affects parts of the human brain where attention and impulsivity are controlled. Along with epinephrine, this compound affects the fight-or-flight response, activating the sympathetic nervous system to directly increase heart rate, release energy from fat, and increase muscle readiness.

nutraceutical: A dietary supplement that provides health benefits.

nystatin: An antifungal medication used especially to treat candidiasis, a common yeast infection.

O

omega-6: Sources include grains, vegetable oils, and grain-fed animal proteins. The biological effects of the omega-6 fatty acids are largely mediated by their interactions with the omega-3 fatty acids—excessive levels of omega-6 acids, relative to omega-3 fatty acids, may increase the probability of a number of diseases. The omega-6s are generally considered to be pro-inflammatory.

omega-3: Sources include fish, flaxseed, and grass-fed animal proteins. Polyunsaturated fatty acids classified as essential because they cannot be synthesized in the body; they must be obtained from food. Important omega-3 fatty acids in human nutrition are: α-linolenic acid (ALA), eicosapentaenoic acid (EPA), and docosahexaenoic acid (DHA). They have anti-inflammatory properties and are a large constituent of cell membranes.

opioids: Any agent that binds to opioid receptors in the central nervous system and GI tract and that mimics some of the pharmacological properties of opiates, including effects on mood and behavior.

organic mercury: Can evaporate and be absorbed by the lungs, and is also well absorbed by ingestion. Since it's lipid soluble, once it enters the body it crosses the blood-brain barrier and the placenta, and it appears in breast milk. It also concentrates in the kidneys and the CNS. Highly toxic.

otitis media: Middle ear infection.

oxidation: A biochemical process defined as the loss of a hydrogen atom, which makes a molecule more reactive to tissues and can lead to oxidative stress.

oxidative stress: Damage to cells (and thereby the organs and tissues composed of those cells) caused by reactive oxygen species (ROS) (includes free radicals, peroxides, and oxygen ions). Occurs when there's an imbalance between free radicals and antioxidants, with the former prevailing.

oxytocin: A hormone that also acts as a neurotransmitter in the brain, it is involved in social response.

P

Paneth cells: Provide defense against microbes in the small intestine. They are functionally similar to neutrophils. When exposed to bacteria or bacterial antigens, they secrete a number of antimicrobial molecules into the lumen, thereby contributing to maintenance of the GI barrier.

paracellular: Between cells.

parasympathetic nervous system: One of three divisions of the autonomic nervous system. Sometimes called the "rest and digest" system, it conserves energy as it slows the heart rate, increases intestinal and gland activity, and relaxes sphincter muscles in the gastrointestinal tract. (The sympathetic nervous system is in charge of the "fight or flight" system.)

parathyroid hormone: Produced in the parathyroid gland; regulates the metabolism of calcium and phosphorus in the body.

paresis: Slight or partial paralysis.

paresthesia: A sensation of pricking, tingling, or creeping on the skin that has no apparent cause.

passive immunity: The transfer of immunity in the form of readymade antibodies in blood or another body fluid, from one individual to another. It can occur naturally, when maternal antibodies are transferred to the fetus through the placenta, and can also be induced artificially, when high levels of antibodies specific for a pathogen or toxin are transferred to non-immune individuals, for instance, via gamma globulin.

pathogen: An agent (such as a bacterium or virus) that causes disease in its host.

peptides: The family of short molecules linking various α-amino acids. When certain food proteins such as gluten, casein, and egg protein are broken down, opioid peptides are formed, mimicking the effects of morphine.

peroxisome proliferator-activated receptors (PPARs): They play a role in cellular functions including lipid metabolism, cell proliferation, differentiation, fat formation, and inflammatory signaling.

perseveration: Continuation of an action or behavior to an exceptional degree or beyond a desired point.

pervasive developmental disorder-not otherwise specified (PDD-NOS): A sub-threshold condition in which some—but not all—features of autism or another pervasive developmental disorder are identified.

phagocytosis: The engulfing and destruction of cells or particles by phagocytes.

pharmacokinetics: The study of a drug's absorption, distribution, metabolism, and excretion in the body.

phenotype: The observable physical or biochemical characteristics of an organism, as determined by both genetic makeup and environmental influences (sometimes refers to an individual or group of organisms exhibiting a particular phenotype).

phenylalanine: An essential amino acid converted in the body to tyrosine, which is a precursor of dopamine and norepinephrine. Phenylalanine uses the same active transport channel as tryptophan to cross the blood-brain barrier, and in large quantities interferes with the production of serotonin.

pink disease (acrodynia): So called because of a painful pink rash-like discoloration on the hands and feet, most often seen in children chronically exposed to mercury. Other symptoms include lethargy, weepiness and avoidance of light sources. The death rate can be as much as 10%; the disease is now considered rare.

polymorphism: A normal variation in a specific DNA sequence.

porphyrins: Pigments found in both animals and plants. They are involved in the formation of many important substances in the body, including hemoglobin, which carries oxygen in the blood.

prevalence: The estimated number of people who have a condition or a disease (such as autism) at any given time. (Not to be confused with incidence, which is the annual rate of diagnosis.)

probiotic: A dietary supplement containing live bacteria that restores beneficial bacteria to the GI system.

prophylactic medication: Medication taken to prevent disease, rather than to cure it.

prospective study: In which a group of subjects is followed over time to assess their disease or outcome status. (An example of a prospective study would be to watch a group of smokers and a group of nonsmokers, measuring incidence of eventual lung cancer.)

psychoactive: Refers to a substance that affects the mind or behavior.

Purkinje cells: Some of the largest neurons in the human brain, with intricately branched dendrites, and axons that extend through the white matter to synapse with the central nuclei of the cerebellum (the only neurons with this capability).

R

reactive oxygen species (ROS): Free radicals, peroxides, and oxygen ions that are byproducts of normal oxygen metabolism, with important roles in cell signaling. However, during times of environmental stress ROS levels can increase dramatically, resulting in significant damage to cell structures, i.e., oxidative stress.

Redox: A process counter to oxidation by which free radicals are converted back to a harmless form.

reflux: Backward flow of the contents of the stomach into the esophagus, due to malfunctioning of a sphincter at the lower end of the esophagus.

relative risk: The risk of an event (for instance, developing a disease) relative to exposure. It's a ratio of the probability of the event occurring in the exposed group versus the control (non-exposed) group. A RR of 1.00 is neutral, a RR of 1.5 means the exposed group is 50% more likely to present than the unexposed group.

retrospective study: A study that looks backward in time, usually using medical records and interviews with patients who are already known to have a disease. Since the gleanings are fore-ordained, subjective, and possibly obscured by retrospection, this study design tends to be less informative than others.

rho(D) immunoglobulin: A shot given to women with Rh-negative blood in order to prevent Hemolytic Disease of the Newborn.

rotavirus: A virus that causes diarrhea, vomiting, and fever, especially in infants and young children.

S

S-adenosylhomocysteine (SAH): A by-product of all methylation reactions, rapidly metabolized to homocysteine.

S-adenosyl methionine (SAMe): A biological compound involved in methyl group transfers, present in all living cells.

scurvy: A disease caused by a lack of vitamin C, characterized by bruises, spongy gums, loosening of the teeth, and bleeding into the skin and mucous membranes.

secretin: A hormone produced in the S cells of the duodenum. It regulates the acid balance (pH) of the duodenal contents.

seizure: The physical manifestations (convulsions, sensory disturbances, loss of consciousness) of abnormal electrical discharges in the brain (as in epilepsy).

selenium: Chemical element that is toxic in large amounts, but traces are necessary for the function of all cells.

sequelae: After-effects of disease, condition, or injury.

serotonin: A neurotransmitter believed to play an important role in the CNS in the regulation of mood, sleep, emesis (vomiting), sexuality, and appetite. Low levels have been associated with depression, migraine, bipolar disorder, and anxiety.

specific carbohydrate diet (SCD): A diet detailed in the book *Breaking the Vicious Cycle* by Elaine Gottschall. The allowed carbohydrates have a molecular structure that is small enough to be transported across the surface of the small intestine into the blood stream. These carbohydrates do not need to be broken down by various processes of the digestive organs such as the pancreas or the intestinal cell surface enzymes.

spironolactone: Used to treat certain patients who produce too much aldosterone (a hormone), patients with low potassium levels, and patients with edema (fluid retention) caused by various conditions, including heart, liver, or kidney disease.

standard of care: A treatment that is provided or recommended universally, with only rare exceptions.

stereotypy: Frequent —almost mechanical— repetition of the same posture, movement, or form of speech.

subacute sclerosing panencephalitis (SSPE): A rare, chronic, progressive encephalitis caused by the measles virus, occurring years after infection.

sulfate: A combination of sulfur and oxygen molecules that forms bonds with other protein structures and accomplishes a variety of tasks, such as detoxification and the formation of cell-to-cell junctions.

sulfation: The addition of sulfate groups to molecules.

superoxide dismutase (SOD): Catalyzes the dismutation of superoxide into oxygen and hydrogen peroxide—an antioxidant defense in nearly all cells exposed to oxygen.

sympathetic nervous system: The part of the autonomic (= automatic) nervous system that readies the body for "fight or flight" responses by raising heart rate, inhibiting digestion and releasing excitatory neurotransmitters. (The part of the nervous system that governs "rest and digest" response is called the parasympathetic.)

systemic: Affecting the body generally, i.e., not localized to a specific body region.

T

T-cells: Members of a group of white blood cells known as lymphocytes, they play a central role in cell-mediated immunity.

T-helpers: A sub-group of lymphocytes that help in establishing and maximizing the capabilities of the immune system. These cells are unusual in that they cannot kill infected host cells or pathogens directly, but stimulate other immune cells to perform this function.

TaqMan RT-PCR: A technique for detecting and quantifying the kind of RNA that carries information that turns protein into a gene product. For example, it can tell the difference between natural measles virus and laboratory-bred measles virus.

theory of mind: The ability to understand that others have beliefs, desires, and intentions that are different from one's own.

Thiamine (vitamin B1): One of the vitamin B complex, all of which are synergistically essential to normal metabolism and nerve function

thimerosal: A combination of ethylmercury (49%), thiosalicylic acid, sodium hydroxide, and ethanol, used as a preservative in some vaccines and other medicinal products. Not used in live vaccines such as MMR because of its toxicity to live organisms.

Thiomersal: Name for thimerosal in some other countries.

tic: A sudden, repetitive, non-rhythmic, involuntary movement or sound that involves a limited group of muscles.

transfer factor: Made up of antigen-specific amino acids, sometimes used to treat specific diseases.

transferrin: A plasma protein for iron ion delivery.

transsulfuration pathway: The part of the detoxification system that involves the formation of glutathione as the primary detoxifier. Cysteine and sulfate are also produced through this pathway. The precursors of transsulfuration are provided by the methylation cycle.

trimethylglycine (TMG): A glycine molecule that holds on to three methyl groups. Like DMG, it's considered a methyl donor.

tumor necrosis factor-alpha (TNF-α): A cytokine involved in systemic inflammation and the "acute phase response".

tyrosine: Amino acid precursor of substances such as epinephrine, norepinephrine, dopamine, thyroid hormones and melanin.

U

ulcerative colitis: A nonspecific inflammatory disease of the colon characterized by diarrhea with discharge of mucus and blood, cramping, abdominal pain, and inflammation and edema of the mucous membrane with patches of ulceration.

V

vaccinal encephalitis: Swelling of the brain caused by a vaccine.

Vaccine Adverse Event Reporting System (VAERS): A joint program of the CDC and the FDA, VAERS is a post-market safety surveillance program, collecting information about adverse events (possible side effects) that occur within a short time after the administration of US licensed vaccines. Does not cover delayed reactions.

valine: An essential amino acid that is one of the building blocks of animal proteins.

vascular pattern: The pattern of blood vessels.

vasopressin: A hormone secreted by the pituitary gland that increases blood pressure and decreases urine flow.

virus: A microscopic particle that can infect the cells of a biological organism and uses the host cell's own genetic structure in order to replicate. Does not respond to antibiotics.

W

white matter: One of the two main solid components of the central nervous system, it is composed of myelinated nerve cell processes, or axons, which connect various grey matter areas (the locations of nerve cell bodies) of the brain to each other and carry nerve impulses between neurons. It's the part of the brain and spinal cord responsible for information transmission. Myelin is whitish, hence the name.

ACKNOWLEDGMENTS

We would like to thank all of the people who have given advice and assistance in the writing of this book: Mark Blaxill, Jill James, Dan Hollenbeck, Anne Van Rensselaer, Laurie Jepson, Andy Wakefield, Anissa Ryland, Jerry Kartzinel, Susie Hiskey, Andrew Botsford, Paul Ashwood, David Kirby, Carolyn and Don Jepson, Caroline Cabot, and Blake Botsford.

PERMISSIONS

CHAPTER 2

Kanner, Leo. "Autistic Disturbances of Affective Contact", *Nervous Child 2* (1943): 217-250. Reprinted by permission of the publisher. From Anne M. Donnellan, *Classic Readings in Autism*, New York: Teachers College Press, © 1985 by Teachers College, Columbia University. All rights reserved.

CHAPTER 4

Table 1, 2: Reprinted from California Department of Developmental Services "Changes in the Population of Persons with Autism and Pervasive Developmental Disorders in California's Developmental Services System: 1987 through 1998." Report to the Legislature March 1, 1999:1-19. Available at: *www.dds.ca.gov:1999*.

Table 3: Reprinted from California Department of Developmental Services "Changes in the California Caseload. An Update: 1999-2002. Available at: *www.dds.ca.gov/autism/pdf/AutismReport2003.pdf.* April, 2003.

Fig 1, 2: Reprinted from California Department of Developmental Services "Changes in the Population of Persons with Autism and Pervasive Developmental Disorders in California's Developmental Services System: 1987 through 1998." Report to the Legislature March 1, 1999:1-19. Available at: *www.dds.ca.gov:1999*.

Fig 3: Reprinted with permission from www.unlockingautism.org.

Fig 4: Reprinted from California Department of Developmental Services "Changes in the California Caseload. An Update: 1999-2002. Available at: *www.dds.ca.gov/autism/pdf/AutismReport2003.pdf.* April, 2003.

Fig 5: Mark F. Blaxill. SafeMinds. The question of time trends in autism. Autism One Conference. May 28, 2006. Reprinted with permission from Mark Blaxill.

Fig 6: Reprinted from California Department of Developmental Services "Changes in the California Caseload. An Update: 1999-2002. Available at: *www.dds.ca.gov/autism/pdf/AutismReport2003.pdf* April, 2003.

CHAPTER 5

Funding table reprinted with permission from Autism Speaks.

CHAPTER 7

Fig. 1. Vojdani A, Campbell AW, Anyanwu E, Kashanian A, Bock K, Vojdani E. Antibodies to neuron-specific antigens in children with autism: possible cross-reaction with encephalitogenic proteins from milk, Chlamydia pneumoniae and Streptococcus group A. *Journal of Neuroimmunology.* © 2002 Aug;129(1-2):168-77. Reprinted with permission from Elsevier.

CHAPTER 8

Fig 1: Taylor B, Miller E, Farrington CP, Petropoulos MC, Favot-Mayaud I, Li J, Waight P. Autism and measles, mumps, and rubella vaccine: no epidemiological evidence for a causal association. *The Lancet.* 1999, vol. 353, pp. 2026-2029. © 2000. Reprinted with permission from Elsevier.

Fig 2: Goldman GS, Yazbak FE. An investigation of the association between MMR vaccination and autism in Denmark. Reprinted with permission from *Journal of American Physicians and Surgeons.* 2004, vol.

9, pp. 70-75.

Fig 3: Lauritsen MB, Pedersen CB, Mortensen PB. The incidence and prevalence of pervasive developmental disorders: a Danish population-based study. *Psychological Medicine.* 2004;34:1339-1346.

Fig 4: Stott C, Blaxill M, Wakefield A. MMR and Autism in Perspective: the Denmark story. Reprinted with permission from *Journal of American Physicians and Surgeons.* 2004;9 (3): 89-91.

Fig 5: Honda H, Shimizu Y, Rutter M. No effect of MMR withdrawal on the incidence of autism: a total population study. *Journal of Child Psychology and Psychiatry.* June, 2005, vol. 46, no. 6, pp. 572-9. Reprinted with permission from Blackwell Publishing.

Table 1, 2: Geier D, Geier M. Pediatric MMR Vaccination Safety. *International Pediatrics.* 2003, vol. 18, no. 2, pp. 203-208. Reprinted with permission from the publisher.

CHAPTER 9

Fig 1, 2: Wakefield AJ, Anthony A, Murch SH, Thomson M, Montgomery SM, Davies S, O'Leary JJ, Berelowitz M, Walker-Smith JA. Enterocolitis in children with developmental disorders. *American Journal of Gastroenterology.* Sept, 2000, vol. 95, no. 9, pp. 2285-95. Reprinted with permission from Blackwell Publishing.

Table 1: Wakefield AJ, Ashwood P, Limb K, Anthony A. The significance of ileo-colonic lymphoid nodular hyperplasia in children with autistic spectrum disorder. *European Journal of Gastroenterology and Hepatology.* Aug, 2005, vol. 17, no. 8, pp. 827-36. Reprinted with permission from Lippincott, Williams & Wilkins, Inc.

CHAPTER 10

Table 1: James SJ, Melnyk S, Jernigan S, Cleves MA, Halsted CH, Wong DH, Cutler P, Bock K, Boris M, Bradstreet JJ, Baker SM, Gaylor DW. Metabolic endophenotype and related genotypes are associated with oxidative stress in children with autism. *American Journal of Medical Genetics Part B, Neuropsychiatric Genetics.* 2006 Aug 17; [Epub ahead of print]. Reprinted with permission from John Wiley & Sons.

CHAPTER 11

Tables 1, 2 Bernard S, Enayati A, Redwood L, Roger H, Binstock T. Autism: a novel form of mercury poisoning. *Medical Hypotheses.* 2001 Apr;56(4):462-71. Reprinted with permission from Elsevier.

Table 3: SafeMinds. *Generation Zero.* www.safeminds.org/ Generation%20Zero%20Syn.pdf. Reprinted with permission from SafeMinds.

Fig. 1, 2, 3: "Analysis and Critique of the CDC's Handling of the Thimerosal Exposure Assessment Based on Vaccine Safety Datalink (VSD) Information." SafeMinds October 2003. www.safeminds.org/ research/library/VSD_SafeMinds_critique.pdf Reprinted with permission from SafeMinds.

Fig. 4, 5: Geier DA, Geier MR. A comparative evaluation of the effects of MMR immunization and mercury doses from thimerosal-containing childhood vaccines on the population prevalence of autism. *Medical Science Monitor.* Mar, 2004, vol. 10, no. 3, pp. PI33-9. Reprinted with permission from Medical Science Monitor.

CHAPTER 12

Fig 1 Stajich GV, Lopez GP, Harry SW, Sexson WR. Iatrogenic exposure to mercury after hepatitis B vaccination in preterm infants. *Journal of Pediatrics.* 2000 May;136(5):679-81. Reprinted with permission from Elsevier.

Fig. 2, 3, 4: James SJ, Slikker W 3rd, Melnyk S, New E, Pogribna M, Jernigan S. Thimerosal neurotoxicity is associated with glutathione depletion: protection with glutathione precursors. *Neurotoxicology.* 2005 Jan;26(1):1-8. Reprinted with permission from Elsevier.

Fig 5, 6: Holmes AS, Blaxill MF, Haley BE. Reduced levels of mercury in first baby haircuts of autistic children. *International Journal of Toxicology.* 2003 Jul-Aug;22(4):277-85. Reprinted with permission from Taylor & Francis, LTD., www.tandf.co.uk/journals.

INDEX

ABOUT THOUGHTFUL HOUSE

In September of 2001, Dr. Andrew Wakefield, along with friends and colleagues, started to formulate a plan for the ideal treatment center for children with developmental disorders. The model combined medical care, behavioral analysis and education, and clinical and laboratory research under one roof.

Thoughtful House opened its doors to patients in January of 2006. Our mission is to fight for the recovery of children with developmental disorders through the unique combination of medical care, education, and research.

Please visit us on the web: www.thoughtfulhouse.org.

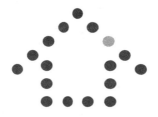

Thoughtful House
Center for Children

ABOUT THE AUTHORS

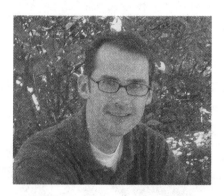

BRYAN JEPSON, M.D., graduated from the University of Utah Medical School in 1995 and completed residency training in Grand Rapids, Michigan in 1998. He is Board certified in emergency medicine. In 2001, his second son was diagnosed with autism. Over the course of that year, he and his wife, Laurie, began exploring treatment options and found that the medical community knew very little about the cause, the treatment, or the prognosis of this disease. After a year of research, the couple established a clinic in Utah where autistic children could receive the most up-to-date care available. From 2002-2005, their non-profit Children's Biomedical Center of Utah raised awareness throughout the intermountain West concerning issues related to autism and other childhood developmental disorders. Dr. Jepson treated hundreds of children on the autism spectrum and enjoyed the experience of watching them improve.

Because he was a leading specialist in the field, Dr. Jepson was recruited to join the team at Thoughtful House Center for Children (www.thoughtfulhouse.org), a multidisciplinary clinic dedicated to caring for children with autism and related conditions. The Thoughtful House is designed to integrate biomedical, gastrointestinal, and educational intervention into a coordinated effort, and to use this model to perform clinical research. Dr. Jepson is now its Medical Director.

He lives in Austin, Texas, with Laurie and their two sons.

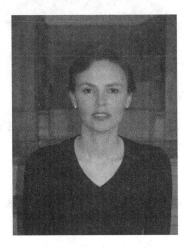

JANE JOHNSON became interested in medical treatment for learning disabilities in 2000, when one of her children was diagnosed with non-verbal learning disorder (NLD). In her effort to educate herself, she became more and more alarmed at the epidemic growth of the prevalence of developmental disorders. She is the Co-Managing Director of the Board of Directors of Thoughtful House. She lives in New York City with her husband and her three children.

Sentient Publications, LLC publishes books on cultural creativity, experimental education, transformative spirituality, holistic health, new science, ecology, and other topics, approached from an integral viewpoint. Our authors are intensely interested in exploring the nature of life from fresh perspectives, addressing life's great questions, and fostering the full expression of the human potential. Sentient Publications' books arise from the spirit of inquiry and the richness of the inherent dialogue between writer and reader.

Our Culture Tools series is designed to give social catalyzers and cultural entrepreneurs the essential information, technology, and inspiration to forge a sustainable, creative, and compassionate world.

We are very interested in hearing from our readers. To direct suggestions or comments to us, or to be added to our mailing list, please contact:

SENTIENT PUBLICATIONS, LLC
1113 Spruce Street
Boulder, CO 80302
303-443-2188
contact@sentientpublications.com
www.sentientpublications.com